Advances in Cardiac Surgery
Volume 3

Advances in Cardiac Surgery

Volume 1

Aortic and Pulmonary Allografts in Contemporary Cardiac Surgery, *by Mark F. O'Brien and David C. McGiffin*

Surgical Treatment of Ventricular Arrhythmias, *by John M. Moran*

Calcium and the Myocardium: Physiologic and Pathologic Processes, *by Glenn A. Langer*

Special Considerations in Mitral Valve and Coronary Artery Disease, *by Robert B. Karp*

Reoperations for Coronary Artery Disease, *by Claude M. Grondin, James C. Thornton, James C. Engle, Helmut Schreiber, and Frederick S. Cross*

Modified Fontan Procedure, *by Gary S. Haas, Hillel Laks, and Jeffrey M. Pearl*

Immunosuppression for Cardiac Transplantation, *by Bruce Reitz*

Current Status of Temporary Circulatory Support, *by D. Glenn Pennington and Marc T. Swartz*

Cardiovascular Grafts and Synthetic Materials, *by Lester R. Sauvage*

Intraoperative Echocardiography: A Practical Approach, *by Bruce P. Mindich and Martin E. Goldman*

Volume 2

Advances in Understanding the Function of the Coronary Circulation in Physiologic and Pathologic States, *by David Drew Gutterman and Melvin Lenard Marcus*

Current Status of Coronary Sinus Interventions, *by Werner Mohl, Philippe Menasche, Harold E. Snyder, and Arthur J. Roberts*

A Rational Approach to the Surgical Treatment of Mitral Valve Disease, *by Tirone E. David*

Effect of Aortic and Mitral Regurgitation on Left Ventricular Structure and Function, *by Henry M. Spotnitz and Maria L. Antunes*

Pulmonary Transplantation in Its Various Forms—1989, *by Bartley P. Griffith*

Coarctation of the Aorta in the Neonate, *by Gary K. Lofland*

Left Ventricular Outflow Tract Obstruction in Children, *by David R. Clarke*

Smart Electronic Devices in the Treatment of Cardiac Arrhythmias, *by Levi Watkins, Jr. and Joseph Levine*

Alternative Conduits for Coronary Artery Bypass Grafting, *by David B. Glick, John R. Liddicoat, and Robert B. Karp*

Cerebral Pathophysiologic Considerations in Patients With Coexisting Carotid and Coronary Artery Disease, *by Andrew H. Foster and David R. Salter*

Advances in
Cardiac Surgery

Editor-in-Chief
Robert B. Karp, M.D.
Professor of Surgery, Chief of Cardiac Surgery, University of Chicago, Pritzker School of Medicine, Chicago, Illinois

Editorial Board
Hillel Laks, M.D.
Professor and Chief, Division of Cardiothoracic Surgery, Director, Heart Transplant Program, UCLA Medical Center, Los Angeles, California

Andrew S. Wechsler, M.D.
Stuart McGuire Professor and Chairman, Department of Surgery, Medical College of Virginia, Virginia Commonwealth University, Richmond, Virginia

Volume 3 · 1992

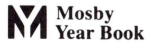
Mosby
Year Book

St. Louis   Baltimore   Boston   Chicago   London   Philadelphia   Sydney   Toronto

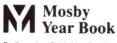

Mosby Year Book

Dedicated to Publishing Excellence

Sponsoring Editor: Linda C. Godbold
Associate Managing Editor, Manuscript Services: Denise Dungey
Assistant Director, Manuscript Services: Frances M. Perveiler
Production Coordinator: Timothy A. Phillips
Proofroom Manager: Barbara M. Kelly

Editorial Office:
Mosby–Year Book, Inc.
200 North LaSalle St.
Chicago, IL 60601

International Standard Serial Number 0889-5074
International Standard Book Number 0-8151-4958-1

RD 598
A 34
vol. 3
1992

Contributors

Anwar S. Abd-Elfattah, Ph.D.

Associate Professor of Surgery and Pharmacology and Toxicology, Division of Cardiothoracic Surgery, Department of Surgery, Medical College of Virginia, Virginia Commonwealth University, Richmond, Virginia

James G. Abel, M.D., M.Sc.

Senior Resident, Cardiovascular Surgery, St. Michael's Hospital; Department of Surgery, University of Toronto, Ontario, Canada

Carl L. Backer

Attending Surgeon, Division of Cardiovascular-Thoracic Surgery, Children's Memorial Hospital; Assistant Professor of Surgery, Northwestern University Medical School, Chicago, Illinois

Leonard L. Bailey, M.D.

Professor of Surgery, Loma Linda University School of Medicine, Loma Linda University Medical Center, Loma Linda International Heart Institute, Loma Linda, California

Gary S. Benton, M.D.

Senior Fellow in Cardiothoracic Surgery, Medical College of Virginia, Richmond, Virginia

James A. Blumenthal, Ph.D.

Associate Professor, Department of Psychiatry; Assistant Professor, Department of Medicine, The Heart Center, Duke University Medical Center, Durham, North Carolina

Mario Chiavarelli, M.D.

Clinical Fellow in Cardiothoracic Surgery, Loma Linda University School of Medicine, Loma Linda University Medical Center, Loma Linda International Heart Institute, Loma Linda, California

Richard Edwin Clark, M.D.

Chief, Surgery Branch, National Heart, Lung, and Blood Institute, National Institutes of Health, Bethesda, Maryland

Javier Alonso De Begoña, M.D.

Research Fellow in Cardiothoracic Surgery, Loma Linda University School of Medicine, Loma Linda University Medical Center, Loma Linda International Heart Institute, Loma Linda, California

Linda L. Demer, M.D., Ph.D.

Assistant Professor of Medicine, Division of Cardiology, Department of Medicine, University of California, Los Angeles School of Medicine, Los Angeles, California

Davis C. Drinkwater, Jr., M.D.

Associate Professor of Surgery, Division of Cardiothoracic Surgery, University of California, Los Angeles Medical Center, Los Angeles, California

Alan M. Fogelman, M.D.

Chief, Division of Cardiology; Professor of Medicine, Department of Medicine, University of California, Los Angeles School of Medicine, Los Angeles, California

Peter Frasco, M.D.

Fellow in Cardiac Anesthesia, Department of Anesthesiology, The Heart Center, Duke University Medical Center, Durham, North Carolina

William J. Greeley, M.D.

Assistant Professor, Department of Anesthesiology; Assistant Professor, Department of Pediatrics, The Heart Center, Duke University Medical Center, Durham, North Carolina

Steven R. Gundry, M.D.

Associate Professor of Surgery, Loma Linda University School of Medicine, Loma Linda University Medical Center, Loma Linda International Heart Institute, Loma Linda, California

Farouk S. Idriss, M.D.

Attending Surgeon, Division of Cardiovascular-Thoracic Surgery, Children's Memorial Hospital; Professor Emeritus of Surgery, Northwestern University Medical School, Chicago, Illinois

Edwin J. Jacobson, M.D.

Associate Clinical Professor, Medicine/Nephrology, University of California, Los Angeles School of Medicine, Los Angeles, California

Frank Kern, M.D.

Assistant Professor, Department of Anesthesiology, Boston Children's Hospital, Boston, Massachusetts

Hillel Laks, M.D.

Professor of Surgery and Chief, Division of Cardiothoracic Surgery, University of California, Los Angeles Medical Center, Los Angeles, California

Samuel V. Lichtenstein, M.D., Ph.D.

Assistant Professor, Cardiovascular Surgery, St. Michael's Hospital; Department of Surgery, University of Toronto, Toronto, Ontario, Canada

Constantine Mavroudis, M.D.

Division Head and A.C. Buehler Professor of Cardiovascular-Thoracic Surgery, Children's Memorial Hospital; Professor of Surgery, Northwestern University Medical School, Chicago, Illinois

Lynn B. McGrath, M.D.
Department of Surgery, Deborah Heart and Lung Center; Department of Surgery, University of Medicine and Dentistry of New Jersey, Robert Wood Johnson Medical School, New Brunswick, New Jersey

Franklin L. Murphy, M.D.
Associate Clinical Professor, Division of Cardiology, Department of Medicine, University of California, Los Angeles School of Medicine, Los Angeles, California

Mark Newman, M.D.
Chief of Cardiothoracic Anesthesia, Department of Anesthesiology, Department of the Air Force, Lackland Air Force Base, Texas

Gary Louis Parenteau, M.D.
Clinical Associate, Surgery Branch, National Heart, Lung, and Blood Institute, National Institutes of Health, Bethesda, Maryland

Jerry G. Reves, M.D.
Professor, Department of Anesthesiology, The Heart Center, Duke University Medical Center, Durham, North Carolina

Saleh Salehmoghaddam, M.D.
Assistant Clinical Professor, Medicine/Nephrology, University of California, Los Angeles School of Medicine, Los Angeles, California

Michael Glenn Siegman, M.D.
Clinical Associate, Surgery Branch, National Heart, Lung, and Blood Institute, National Institutes of Health, Bethesda, Maryland

Darryl G. Stein, M.D.
Research Fellow, Division of Cardiothoracic Surgery, University of California, Los Angeles Medical Center, Los Angeles, California

Ross M. Ungerleider, M.D.
Assistant Professor, General and Thoracic Surgery; Chief, Pediatric Cardiac Surgery, Department of Surgery, Duke University Medical Center, Durham, North Carolina

Richard Van Anderson, M.D.
Clinical Associate, Surgery Branch, National Heart, Lung, and Blood Institute, National Institutes of Health, Bethesda, Maryland

Sheel Kumar Vastia, M.D.
Clinical Associate, Surgery Branch, National Heart, Lung, and Blood Institute, National Institutes of Health, Bethesda, Maryland

Robert E. Vigesaa, M.D.
Chief Resident in Cardiothoracic Surgery, Loma Linda University School of Medicine, Loma Linda University Medical Center, Loma Linda International Heart Institute, Loma Linda, California

Andrew S. Wechsler, M.D.
Stuart McGuire Professor of Surgery; Chairman, Department of Surgery, Professor of Physiology, Medical College of Virginia, Virginia Commonwealth University, Richmond, Virginia

Preface

For this third edition of *Advances in Cardiac Surgery,* the editors have assembled a splendid group of authors who have among them contributed 12 chapters covering a wide scope of cardiac surgical issues. The volume is introduced by discussion of atherosclerosis by Dr. Fogelman and his associates and appropriately deals with some of the basic science associated with a process, atherosclerosis, that leads to perhaps 333,000 operations and a similar number of angioplasties in the United States per year. To accompany that in Chapter 3, Drs. Benton and Wechsler review the place of coronary revascularization in the setting of acute myocardial infarction with comments relevant to all types of medical and surgical reperfusion and myocardial protection.

The second, fourth, fifth, and sixth chapters deal with new or controversial concepts in cardiopulmonary bypass and myocardial protection from the cellular to the operative level. Cardiac surgery in children is brought up to date by Leonard Bailey and his associates who discuss heart transplantation in the pediatric age group, Lynn McGrath, who discusses tetralogy of Fallot, and Constantine Mavroudis and his associates who describe their experience with the arterial switch operation for transposition. Echocardiography in one form or another can be found in most cardiac surgical operating rooms presently. Ungerleider discusses its use during repair of congenital heart defects.

Finally, two ever present complications that perhaps are seen more frequently, especially in elderly patients these days are covered in the tenth chapter by Dr. Reves and his associates for the central nervous system and by Drs. Salehmoghaddam and Jacobson for the kidneys.

The editors wish to express their appreciation to our authors who have so generously given of their time and expertise, and also to Mosby-Year Book, Inc., who again have produced an exciting volume.

Robert B. Karp, M.D.

Contents

Central Nervous System Dysfunction After Cardiac Surgery.

By Mark Newman, Peter Frasco, Frank Kern, William J. Greeley, James A. Blumenthal, and J.G. Reves.

Epicardial Echocardiography During Repair of Congenital Heart Defects.

Renal Failure in the Perioperative Patient.

Pathogenesis and Treatment of Atherosclerosis

Linda L. Demer, M.D., Ph.D.

Assistant Professor of Medicine, Division of Cardiology, Department of Medicine, University of California, Los Angeles School of Medicine, Los Angeles, California

Franklin L. Murphy, M.D.

Associate Clinical Professor, Division of Cardiology, Department of Medicine, University of California, Los Angeles School of Medicine, Los Angeles, California

Alan M. Fogelman, M.D.

Chief, Division of Cardiology; Professor of Medicine, Department of Medicine, University of California, Los Angeles School of Medicine, Los Angeles, California

Pathogenesis

During the past decade, much progress has been made in understanding the pathogenesis of atherosclerosis. In this chapter, we will present our view of this process based on our interpretation of clinical, epidemiological, pathological, and experimental (both in vivo and in vitro) data.

The earliest event in the development of an atherosclerotic lesion appears to be the retention of apolipoprotein B–containing lipoproteins in the subendothelial space.[1, 2] These lipoproteins accumulate particularly at sites of predilection. Such sites probably are determined by mechanical factors with related patterns of distribution, such as stretch and bending forces acting within the artery wall and frictional flow forces (shear) acting on the artery wall.[3] The role of these forces in atherogenesis currently is under investigation. In the subendothelial space, the lipoproteins are intimately associated with a three-dimensional cage-work created by bundles of collagen and connecting fibrils.[4] The partial pressure for oxygen in this space is nearly identical to that in the arterial lumen,[5] which is essentially the same as in the alveolus. Additionally, the endothelial cells and smooth muscle cells produce and release into the microenvironment reactive oxygen species. It currently is thought that the lipid contained in the lipoproteins that are trapped within the subendothelial space becomes mildly oxidized. This oxidized lipid then stimulates the overlying endothelial cells to express a protein on their luminal surface that binds monocytes but not neutrophils.[6] It also stimulates the endothelial cells (and the few smooth muscle cells that normally reside in the subendothelial space) to produce a chemotactic factor for monocytes (monocyte chemotactic protein-1 [MCP-1]).[7] The endothelial cells are stimulated in addition by the oxidized lipid to produce colony-stimulating factors (granulocyte-monocyte colony stimulating factor [GM-CSF], monocyte colony stimulating factor [M-CSF]) that favor the conversion of monocytes into macrophages and promote monocyte-macrophage growth and proliferation.[8] As a result, monocytes bind to the endothelial cells, migrate into the subendothelial space, convert into macrophages, and proliferate.

The macrophages have a very active arachidonic acid metabolism, especially via the lipoxygenase and cyclooxygenase pathways. The by-products of this metabolism include a number of aldehydes (malondialdehyde, 4-hydroxynonenal, and others).[9] These aldehydes are quite reactive and form Schiff's bases with the epsilon amino groups of the lysines in the protein portion of the lipoproteins that are trapped in the microenvironment of the subendothelial space. These, together with other oxidative products released by the macrophages, modify the trapped lipoprotein so that it is no longer recognized by the usual lipoprotein receptor, the low-density lipoprotein (LDL) receptor. This receptor is tightly regulated by the cholesterol content of the cells. As cells increase their cholesterol content, they decrease their LDL receptor numbers and thus are protected from an overaccumulation of cholesterol. However, the modified lipoproteins are not recognized by the LDL receptor, but are recognized by the scavenger or acetyl LDL receptor. This receptor is not regulated by the cholesterol content within the cell. Consequently, the modified lipoproteins are taken up at a rate that does not change appreciably as the cholesterol content of the cell increases. The result is an overaccumulation of cholesterol.

By mechanisms not yet fully understood, some of the lipoproteins that enter into the subendothelial space appear to coalesce, forming large lipid-rich aggregates. These can be taken up by the macrophages also, perhaps by phagocytosis. This also leads to an overaccumulation of cholesterol within the macrophages. The accumulated lipid gives the macrophages' cytoplasm a foamy appearance that led histologists to name these cells "foam cells." Unlike the apolipoprotein B−containing lipoproteins, high-density lipoproteins (HDL) are not retained in the subendothelial space, but readily enter and leave it. Thus, levels of HDL are inversely related to risk for clinical atherosclerotic events. There is evidence that HDL may serve at least two functions in limiting lesion progression. It may prevent the oxidative modification of the apolipoprotein B−containing lipoproteins and it may function to remove excess cholesterol from lesions and prevent foam cell formation.

In addition to the oxidative products released by the macrophages, growth factors are also given off, particularly the B chain of a protein that was originally from platelets isolated and hence was named platelet-derived growth factor (PDGF).[10] The gene encoding the human PDGF B chain is the normal counterpart of the v-sis oncogene. The PDGF B chains released by the macrophages into the microenvironment stimulate the migration of smooth muscle cells from the media into the subendothelial space and promote their proliferation. As some of the foam cells die, they release their lipid droplets into the microenvironment; these are taken up by the adjacent smooth muscle cells, causing them to become foam cells.

Initially, the lesion expands toward the adventitia and the artery actually enlarges in order to preserve the luminal size.[11] However, after approximately 40% of the area contained between the endothelial monolayer and the internal elastic lamina has become involved with the atherosclerotic plaque, the compensatory enlargement ceases and lesion expansion begins to impinge on the lumen. It is not clear why the compensatory enlargement ceases. It may be due to cellular events in response to mechanical factors and/or calcification of the lesion. Mechanical forces affect many activities of the artery wall, including endothelial turnover,[12] and the synthesis and release of vasoactive substances such as endothelin,[13] endothelium-derived relaxing factor,[14] prostacyclin (PGI_2, which also inhibits platelet aggregation),[15] and structural proteins such as collagen[16] and fibronectin.[17] As lesions advance, calcification often occurs within the lesion and in the midwall of the artery, progressing in some cases to the formation of bone. Unless the lesion protrudes into the lumen, it is highly unlikely to be clinically important. Therefore, determining which factors limit the compensatory response may provide important new therapeutic avenues for altering the clinical outcome.

As the lesion expands into the lumen, the normal laminar blood flow is disrupted and microbreaks in the endothelium appear. These expose the underlying cells and matrix and provide the nidus for platelet deposition. (Atherosclerotic arteries appear to have impaired production of prostacyclin, an inhibitor of platelet aggregation.) In addition, the normal, protective arterial dilation in response to platelet aggregation is impaired in atherosclerosis, possibly through the loss of endothelium-derived relaxing factors (EDRF) related to nitric oxide.[18] High shear forces also directly influence platelet aggregation.[19] Products released from the platelets, including PDGF, further stimulate lesion progression.

There are several consequences of lesion formation. Normally, the artery relaxes and contracts in response to stimuli such as exercise, thrombin deposition, and stress. These periodic dilations and contractions are mediated in part by EDRF, a natural analogue of nitroglycerin, and possibly by endothelin, a homologue of a protein in viper venom that causes intense vasoconstriction. The normal response to exercise and thrombin deposition is arterial dilation mediated in part by EDRF. Teleologically, dilation is appropriate to produce the increased blood flow required for exercise, and dilation upon the formation of thrombin would be beneficial in washing out an early clot and preventing intravascular thrombosis. However, atherosclerotic arteries show an impairment of this EDRF response and actually may contract in response to stimuli that would dilate normal arteries. Stress causes norepinephrine release, which favors contraction, and this vasospastic response is potentiated by endothelin. It appears that in atherosclerotic lesions, the normal balance between vasodilation and vaso-contraction is altered in favor of the latter.

The cyclic deposition of platelets at the sites of microbreaks in the endo-thelium results in the release of serotonin and thromboxane A_2 and leads to vasospasm and transient arterial occlusion, which produces the acute coronary syndromes that can lead to permanent thrombosis in some cases.

It is clear that many lesions that are found to be 100% occluded by thrombus actually obstructed less than 50% of the lumen at the time of thrombus initiation. It may be that these lesions, which do not limit flow, produce as yet unknown mechanical changes that make them more vul-nerable to rupture or fissure at specific sites. The release of lipids from the core of the plaque or the induction of tissue factor then may lead to throm-bus formation.

Recently, the structure of a lipoprotein known as Lp(a) was determined. This lipoprotein turns out to be LDL connected to a remarkable duplica-tion of portions of plasminogen. Because of this homology, it may com-pete for fibrin binding sites and thus interfere with fibrinolysis. Patients with elevated levels of Lp(a) have long been known to be at very high risk for myocardial infarction and this link to thrombosis may be the explanation.

Treatment

Since the apolipoprotein B-containing lipoproteins appear to be required for lesion initiation, it seems prudent to lower their plasma levels. Current recommendations by the American Heart Association and the National In-stitutes of Health[20] include the reduction of plasma cholesterol levels to be-low 200 mg/dL and LDL cholesterol to below 160 mg/dL with diet. Ther-apy should be directed toward the reduction of dietary saturated fat and cholesterol and the reduction of body weight to lean body mass. The latter may be particularly important because of the association of intra-abdomi-nal fat with increased risk for atherosclerosis. The fatty acids released from these fat stores pass directly into the portal vein and, upon reaching the liver, stimulate apolipoprotein B-containing lipoprotein synthesis and secre-tion.

Unsaturated fat from land plants (such as corn oil or safflower oil) will reduce LDL levels without reducing the triglyceride-rich very-low-density lipoprotein (VLDL) (both LDL and VLDL contain apolipoprotein B). Un-saturated fat from the food chain beginning with plankton (omega-3 fatty acids) will tend to lower both LDL and VLDL and also to prolong the bleeding time by inhibiting thromboxane A_2 synthesis. Omega-3 fatty acids also may inhibit monocyte adherence and migration into the subendothe-lial space. Use of the omega-3 fatty acids for the latter purposes may be helpful; however, the use of unsaturated fat to lower lipoprotein levels is probably not indicated in most cases. These fats are useful not as a supple-ment, but as substitutes for saturated fat when dietary fat is required. Mo-nounsaturated fat such as that found in olive oil will lower plasma concentrations of LDL and also may raise HDL levels.[21] Aerobic exercise is a valuable adjunct to diet, especially with weight loss. LDL and VLDL levels will fall and HDL levels will rise in most people who diet and exercise regularly.

Smoking contributes to atherosclerosis by rendering the lipoproteins more susceptible to oxidation, lowering HDL levels, increasing the tendency for clotting, and contributing to vasospasm and, therefore, is absolutely contraindicated.

For those persons who fail to respond sufficiently to smoking cessation, diet, and exercise, one must consider drug therapy.[22] Currently, the recommendation is to initiate drug therapy if the LDL level exceeds 190 mg/mL after smoking cessation, diet, and exercise in patients without risk factors other than hyperlipidemia. In those with additional risk factors or proven atherosclerosis, the recommendation is to initiate drug therapy if the LDL levels cannot be brought below 160 mg/dL with these measures. The drugs that are commonly used include niacin, bile sequestrating agents, fibric acid derivatives, and HMG-CoA reductase inhibitors. Niacin at a dose of 1 to 3 g daily will lower both LDL and VLDL levels and raise HDL levels in many patients. The major side effects to niacin therapy include flushing, pruritus, exacerbation of glucose intolerance, hyperuricemia, and liver dysfunction including, rarely, cirrhosis. Bile acid sequestrants will lower LDL levels and may raise HDL levels very modestly while increasing VLDL levels. These agents have been shown in clinical trials to reduce the incidence of clinical atherosclerotic events. The main side effects of these agents relate to their propensity to cause gastrointestinal discomfort, their association with an increased incidence of gallstones, and their ability to interfere with the absorption of several other drugs, most notably warfarin (which cannot be given safely with a bile acid sequestrant). The major fibric acid derivative available today is gemfibrozil. This agent has been shown to lower VLDL levels and raise HDL levels and has been associated with increased survival after myocardial infarction. It has relatively little effect on LDL levels. Its main side effects are gastrointestinal, but it is usually well tolerated. HMG-CoA reductase inhibitors competitively inhibit the key enzyme in cholesterol biosynthesis (HMG-CoA reductase). As a result, these agents raise LDL receptor levels and lower plasma LDL and, to a much lesser extent, VLDL. There is often a modest increase in HDL levels as well. These agents are well tolerated and their main side effects relate to hepatotoxicity and rarely myositis.

The combination of an HMG-CoA reductase inhibitor (lovastatin) with either niacin or gemfibrozil increases the risk of myositis from about 0.2% to 2.0%. The combination of a bile sequestrating agent and an HMG-CoA reductase inhibitor is especially effective in lowering LDL levels and does not appreciably increase the risk from either drug. Probucol is a hypocholesterolemic agent that has a minimal effect on LDL levels but in vitro inhibits LDL oxidation and in one animal model has been shown to retard the development of aortic atherosclerosis. Unfortunately, probucol lowers HDL levels substantially and, consequently, its role in therapy remains to be determined. It seems likely that some antioxidant therapy will be useful and beta carotene may be one such agent, but proof of efficacy is lacking at present. Since the final common pathway for clinical events is often a thrombus, antiplatelet therapy is appropriate and aspirin is the best-studied agent. Doses of 160 mg daily have been shown to decrease the incidence of clinical atherosclerotic events.

Conclusion

Every patient who undergoes a surgical procedure for atherosclerosis should be evaluated for risk factors. Smoking must be stopped; total cholesterol, LDL cholesterol, triglycerides, and HDL cholesterol levels should be determined, and appropriate therapy should be initiated. Our progress in understanding the pathogenesis of atherosclerosis has led to more rational and effective therapies and provides great promise for the future prevention and control of this disease process.

References

1. Schwenke DC, Carew TE: Initiation of atherosclerotic lesions in cholesterol-fed rabbits. I. Focal increases in arterial LDL concentration precede development of fatty streak lesions. *Arteriosclerosis* 1989; 9:895–907.
2. Schwenke DC, Carew TE: Initiation of atherosclerotic lesions in cholesterol-fed rabbits. II. Selective retention of LDL vs. selective increases in LDL permeability in susceptible sites of arteries. *Arteriosclerosis* 1989; 9:908–918.
3. Thubrikar MJ, Baker JW, Nolan SP: Inhibition of atherosclerosis associated with reduction of arterial intramural stress in rabbits. *Arteriosclerosis* 1988; 8:410–420.
4. Frank JS, Fogelman AM: Ultrastructure of the intima in WHHL and cholesterol-fed rabbit aortas prepared by ultra-rapid freezing and freeze-etching. *J Lipid Res* 1989; 30:967–978.
5. Crawford DW, Back LH, Cole MA: In vivo oxygen transport in the normal rabbit femoral arterial wall. *J Clin Invest,* 1980; 65:1498–1508.
6. Berliner JA, Territo MC, Sevanian A, et al: Minimally modified LDL stimulates monocyte endothelial interactions. *J Clin Invest* 1990; 85:1260–1266.
7. Cushing SD, Berliner JA, Valente AJ, et al: Minimally modified low density lipoprotein induces monocyte chemotactic protein 1 in human endothelial cells and smooth muscle cells. *Proc Natl Acad Sci U S A* 1990; 87:5134–5138.
8. Rajavashisth TB, Andalibi A, Territo MC, et al: Modified low density lipoproteins induce endothelial cell expression of granulocyte and macrophage colony stimulating factors. *Nature* 1990; 344:254–257.
9. Steinberg D, Parthasarathy S, Carew TE, et al: Beyond cholesterol. Modifications of low-density lipoprotein that increase its atherogenicity. *N Engl J Med* 1989; 320:915–924.
10. Ross R: The pathogenesis of atherosclerosis—an update. *N Engl J Med* 1986; 314:488–500.
11. Glagov S, Weisenberg E, Zarins CK, et al: Compensatory enlargement of human atherosclerotic coronary arteries. *N Engl J Med* 1987; 316:1371–1375.

12. Davies PF, Remuzzi A, Gordon EJ, et al: Turbulent fluid shear stress induces vascular endothelial cell turnover in vitro. *Proc Natl Acad Sci U S A* 1986; 83:2114–2117.
13. Yoshizumi M, Kurihara H, Sugiyama T, et al: Hemodynamic shear stress stimulates endothelin production by cultured endothelial cells. *Biochem Biophys Res Commun* 1989; 161:859–864.
14. Rubanyi GM, Romero JC, Vanhoutte PM: Flow-induced release of endothelium-derived relaxing factor. *Am J Physiol* 1986; 250:H1145–1149.
15. Pohl U, Busse R, Kuon E, et al: Pulsatile perfusion stimulates the release of endothelial autacoids. *J Appl Cardiol* 1986; 1:215–325.
16. Glagov S, Grande JP, Xu C, et al: Limited effects of hyperlipidemia on the arterial smooth muscle response to mechanical stress. *J Cardiovasc Pharmacol* 1989; 14:S90–97.
17. Gupte A, Frangos JA: Effects of flow on the synthesis and release of fibronectin by endothelial cells. *In Vitro Cell Dev Biol* 1990; 26:57–60.
18. Guerra R Jr, Brotherton AFA, Goodwin PJ, et al: Mechanisms of abnormal endothelium-dependent vascular relaxation in atherosclerosis: Implications of altered autocrine and paracrine functions of EDRF. *Blood Vessels* 1989; 26:300–314.
19. Zwaginga JJ, Sixma JJ, deGroot PG: Activation of endothelial cells induces platelet thrombus formation on their matrix: Studies of new in vitro thrombosis model with low molecular weight heparin as anticoagulant. *Arteriosclerosis* 1990; 10:49–61.
20. Report of the National Cholesterol Education Program Expert Panel on Detection, Evaluation, and Treatment of High Blood Cholesterol in Adults. *Arch Intern Med* 1988; 148:36–69.
21. Grundy SM, Getz G: Dietary influences on serum lipids and lipoproteins. *J Lipid Res* 1990; 31:1149–1172.
22. Havel RJ: Lowering cholesterol, 1988. Rationale, mechanisms, and means. *J Clin Invest* 1988; 81:1653–1660.

New Concepts in Cardiopulmonary Bypass

Gary Louis Parenteau, M.D.

Clinical Associate, Surgery Branch, National Heart, Lung, and Blood Institute, National Institutes of Health, Bethesda, Maryland

Richard Van Anderson, M.D.

Clinical Associate, Surgery Branch, National Heart, Lung, and Blood Institute, National Institutes of Health, Bethesda, Maryland

Micheal Glenn Siegman, M.D.

Clinical Associate, Surgery Branch, National Heart, Lung, and Blood Institute, National Institutes of Health, Bethesda, Maryland

Sheel Kumar Vastia, M.D.

Clinical Associate, Surgery Branch, National Heart, Lung, and Blood Institute, National Institutes of Health, Bethesda, Maryland

Richard Edwin Clark, M.D.

Chief, Surgery Branch, National Heart, Lung, and Blood Institute, National Institutes of Health, Bethesda, Maryland

Metabolism

The relationship of plasma proteins to immune function following cardiopulmonary bypass (CPB) is a new area of investigation. A recent report examined the suppressive effects of ulinastatin, a human urinary trypsin inhibitor, on plasma fibronectin. Plasma fibronectin is an opsonic glycoprotein that modulates the reticuloendothelial phagocytic clearance of foreign protein. There is general agreement that there is a decrease of plasma fibronectin after CPB. It was thought previously that this was due to consumption. The new report showed that the administration of ulinastatin to animals not only inhibited the postoperative depression, but maintained the plasma fibronectin concentration in the normal range. It also showed that its effect was by inhibition of proteolytic enzymes, challenging the currently accepted idea of how fibronectin is metabolized. Therefore, the administration of ulinastatin will have a favorable effect on the reticuloendothelial phagocytic system.[1] This study gained more importance after Anderson and colleagues reported the detection of endotoxins in ten consecutive patients undergoing CPB. Preoperatively, there was no detectable endotoxin. The endotoxin content was lower 6 hours after CPB and decreased further by the seventh postoperative day. The source of endotoxin arises in the extracorporeal circuit from bacteria entrained by the cardiac suction lines.[2] None of the patients had positive blood cultures. This information indicates that transient bacteremia is common, but controlled by an intact phagocytic system.

Platelet function and products as well as prostacyclins are coming under intense scrutiny now. CPB has been shown to cause significant prostaglandin imbalance. Prostaglandin E_2 (PGE_2) concentration increased during CPB and decreased with reperfusion of the lung, whereas prostacyclin, which increased after heart cannulation and aortic clamping, was not influenced by lung reperfusion. Thromboxane B_2 concentrations were found to rise at the end of CPB, which reflected thromboxane A_2 release from sequestered pulmonary platelets and pulmonary microemboli.[3] Significant alterations in thromboxane A_2 and prostacyclin synthesis were demonstrated during pediatric cardiovascular surgical procedures.[4] Increased levels of thromboxane A_2, as determined by measuring its stable metabolite thromboxane B_2, were not significantly correlated with alterations in pulmonary vascular resistance, platelet loss, duration of CPB, or cross-clamp time. The authors speculated that the increased production of prostacyclin may exert protection against the effects of thromboxane. Consequently, some groups have begun to look at the inhibition of thromboxane and its clinical effects in cardiac surgery. When patients were given CGS-13080, a thromboxane synthetase inhibitor, their pulmonary pressure and pulmonary resistance were reduced significantly as compared to controls. There was no effect on the systemic values. Serum thromboxane B_2 levels also were significantly reduced, with no apparent side effects in the patients.[5] The use of another thromboxane inhibitor, U63,557A, during coronary occlusion in dogs demonstrated decreased production of thromboxane A_2, with a lesser reduction in myocardial shortening and decreased frequency of premature ventricular contractions as compared to controls.[6]

Atrial natriuretic factor (ANF), a hormone secreted by the atria, participates in the regulation of vascular volume by increasing renal sodium excretion, decreasing vasomotor tone, and modulating aldosterone and catecholamine synthesis. The primary stimulus for ANF release is stretching of the atrial wall. Investigation of ANF and its effects during and after CPB have begun because of the changes that occur during CPB in regard to volume of the atria. Dewar et al. showed an interesting paradoxic rise of ANF during CPB and a lack of correlation between atrial filling pressure and ANF secretion in the early postoperative period. The ANF response to pulmonary wedge pressure began to normalize 24 hours postoperatively.[7] It was concluded that the usual physiologic regulatory mechanisms of ANF release were disturbed by CPB, resulting in paroxysmal hypertension and fluid retention. Further studies of the relationship of ANF, antidiuretic hormone, and aldosterone have been done. Schaff and associates made the conclusion that the early natriuresis during CPB occurred in the presence of a high antidiuretic hormone concentration with no significant increase in plasma ANF. This may be a paradoxic response to supraphysiologic levels of antidiuretic hormone. The natriuresis after CPB appeared to be associated strongly with increased ANF present for at least 30 minutes after CPB, which could reflect ANF release from atrial distention during volume loading.[8]

Systemic hypertension is common in patients after coronary artery bypass operations. Some have thought that the renin-angiotensin system may be responsible. However, in a prospective study of patients undergoing coronary artery bypass grafting, there were no differences in plasma levels of renin activity, angiotensin II, or aldosterone between normotensive and hypertensive patients postoperatively.[9] Changes of angiotensin converting enzyme have been evaluated. After lung exclusion during CPB, angiotensin converting enzyme concentrations fell rapidly, and then rose almost to baseline levels after lung reperfusion. These subsequently fell, remained stable for several hours, and then returned to baseline 24 hours after operation. The authors concluded that angiotensin converting enzyme fluctuates rapidly and is cleared from serum at a site distant from the lung, most likely the liver.[10] The association to hypertension remains unclear at present.

Thyroid hormone influences many metabolic processes, and investigative work indicates that it may have a beneficial effect on the myocardium in the postoperative period. The effects of hypothermic bypass on thyroid hormone concentrations showed a marked decrease of thyroxine (T_4) and triiodothyronine (T_3) concentrations, with a concomitant increase of reverse T_3. Thyroid-releasing hormone (TRH) has been administered to patients during CPB, and a blunted thyroid-stimulating hormone (TSH) response was observed. Increases of free T_4 and free T_3 were thought to be due to large doses of heparin. Thus, the blunted response of TSH to TRH might be the consequence of the elevated free T_4 and free T_3.[11] It was shown further that T_3 has an inotropic effect on the heart following CPB by the restoration of adenosine triphosphate. T_3 increases intracellular calcium, which stimulates pyruvate dehydrogenase. This, in turn, stimulates the transport of adenosine triphosphate into the cytoplasm, yielding increased contractility.[12] This has been demonstrated experimentally in baboons on bypass.[13] In clinical trials, the administration of T_3 improved postpump cardiac performance compared to no T_3 only for patients with a preoperative ejection fraction of >40%. End points were improved stroke volume, cardiac output, and reduced systemic and pulmonary resistances.[14, 15]

The changes in concentrations of the major and trace elements during and after CPB have been elucidated recently. In one study of patients on CPB with the pH held constant, the start of CPB was associated with increases in total ionized calcium of 25% and decreases in magnesium and phosphorus of 29% and 40%, respectively. At the end of blood cooling, ionized calcium was still 11% above control, magnesium was 50% above, and phosphorus was 39% below. Before weaning, calcium remained 10%

below baseline values, magnesium remained 41% below, and phosphorus remained 26% below. After CPB, the different divalent ions returned to the initial levels within 1 hour for ionized calcium, within 6 hours for phosphorus, and within 9 hours for magnesium. One day after operation, ionized calcium was at its starting level, magnesium was 13% lower, and phosphorus was 36% higher.[16] Another study found that calcium remained essentially normal during CPB, while copper increased, then returned to normal on the fifth postoperative day. Zinc concentrations increased during surgery, fell below preoperative values in the postoperative period, and then returned to baseline on the fifth postoperative day. It should be noted that in this latter study, all patients had reduced levels of trace elements preoperatively.[17] Serum levels of zinc and copper, without controlling for pH or acid/base, fell immediately after surgery and returned to preoperative levels on the second and seventh days postoperatively, respectively. The changes in plasma magnesium were not pronounced, and there was only a slight fall postoperatively.[18] Although there was not agreement among these three studies, they give an indication of the dynamic changes that occur in trace elements during CPB and in the postoperative period. This eventually will lead to better postoperative management, since there is evidence that both atrial and ventricular arrhythmias are related to calcium and magnesium concentrations.

Little investigation has dealt with the effects of low flow and pressure during CPB on cell metabolism. Since this a common form of bypass employed in cardiac surgery and it limits peripheral perfusion, two recent studies are pertinent. Immediately following CPB, patients had a metabolic acidosis with a superimposed respiratory alkalosis. There was an increased anion gap secondary to increased lactate production. The pH did not change, nor did the intracellular acid/base indexes. There was increased water content in all patients examined, although intracellular water content did not change. There was a consumption of bicarbonate in all patients, indicating its use to maintain pH.[19] The extracellular metabolic acidosis was linked to muscle cell anaerobic metabolism. The authors concluded that altered metabolism was the result of hypothermia and vasoconstriction caused by catecholamine release during CPB. The implications of these data on the postoperative return of function are self-evident and suggest possible interventions to manage acid/base status.[20]

Platelets/Bleeding

Excessive bleeding has remained a significant complication of CPB since its clinical inception by John Gibbon in 1953. This is a result of the hemostatic changes secondary to CPB and alterations due to systemic anticoagulation with heparin. Hemostatic changes during CPB and their modulation remain the focus of much recent investigation.

The exposure of blood to nonendothelial surfaces and high shear stresses in the bypass circuit accounts for many of the changes that occur in the blood and blood components.[21] Platelet dysfunction and thrombo-cytopenia seem to be primarily responsible for bleeding associated with CPB,[22] although changes in the coagulation and fibrinolytic systems are incurred also. Other factors implicated in bleeding include hypothermia, heparin and protamine excess, heparin rebound, low fibrinogen, primary fibrinolysis, abnormal fibrin polymerization, and disseminated intravascular coagulation.[23-25] Clotting factors are diluted to about one half of normal levels when a nonblood prime is used in the oxygenator. These levels are generally adequate for hemostasis.[22] Studies also have shown that the increased fibrinolytic activity observed during CPB returned to normal at its conclusion.[26] Heparin and protamine have been found individually to contribute to increased fibrinolysis, in addition to the fibrinolytic activity induced within the bypass circuit itself.[23, 27]

Platelets undergo a number of qualitative and quantitative changes during CPB, resulting in platelet dysfunction and thrombocytopenia. These changes are related primarily to platelet activation in the bypass circuit, especially within the oxygenator. Observed changes include alpha granule release, decreased fibrinogen and α_2-adrenergic receptors, and reduced sensitivity to soluble platelet agonists.[22, 28] Thrombocytopenia during CPB, although hemodilutional to some extent, is related also to adhesion in the circuit and to the formation of platelet aggregates and their removal with subsequent filtration. The adherence of platelets to synthetic surfaces requires platelet activation, with adsorption of fibrinogen onto the surface and platelet membrane fibrinogen receptors.[29]

The platelet membrane glycoprotein (GP) receptors have been the focus of much recent investigation. The exposure of platelet fibrinogen receptors associated with GPIIb-GPIIIa complex has been shown to contribute to platelet consumption during CPB.[30] In addition, fragmentation of platelet membranes, degradation of platelet GPIIIa, and a reduction in the number of membrane fibrinogen receptors of circulating platelets have been demonstrated during CPB.[29] On the basis of these studies, it was concluded further that a heterogenous population of platelets is present at the termination of CPB. This population consists of new intact functional platelets, partially degranulated platelets, platelets with damaged membranes that have resealed, and platelet fragments. Subsequent replacement of damaged platelets probably results in the recovery of platelet function and the return of normal bleeding times after CPB.[29]

Alterations in platelet size and mass, specifically mean platelet volume and plateletcrit, have been noted to occur during CPB.[31] Studies have revealed decreased mean platelet volumes and plateletcrit to be associated with a greater incidence of postoperative hemorrhage. A plateletcrit of less than 0.1% was found to be predictive of the risk of bleeding after CPB. Many studies have demonstrated a relative lack of larger and functionally more active platelets at the termination of CPB.

CPB-induced platelet activation and damage relate not only to hemostatic changes, but also to the associated release of vasoactive substances such as thromboxane, and resultant adverse hemodynamic effects.[32] In addition, there is evidence of myocardial deposition or sequestration of platelets upon reperfusion, which may contribute to perioperative myocardial ischemia and dysfunction.[33] Hence, strategies aimed at the prevention of platelet activation have been pursued intensely. This may be achieved by making platelets reversibly nonfunctional or by reducing the platelet-stimulating properties of the nonbiologic surfaces during CPB.

Among the agents recently investigated for use in making platelets reversibly nonfunctional are prostanoid compounds and dipyridamole. The clinical results with these agents are discussed later. Attempts to reduce the platelet-stimulating properties of the bypass circuit include precoating the nonbiologic surfaces with albumin.[34] In addition, canine experiments have shown the feasibility of heparin-coated systems, obviating the need for systemic heparinization, during high-flow CPB.[35]

Other agents have been used to reduce blood loss during CPB. The beneficial effect of desmopressin acetate on hemostasis was related to an increase in von Willebrand factor concentration.[25, 36] The administration of desmopressin has been shown to reduce blood loss in patients undergoing complex cardiac operations,[25] and in those who recently have ingested aspirin.[37]

The majority of patients who undergo elective cardiac surgery receive no hemostatic benefit from the use of this agent, however.[38] Desmopressin does not reduce blood loss after cardiac operations in children.[39] Significant hypotension has been associated with its use,[40] and studies have even demonstrated increased blood loss with its administration, possibly related to increased tissue plasminogen activator release.[41] When desmopressin was administered after CPB, the best results were seen when it was given within the first 60 to 90 minutes. Subsequent additional administration did not give a comparable improvement in the bleeding time until the next 12 to 24 hours.[42]

Aprotonin, a serum proteinase inhibitor, also has been used to reduce the blood loss associated with CPB. This agent has inhibitory effects on human plasmin, trypsin, and plasma and tissue kallikrein. In this setting, it seems to act by preservation of adhesive platelet receptors. Preservation of the CPIb receptor also has been demonstrated.[42, 43] Adding aprotonin to the prime has revealed improved hemostasis during and after CPB, with the platelets being affected in the first pass of blood through the bypass circuit.[42] In one study, a 40% reduction in blood loss and transfusion requirement was noted. A randomized, double-blind study found beneficial hemostatic effects in primary, reoperative, and infective endocarditis–related cardiac surgery.[43] Aprotonin had the greatest benefit in the latter two high-risk groups. Studies also show that aprotonin does not reduce platelet consumption, with no preservation of platelet numbers.

Dipyridamole also has been found to reduce postoperative blood loss and transfusion requirements. One study showed the preservation of platelets, leukocytes, and red cells after preoperative dipyridamole administration.[44] The intravenous route yielded more stable plasma levels and higher postoperative platelet and red blood cell counts. In addition, dipyridamole use has been demonstrated to decrease myocardial platelet and leukocyte deposition, and thus may reduce perioperative ischemic injury.[33]

Prostacyclin (PGI_2), the most potent endogenous inhibitor of platelet aggregation known, has shown little benefit in reducing bleeding during randomized, double-blind study.[45] Its use is limited also by virtue of potent vasodilatory effects. However, the hypotensive action of PGI_2 is easier to control once on bypass.[46] Despite the disappointing results of this prostanoid in this situation, Iloprost, a prostacyclin analogue, has been found to be very effective in preventing platelet activation in patients with heparin-induced thrombocytopenia.[47]

Heparin-induced thrombocytopenia appears to be an immune-mediated platelet activation, resulting in a falling platelet count and thrombosis after heparin administration.[22] Significant morbidity and mortality are associated with this syndrome. In patients who are sensitized, the administration of heparin for CPB may have catastrophic results. Prostacyclin (Iloprost) has been shown to prevent heparin-induced platelet activation while preserving platelet function in these patients,[47] thereby allowing uneventful CPB. Although prostacyclin has been very effective and is used widely, several other agents also have been employed in this situation. Combined aspirin and dipyridamole have allowed uneventful exposure to heparin by inhibiting platelet aggregation.[48] Ancrod, a defibrinating agent derived from Malayan pit viper venom, has been used successfully as an alternative anticoagulant in patients with heparin-induced thrombocytopenia.[49]

In the context of thrombosis and bleeding during CPB, expedient and accurate monitoring of systemic anticoagulation with heparin is essential. The whole blood activated clotting time currently is employed for this purpose, with the empiric maintenance of a value just exceeding 400 seconds for safe CPB. Doses of heparin and protamine administered during CPB are given on the basis of measured activated clotting time. There is evidence that, in addition to the circulating plasma heparin level, the wide variations in platelet number, platelet function, and packed cell volume that frequently are observed during CPB also may influence the activated clotting time value.[50] Also, a minimum activated clotting time value for adequacy of heparinization has not been defined, although there is evidence that it may be less than 400 seconds.[51] In the assessment of the coagulation status during CPB, alternative methods have been found to be useful. It has been demonstrated that the viscoelastic determinants of clot strength may be abnormal after CPB; therefore, thromboelastography and Sonocot analysis are more useful than routine clotting tests for the detection and management of coagulation defects associated with CPB.[52]

In the management of excessive bleeding after CPB, the hemostatic effect of 1 unit of fresh whole blood has been found to be at least equal, if not superior, to the effect of 10 units of platelets.[53] This is consistent with the finding that the effect of 1 unit of fresh whole blood on platelet aggregation similarly was just as good, if not better, than the effect of 8 to 10 units of platelets.[54] Autologous blood transfusion has resulted in decreased use of homologous transfusion, as well as fresh-frozen plasma and platelets.[55] It also has been demonstrated that routine prophylactic transfusion of fresh-frozen plasma after CPB does not prevent postoperative bleeding.[56]

Protamine

Composition and Action

Protamine is a strongly basic protein derived from the sperm of salmon and other species of fish. This cationic protein reacts rapidly with anionic heparin to form an inactive complex, thereby neutralizing the anticoagulant activity of heparin. Each milligram of protamine sulfate neutralizes approximately 90 *USP* units of heparin activity derived from bovine lung tissue or about 115 *USP* units of heparin derived from intestinal mucosa.[57]

Dosage and Methods of Determination

The requirement for protamine varies from patient to patient. It is affected not only by both the source and method of preparation of both heparin and protamine, but by a variety of other factors as well, including the duration of CPB, body temperature, repeated heparin doses at varying intervals, arterial line heparin flushes, and reinfused perfusate at the completion of CPB.[58] The importance of determining a precise dose of protamine for heparin neutralization following CPB relates to the need for effective hemostasis, as well as the desire to avoid possible adverse effects associated with overdosage.

In practice, it is common for activated clotting time assays to be performed with a control sample of the patient's blood being obtained both before and after heparinization. A heparin dose-response curve is constructed, enabling the determination of subsequent heparin levels on bypass.[59] Alternate methods of determining heparin reversal dosage have been developed. Protamine titration assays have been used clinically and have been shown to decrease the dosage of protamine sulfate significantly when compared to a quantitative estimation of heparin level based on activated clotting time and arbitrary conventional formulas.[58, 60, 61] In addition, it has been demonstrated that the activated clotting time assay, reflecting both the coagulation cascade and platelet function, may be misleading as a measure of protamine reversal of heparin.[62, 63]

In contrast to these assays, which use biologic end points (i.e., coagulation of a specimen), a rapid chemical measurement of plasma heparin has been developed.[59, 64, 65] This method makes use of the metachromatic activity of the biologic dye azure A in the presence of heparin. It is based on the reversible competitive binding of protamine and azure A dye to heparin. This assay has been shown to provide greater accuracy in determining the heparin reversal dose of protamine compared to either automated protamine titration or activated clotting time methods.[59] The effects of divided dosing of protamine on heparin levels have been investigated. When 75% of the total calculated amount of protamine was given after the termination of CPB and 25% was given after the transfusion of all blood in the heart-lung machine, a significantly lower plasma heparin level was obtained 5 minutes after the transfusion of all blood from the heart-lung machine, as well as 60 minutes following the termination of CPB.[66]

Heparin Rebound

"Heparin rebound" refers to the reappearance of circulating heparin following reversal by protamine sulfate. It is considered a major cause of excessive blood loss following CPB. In a study by Kesteven et al. the effect was observed in 29% of patients undergoing open heart surgery and found to correlate with both the total circulating level of heparin requiring reversal and higher postoperative drainage.[67] It has been suggested, based on in vitro experimentation, that it is the breakdown of excess free protamine, necessary for the stability of the heparin-protamine complexes, that leads to "heparin rebound."[68] If excess protamine is lost, the delicate equilibrium developed between heparin, antithrombin III, and protamine becomes more sensitive to any element that will create a shift toward the reactivation of antithrombin III. This would include any increase in free heparin or added antithrombin III through production by the liver or the transfusion of blood products. In addition, it is suggested that the large complexes formed between heparin and protamine and excess protamine may activate antithrombin III.[68]

Adverse Reactions

There exist significant undesirable effects of protamine that involve important hemodynamic, pulmonary, and hematologic alterations. There are three distinct types of adverse cardiovascular responses to protamine.[69] First, there are reactions involving transient hypotension related to rapid drug administration, which appear to occur in most patients. Second, there are anaphylactoid responses, which, based on estimates from published reports, occur in greater than 5% of patients who receive protamine. Last, there are those rare reactions characterized by catastrophic pulmonary vasoconstriction that appear to be especially likely to occur in patients with abnormal pulmonary hemodynamics.[69]

Adverse hemodynamic alterations include hypotension, increased pulmonary pressures secondary to increased pulmonary vascular resistance, decreased cardiac contractility of the right and left ventricles, augmented right ventricular work, and decreased cardiac output, all of which were found following the administration of protamine sulfate in dogs undergoing CPB.[70] The augmented right ventricular work may account for the appearance of edema in that ventricle observed in one study. The mechanisms involved in these hemodynamic changes, as well as the pulmonary and hematologic alterations also observed following the administration of protamine, appear to be intimately related and are the subject of much research. Many areas have been studied, several of which include (1) the role of platelets, specifically, pulmonary sequestration,[71] aggregate formation,[62, 63] and platelet-associated humoral events, including the role of arachidonic acid metabolites[72-75]; (2) the role of complement activation[72, 75-77]; (3) direct cardiac toxicity of protamine[78]; and (4) the role of other humoral mediators, including coagulation factor XII and kallikrein.[79]

A marked decrease in both platelet number and function was demonstrated in a canine model with an overdose of protamine.[62] These investigators found a protective effect of prostacyclin on platelet number and function. Prostacyclin inhibited the platelet aggregating effect of protamine. The anticoagulant action of protamine sulfate was investigated in both the presence and the absence of prior heparin administration in a canine model.[63] Decreased platelet counts and progressive inhibition of platelet aggregation to adenosine diphosphate with increasing doses of protamine were demonstrated. A greater effect of partial thromboplastin time as compared to prothrombin time also was shown, suggesting that the enzymes or cofactors of the intrinsic pathway were more sensitive to protamine sulfate.

Excessive thromboxane A_2 production has been implicated as a cause of pulmonary hypertension and bronchospasm in cardiac surgery patients following protamine infusion.[72] A significant increase in the plasma concentration of thromboxane B_2, the biologic inactive form of thromboxane A_2, and the inhibition of adverse hemodynamic side reactions were seen in pigs following pretreatment with a thromboxane receptor antagonist, BM 13.177.[73] This provided further support for the hypothesis that the adverse pulmonary hemodynamic effects following protamine antagonization of heparin are mediated largely by thromboxane A_2. The hemodynamic alterations in this study were not found to be related directly to changes in leukocyte or platelet counts. In a similar model, pretreatment with indomethacin, a cyclooxygenase inhibitor, prevented hemodynamic and blood gas alterations.[74] Pretreatment with either indomethacin or dimethylurea, a hydrogen peroxide scavenger, effectively blocked increases in thromboxane levels, as well as the pulmonary vasoconstriction seen in heparinized sheep following protamine injection.[75]

Kirklin et al. demonstrated that human serum containing a mixture of protamine sulfate and heparin results in marked activation of complement via the classic pathway. This complement-activating effect is hypothesized to be the result of a combination of protamine with both heparin as well as products of "whole body inflammation" believed to be due to CPB. It is speculated that the more pronounced response to protamine sulfate–heparin–induced activation of the classic pathway could cause some or all of the hemodynamic derangements that can occur after protamine administration.[76] When protamine reversal of heparin was investigated in complement-depleted dogs, adverse hemodynamic and hematologic responses still occurred, suggesting that complement activation may be a secondary event rather than a cause of major hemodynamic and hematologic changes.[77]

Factor XII activates both the first component of complement and prekallikrein during CPB in the presence of heparin. This could lead to the activation of plasma kallikrein and the release of bradykinin, which may contribute to the systemic hypotension noted in the protamine reversal syndrome.[79] The human plasma enzyme, carboxypeptidase N inactivates bradykinin as well as the anaphylatoxins C3a, C4a, and C5a of the complement system. Protamine has been found to be a potent inhibitor of carboxypeptidase N and, as such, may be partially responsible for many of the adverse effects seen to occur in some patients following its administration.[80]

A prospective study examining the incidence of immediate adverse reactions following protamine administration to patients undergoing CPB showed 11% of patients exhibiting significant or precipitous falls in blood pressure.[81] In an attempt to examine the role of type I hypersensitivity reactions, investigators found that immediate adverse reactions occurred predominantly in patients with previous exposure to protamine and demonstrated a significant relationship between immediate reaction to protamine and both a history of diabetes mellitus as well as prior use of insulin-containing protamine sulfate. They failed to show any statistically significant relationship between a hypotensive event and a positive skin test or the presence of an antiprotamine IgE antibody, despite the high incidence of antiprotamine IgE found in diabetic patients exposed to very small doses of protamine.[82] Other studies also have shown an increased incidence of adverse reactions to protamine in patients with insulin-dependent diabetes.[83]

Data obtained from an in vitro mock circulation model provided support for the concept that macromolecular complexes formed between protamine and heparin or other plasma components caused obstruction in the pulmonary vascular bed.[84] This transient mechanical obstruction, which occurred immediately after the administration of protamine, may be primarily responsible for some of the hemodynamic alterations described previously.

No advantage to intra-aortic administration of protamine was found compared to intravenous administration in anesthetized dogs in relation to hemodynamic effects.[85] When studied in patients undergoing coronary artery bypass grafting, the route of administration had no effect on the hemodynamic changes associated with protamine administration.[86]

Prevention of Adverse Side Effects

Much research has involved a search for methods to prevent the severe protamine-heparin reaction. Several studies using thromboxane receptor inhibition,[73] cyclooxygenase inhibition,[74, 75] and hydrogen peroxide scavengers[75] in an attempt to attenuate adverse effects associated with protamine administration have been referred to earlier. The use of SQ30,741, a thromboxane A_2 receptor–specific antagonist, in sheep undergoing hypothermic CPB completely prevented prolonged, significant rises in the pulmonary vascular resistance index as well as the decreases in left and right ventricular function seen with protamine neutralization of heparin.[87] The infusion of nafamstat mesilate (FUT-175), a protease and complement pathway inhibitor, prior to protamine administration in heparinized sheep reduced protamine-induced rises in arterial plasma thromboxane B_2, pulmonary vascular resistance, pulmonary artery pressures, and C3a levels.[88]

It has been shown that platelet depletion in sheep does not prevent either acute or severe pulmonary hypertension or rises in plasma thromboxane B_2 levels induced by heparin-protamine administration.[89] A cellulosic, hollow-fiber filter device containing protamine has been designed and tested. The filter binds and selectively removes heparin before blood is returned to the patient, thereby permitting an external protamine reaction.[90] It has been shown to remove greater than 80% of the anticoagulant activity of heparin without causing a clinically significant hemodynamic response when tested in dogs. The filter theoretically minimizes adverse effects by obviating the direct interaction of protamine with cells in the lungs and other tissues of the body.[90, 91]

Protamine sulfate pretreatment, immediately prior to heparinization, was found to attenuate the adverse hemodynamic alterations associated with the rapid administration of protamine to dogs that had undergone aortic graft placement.[92] In patients undergoing aortic reconstructive surgery, low-dose protamine pretreatment was shown to attenuate the adverse hemodynamic effects of the intravenously administered protamine used to reverse heparin anticoagulation.[93] Pretreatment with protamine compared with saline solution prevented the hypotension and increasing pulmonary artery pressure observed with protamine reversal of heparin. The investigators suggest cell membrane alterations as a possible mechanism.

Alternatives to Heparin/Protamine

In an attempt to avoid exposure to protamine, alternatives to this agent for reversal of heparin have been sought. Two agents that were studied previously include hexadimethrine and toluidine blue. Hexadimethrine has been shown to be clinically effective as a heparin antidote and has been used successfully when protamine was contraindicated. Toluidine blue is less efficacious and has been found to cause methemoglobin formation.[69] Several other agents, including vancomycin, polybrene, polylysine, and histones, have been studied and shown to neutralize heparin.[94] Unfortunately, each has exaggerated protamine-like side effects. Platelet factor 4, which neutralizes heparin's anticoagulant activity; heparinases that selectively destroy heparin; and the removal of heparin in the extracorporeal circuit by adsorption require additional research before they can become clinically applicable.

Alternatives to heparin have been investigated also. Ancrod, a defibrinating enzyme prepared from the venom of the Malayan pit viper, has been used clinically in patients undergoing CPB and found to be an effective method of anticoagulation.[95, 96] When it was used in 20 patients undergoing elective aortocoronary bypass surgery, there was no difference in the postoperative courses or recovery periods compared to 20 matched controls. However, there was an increased requirement for blood product administration in the ancrod-treated patients.[96] Org 10172, an experimental heparinoid (nonprotein glycosaminoglycan), has been used successfully in a patient undergoing CPB.[97] Its use may prove to be limited, though, because of its long half-life (18 hours) and lack of means of pharmacologic reversal.

Complement-Mediated Effects

Much of the recent investigation of the effects of CPB on the immune system has focused on complement fractions and products of granulocytes. Lactoferrin, a component of the specific granules elastase and myeloperoxidase, which are components of the azurophil granules, all increased severalfold during CPB. The plasma levels of lactoferrin returned to normal 24 hours postoperatively.[98–101] To study the relationship of complement to granulocyte degranulation further, it was shown that the continuous infusion of nifedipine causes significant lowering of elastase and lactoferrin concentrations compared to controls. The clinical implication of these studies is that calcium channel blockers may be efficacious in preventing granulocyte degranulation and hence decreased effects of leukotrienes on vascular beds.[98] No recent studies have compared patients who received calcium channel blockers to those who did not. Others have demonstrated that lidocaine will inhibit the release of lactoferrin and elastase.[102] Colman has also found that prostaglandin E_1 will prevent neutrophil alterations.[99]

The effects of CPB on neutrophil function have been studied. It was found that chemotaxis, random migration, and a phagocytic index were unaffected, but bactericidal capacity decreased and remained depressed for 48 hours.[100] Various investigators have shown that C5a, kallikrein, and factor XII activated neutrophils.[103, 104] Increasing evidence suggests that it is the release of toxic substances from these activated neutrophils, which are sequestered in the lung, that results in the pulmonary injury associated with CPB.[105] Histologic studies have shown clearly that there is trapping of polymorphonuclear leukocytes in the capillaries of the lung.[106, 107] In theory, activated neutrophils may release a number of substances, including proteolytic enzymes, oxidant free radical species, and products of arachidonic acid metabolism such as thromboxane A_2. All of these substances are capable of causing tissue injury with alterations in permeability and the accumulation of extravascular fluid. Bando and associates showed that pulmonary function was preserved better in dogs placed on CPB when leukocytes were depleted by a special filter.[108] Pretreatment with methylprednisolone was shown to attenuate complement-mediated neutrophil activation when studied in pediatric patients undergoing CPB.[109] This was indicated by improvement in associated parameters, including neutropenia, altered neutrophil chemotactic responses, and neutrophil degranulation. The investigators hypothesize that this form of pretreatment may ameliorate complement-mediated pulmonary microvascular injury in CPB.

The effect of CPB on the lymphocyte population and subgroups has been studied extensively. Lymphocytopenia occurs in the early postoperative period and disappears within the first week after operation. Further analysis of the cell subpopulations showed that the T cell ratio (T4/T8) decreased significantly on the first 3 postoperative days, while the B cell ratio decreased only on the operative day. Analysis of bone marrow aliquots showed that there was a redistribution to the marrow, since there was a slight increase of T4 cells in the marrow.[110] Characterization of in vivo activation of lymphocytes by 3H-thymidine uptake demonstrated an increase on the second postoperative day that peaked on the seventh postoperative day and was found predominantly in B cells. IgA-secreting cells were the most elevated fraction. Contrary to the aforementioned study, the percentage of helper and suppressor cells in the postoperative period was not significantly different from preoperative values.[111] Brody and associates demonstrated an absolute lymphopenia, with a reduction in the T4 subset and a significant reversal of the T4/T8 ratio. A return of the normal T4 subset and T4/T8 ratio occurred 24 hours after CPB. A third study by Pollock et al. demonstrated a significant decline in the T4/T8 ratio during CPB that remained until the sixth postoperative day. This sustained depression of the ratio was attributed to a persistent increase in the proportion of T8 subset.[112] These investigators demonstrated a depression of T cell numbers, which suggested an increased susceptibility of postoperative patients to viral infection, in particular, the human immunodeficiency virus. However, mechanisms of the changes in T cell concentrations and ratios have not been determined. These insights add a new and important aspect to how CPB may change patient susceptibility to viral infection.

Hemolysis and leukopenia develop during and after CPB. It has been demonstrated recently that the terminal C5b-9 complement complexes are deposited on erythrocytes and polymorphonuclear neutrophilic leukocytes during CPB. Furthermore, the appearance of ghost erythrocytes carrying the C5b-9 complex cause pore formation in cell membranes. There also was evidence that the complexes were located on leukocytes, suggesting a means of activation or explanation for leukopenia.[113] A recent article reports that interleukin-1, an endogenous pyrogen and key mediator of inflammation, is generated transiently and consistently in vivo by circulating monocytes within hours after CPB.[114]

The complement cascade is only starting to be understood now in terms of its complexity and effects. Much of the recent literature investigates the activation, effects, and attenuation of complement activation during CPB. C3a increases significantly during CPB, while C5a remains constant. It has been demonstrated in vitro that C5a binds to neutrophils, activating them and increasing the surface concentration of C3b receptors.[104, 115] C4a levels increase as well during CPB.[116] Great interest has been shown in the literature regarding the effects of membrane vs. bubble oxygenators. Recent work suggests that complement is activated by the classic pathway in a bubble oxygenator and via the alternative pathway in a membrane oxygenator. This was determined by measuring levels of complement byproducts (C3a and C5a) in the serum. There were higher anaphylatoxin levels in the bubble group.[116] Since the active component of C5 is common to both pathways, the elevation of C3a during CPB has led investigators to implicate the alternative pathway. However, the classic complement pathway must be considered now, since levels of C1s-C1-inhibitor complex unique to the classic system are elevated as a result of extracorporeal circulation.[103] Wachtfogel and associates further implicate factor XII on the surface of the bypass circuit for the activation of both pathways.[103] Despite the fact that the formation of heparin-protamine complexes in vitro activated the classic pathway, a heparin-coated bypass circuit reduced the activation of complement.[117] The work of Moore and colleagues points to the conclusion that hypothermia, dilution, and heparin reduce the generation of C3a, C5a, and the subsequent cellular response from neutrophils.[104] Therefore, the conditions employed during CPB offer ways of attenuating the generation of the complement cascade. The addition of steroids as pretreatment did not alter the production of complement.[109]

Complement activation during CPB has been studied using dextran or plasma prime. There was a significant increase of C3 activation demonstrated by measured levels of C3d and C3dg in both groups. There was no difference in the concentration of terminal complement complexes SC5b-9.[118] From a pathophysiologic view, it can be argued that dextran should be preferred over plasma in order to minimize C3 conversion, although the clinical data are lacking.

The time course of histamine release has been shown to begin in the early phase of the operation, continue to rise during the first 30 minutes of CPB, slowly fall during the operation, and then exhibit a second rise at the conclusion of bypass.[119] Studies of a pediatric population demonstrated that there was a rise in histamine during pump priming that continued throughout the operation. These data suggested that the prime of stored blood was a major contributing source of histamine. It is well known that histamine contributes to leaky capillary syndrome, contributing to pulmonary edema. It is suggested that the addition of $histamine_1$ and $histamine_2$ blockers may attenuate this response.[120, 121] However, the authors did not compare blood prime to crystalloid prime in terms of histamine levels. To date, there are no reports of blinded, randomized, clinical studies using $histamine_1$ and $histamine_2$ blockers during CPB.

Oxygen free radicals are known to disrupt phospholipid membranes, thereby altering cellular function. The complement-derived chemotactic factor C5a can activate polymorphonuclear neutrophils, which are able to liberate excessive quantities of oxygen free radicals, in particular, superoxide anion and hydrogen peroxide. The relationship of free radical production and lung injury has been demonstrated by many.[104, 108, 107, 122, 123] Significant rank correlation was demonstrated between transvascular lung protein flux measured after CPB and both net lung lipid peroxidation and neutrophil sequestration during the time period after pulmonary perfusion recommenced.[107] This correlation between lipid peroxidation, used as an index of free radical activity, and neutrophil sequestration in the lung was confirmed further in patients undergoing CPB.[124] Others have demonstrated a correlation between pulmonary leukosequestration and increased oxygen free radical generation as indicated by a rise in plasma hydrogen peroxide levels.[125] It was suggested that oxygen free radical generation, perhaps by activated leukocytes trapped in the pulmonary circulation, exceeded the capacity of the endogenous free radical scavenging systems.

When given intravenously and in cardioplegia, deferoxamine, by inhibiting iron-catalyzed free radical production, has been shown to decrease neutrophil production.[122] Pretreatment with allopurinol or mannitol, both known inhibitors of oxygen free radical production, decrease oxygen free radical concentrations during CPB as measured by the degradation end products (dienes).[123] Pretreatment with vitamin E also has been shown to decrease oxygen free radical production in a clinical setting.[126]

Cerebral Protection During Cardiopulmonary Bypass

From their inception, both extracorporeal circulation and hypothermia were envisioned as techniques to protect organs from ischemia during arrest of the circulatory system. While serving as a research fellow at Massachusetts General Hospital in 1931, John Gibbon observed a young woman slowly dying from a massive pulmonary embolism. Once she became pulseless, surgery was attempted, but the effort was in vain. During the experience, it occurred to Gibbon "that it might be possible to remove venous blood from the patient, oxygenate it, allow carbon dioxide to escape from it, and then to reinfuse it into the body."[127]

Similarly, while serving as a research fellow at Johns Hopkins in 1946, Wilfred Bigelow observed that "surgeons would never be able to correct or cure heart conditions unless they were able to stop the circulation of the blood through the heart, open it, and operate in a bloodless field under direct vision."[128] His solution to this problem was to "cool the body, reduce oxygen requirements, and interrupt the circulation and open the heart."

In 1959, Frank Gollan demonstrated that extracorporeal circulation and hypothermia could be used safely simultaneously.[129] Although many surgeons were reluctant to combine these techniques, Dr. Glenn Young employed deep hypothermia and intermittent circulatory arrest to repair successfully a tetralogy of Fallot in 1959.[130] Over the following 3 decades, many advances and refinements would result in hypothermic CPB becoming a routine procedure.

The Extent of the Problem

Improvements in surgical technique, anesthesia delivery, and CPB have resulted in decreased morbidity and mortality. Attention now has shifted toward the physiologic and pathophysiologic responses of individual organ systems to CPB. It is well known that the brain is the organ most sensitive to ischemia. Although the incidence of fatal cerebral injury has decreased to 0.3% to 2.0%,[131] postoperative neurologic morbidity remains a disabling and costly complication. Furthermore, as more prospective studies using detailed neuropsychologic assessments are performed, the percentage of patients with detectable neurologic complications increases. In general, retrospective studies report a 1% to 5% incidence of postoperative neurologic dysfunction.[131] Prospective studies employing neuropsychologic testing as part of the neurologic assessment have detected postoperative complications ranging from 30% to 61%.[131] Retrospective studies most likely detect only the most overt complications, such as coma or paralysis, whereas detailed preoperative and postoperative evaluations detect more subtle disorders.[132]

As the equipment and techniques of CPB have advanced to a more sophisticated level, "brain protection" has become a high priority. The perfusion, anesthesia, and cardiac surgery literature contain a large body of work investigating mechanic, pharmacologic, and metabolic interventions intended to prevent neurologic insult.

Cerebral Protection and Bypass Equipment

Embolic phenomena associated with cardiac surgery and CPB generally are classified as macroembolization and microembolization. It is agreed that macroembolization from the surgical field (e.g., calcium fragments, air, valve vegetations, mural thrombus) is the most common cause of cerebral injury and often results in focal neurologic deficits.[133] Improved neurologic assessment and increased recognition of subtle neurologic and neuropsychologic deficits have given rise to new questions regarding the role of microembolism in diffuse cerebral injury.

The majority of microemboli reaching the brain are platelet-fibrin aggregates and gaseous microemboli. Over the past several years, new techniques have been developed that aid in the study of cerebral microembolization. Recently, several studies have examined the influence of oxygenator type on microembolism using retinal fluorescein angiography. Transcranial Doppler ultrasound is being used to detect microemboli in the middle cerebral artery. This technique has been used to evaluate the effectiveness of arterial line filtration.

Using the retinal circulation as an extension of the cerebral microcirculation, specifically the internal carotid artery distribution, Blauth and associates have adapted the technique of retinal fluorescein angiography to the study of microembolic events in vivo during CPB.[134-138] Forty patients who underwent coronary artery bypass surgery had retinal fluorescein angiograms 5 minutes before CPB was discontinued. Each patient also underwent a battery of neuropsychologic tests before and after surgery. A bubble oxygenator (Harvey H1700) was used for 23 patients and a sheet membrane oxygenator (Cobe CML) was used for 17 patients. Arterial line filtration (Pall EC-Plus, 40-μm) was used in all cases. All 23 (100%) patients in the bubble oxygenator group had microvascular occlusions consistent with microembolization. Only 8 of 17 (47%) patients in the membrane oxygenator group demonstrated evidence of microembolization ($P <$

.001). In those retinas with occlusions, the mean area of nonperfusion was less in the membrane oxygenator group (0.11 mm^2) than in the bubble oxygenator group (0.29 mm^2; $P < .01$). Neuropsychologic deficits were more severe following bubble oxygenation, but the difference was not statistically significant ($P < .11$, Mann-Whitney test).[136]

In order to quantify the extent of retinal ischemia more accurately, Blauth and colleagues[138] performed a similar study using digital image analysis. Oxygenators and arterial line filters were identical to those used in the previous study. Microembolic perfusion defects were identified by digital subtraction of preoperative and end-CPB retinal fluorescein angiograms, and total area was computed. The results were similar. All 30 patients in the bubble oxygenator group demonstrated perfusion defects indicating microembolization. In contrast, 66% of patients in the membrane oxygenator group had no perfusion defects ($P < .001$). In addition, patients in the membrane group had significantly fewer lesions (Fig 1) and notably smaller total areas of retinal ischemia as determined by digital image analysis. Although fluorescein angiography cannot distinguish between

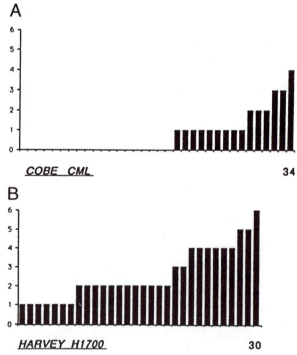

FIG 1.
Histograms showing the number of perfusion defects per patient in the Harvey H1700 bubble **(B)** and COBE CML membrane oxygenator groups **(A)**. Each column represents one patient. (From Blauth CI, Smith P, Arnold J, et al: *J Thorac Cardiovasc Surg* 1990; 99:61–69. Used by permission.)

gaseous and particulate microemboli, these studies indicate that a significant proportion of microemboli reaching the brain may be microbubbles originating from oxygenators, specifically bubble oxygenators.

Once emboli from any source enter the arterial circuit, it is desirable that they be filtered from it. Even though arterial line filters are used in most centers in the United States and are gaining popularity in Europe,[139] there is continuing debate over the effectiveness and importance of microembolus filtration. As it becomes increasingly apparent that microembolization plays an important role in postoperative neurologic morbidity, the question becomes one of arterial line filter effectiveness.

Doppler ultrasonic techniques have been used to detect emboli in the CPB circuit since 1965.[140] Recently, this technology has been used to study microembolism directly within the cerebral circulation. Pugsley[140] and coworkers tested the ability of a transcranial Doppler system to detect microemboli using a closed CPB circuit. The circuit was injected with either blood, blood agitated with air, or water containing either 30- to 90- or 90- to 200-μm plastic microspheres. Injecting blood free of air bubbles did not alter the steady-state blood velocity signals. When blood containing microbubbles was injected, high-amplitude flow disturbance signals (microembolic events) were obtained. Similar signals were obtained when the microspheres were injected. Signals obtained from the bubbles and spheres were indistinguishable. Despite injecting equal numbers of spheres, the number of microembolic events recorded for the smaller spheres was consistently lower when compared with the larger spheres. Diluting the concentration of microspheres by 50% reduced the number of microembolic events by approximately one half. This held true for both sizes of spheres, although the total number of microembolic events again was lower for the smaller particles.

Treasure, Pugsley, and associates[139, 140] used transcranial Doppler ultrasound to compare arterial line filtration with no filtration. Patients undergoing elective coronary artery bypass surgery were randomized into two groups. CPB using bubble oxygenators was standardized, except for the presence of an arterial line filter (40-μm Pall EC-Plus) in one group. In both groups, microembolic events occurred at the time of aortic cannulation and at the commencement of perfusion. The actual microembolic event count for the two groups did not differ significantly. Once CPB was established, a major difference in the microembolic event count between the filtered and nonfiltered groups was noted (Table 1).

All 40 patients underwent preoperative neuropsychologic testing and postoperative testing at 8 days and again at 8 weeks. During the course of the testing, a small learning effect was not unexpected. In the unfiltered group, 5 out of 20 patients demonstrated a small improvement, 6 out of 20 were unchanged, and 9 out of 20 showed deterioration. In the filtered group, 15 out of 20 patients improved their score, 2 out of 20 were unchanged, and 3 out of 20 deteriorated ($P < .01$).

Padayachee and colleagues[141] also used transcranial Doppler ultrasound to compare the effect of no arterial line filtration with filtration using

TABLE 1.
Microembolic Events in 20 Patients With Filters and 20 Patients Without Filters*

Time of Event†	Filtered	Nonfiltered	Significance (Wilcoxon)
Cannulation			
Median (MEE/1.5 min)	12	10	$P > .1$
Range (per 1.5 min)	1–25	2–20	
Inception CPB			
Median (MEE/2.5 min)	36	45	$P > .1$
Range (per 2.5 min)	5–82	5–100	
During CPB			
Median (MEE/30 min)	6	243	$P > .001$
Range (per 30 min)	0–10	30–768	

*From Pugsley W: *Perfusion* 1989; 4:115–122. Used by permission.
†MEE = microembolic events; CPB = cardiopulmonary bypass.

25-μm and 40-μm filters. In addition, oxygen flow rates were varied (2 to 5 L/min). Unfiltered patients had the highest microembolic index at high and low oxygen flow rates. Group 2 patients (40-μm filters) had a significantly lower microembolic index, particularly at lower flow rates. Group 3 (25-μm filters) had the lowest microembolic index. No microemboli were detected at low oxygen flow rates, and only 0.1% of the samples demonstrated detectable microemboli at high oxygen flow rates. Neuropsychologic testing was not performed.

These studies demonstrate that embolism of the cerebral microvasculature is a significant problem that, at least in part, contributes to postoperative neurologic morbidity. Moreover, they illustrate the usefulness of retinal fluorescein angiography and transcranial Doppler ultrasound for the study of cerebral microembolization. Additional studies need to be performed in order to confirm these preliminary findings, and to determine the long-term effects of cerebral microembolization.

Cerebral Protection—Pharmacologic and Metabolic Interventions

As stated earlier, the brain is the organ most sensitive to ischemia. It has been shown that the normothermic brain will exhaust all free energy stores after as little as 2 minutes of complete ischemia.[142] Following adenosine triphosphate depletion, anaerobic glycolysis is activated, converting each glucose molecule into two lactate molecules and two hydrogen ions and resulting in intracellular acidosis. Hyperglycemia will potentiate this reaction, resulting in increased lactic acidosis and further decreases in intracellular pH.[143] Ion-pumping enzyme systems fail, with the disruption of ion gradients and changes in membrane permeability allowing, among other things, intracellular calcium accumulation. This may result in the liberation of membrane fatty acids, alterations in protein phosphorylation, and the release of proteinases.[144] The metabolism of free fatty acids, specifically arachidonic acid, produces oxygen free radicals, which are important in mediating vascular injury.[145–147]

During reperfusion, injured vascular endothelium will attract neutrophils and platelets that also can release free radicals, proteinases, and arachidonic acid derivatives such as thromboxane (a vasoconstrictor) and leukotrienes (which increase membrane permeability). In addition to releasing cytotoxic agents, the accumulation of platelets and neutrophils may occlude vessels, resulting in reduced perfusion and further ischemia.[147] Once irreversible membrane damage has occurred, neuronal death will follow. If the ischemic insult is severe enough, the surrounding astrocytes are damaged also, resulting in progressive cerebral edema and infarction.[143]

Cerebral ischemia during CPB may be caused by either embolization or hypoperfusion. The advent of inert-gas clearance techniques has made possible the in vivo study of cerebral blood flow. Recently, ^{133}Xe washout techniques have been applied to the study of cerebral blood flow and autoregulation during CPB. Cerebrovascular autoregulation, which functions to couple oxygen delivery and utilization, can be altered by many factors, including anesthetic agents, acid-base alterations, intracerebral pathology, and a variety of metabolic and endocrine disorders.[148] During hypothermic CPB, as under normothermic conditions. $Paco_2$ plays an important role in the control of cerebral autoregulation.

It has been established clearly that $Paco_2$ levels during CPB have a direct effect on autoregulation.[148–154] The pH-stat scheme of acid-base management, which maintains the temperature-corrected $Paco_2$ and pH at 40 mm Hg and 7.40, respectively, results in hypercapnia (uncorrected $Paco_2$ approximately 60 mm Hg), which gives rise to impaired autoregulation, pressure-dependent flow, and the uncoupling of cerebral blood flow and metabolism. The alpha-stat strategy of acid-base management, which maintains the non–temperature-corrected $Paco_2$ and pH at 40 mm Hg and 7.40, respectively, maintains a physiologic $Paco_2$ and pH and thus preserves cerebral autoregulation. Theoretically, the increased cerebral blood flow, associated with pH-stat management could result in an increased opportunity for cerebral embolization of gaseous or particulate matter.[148] Moreover, increased global cerebral blood flow may redirect flow away from potentially ischemic areas, the so-called "steal phenomenon."[148] In contrast, the decreased cerebral blood flow that may occur with alpha-stat management might lead to critical hypoperfusion in selected patients.[155] Not until recently have clinical studies been undertaken to address these hypothetical concerns.

Bashein and associates[156] recently reported the results of a clinical study comparing alpha-stat and pH-stat management of acid-base balance during hypothermic CPB. This study is unique in that all patients underwent comprehensive neuropsychologic testing preoperatively and postoperatively. Eighty-six patients undergoing coronary artery bypass grafting or open heart procedures were randomized into two groups. Neuropsychologic testing was performed the day before surgery, just prior to discharge (mean 8 days), and 7 months later. Testing at 8 days demonstrated a wide variability of scores and generalized impairment unrelated to $Paco_2$ management. By 7 months, most deficits had resolved and still no significant difference between groups was noted.

The investigators concluded that neuropsychologic outcome following hypothermic CPB was not related to acid-base management strategy. Indeed, for most patients, the specific method used probably is not crucial. However, there may be certain groups of patients in whom major alterations of CPB may be critical, specifically, those with diabetes mellitus, hypertension, and cerebrovascular disease.[148]

Gravlee et al.[157] recently performed a study to determine if hypercapnia during CPB resulted in the redistribution of cerebral blood flow from marginally perfused regions to well-perfused regions (intracerebral steal). Patients with documented cerebrovascular disease were subjected to alterations of arterial $Paco_2$ (from 40 to 60 mm Hg, uncorrected for temperature) during CPB. Cerebral blood flow studies using ^{133}Xe clearance techniques failed to demonstrate intracerebral steal during increased arterial CO_2 tension. Neuropsychologic testing was not performed.

In summary, both experimental and clinical data support the conclusion that alpha-stat acid-base management during hypothermic CPB closely approximates normal physiology, thus preserving cerebral autoregulation. The clinical relevance of this information remains to be determined. The two studies previously described conclude that increased arterial CO_2 tension may not be clinically significant. However, the results of these studies must be corroborated by further investigation before definite conclusions can be made. Furthermore, the study of patients with preexisting cerebrovascular disease and derangements of autoregulation, i.e., those with hypertension or diabetes mellitus, needs to be pursued. Undoubtedly, neuropsychologic testing will play a major role in future investigations. As previously described, ischemia in normothermic brain tissue quickly gives rise to intracellular acidosis, which, if severe enough, will lead ultimately to cell death. Animal studies have demonstrated that cerebral ischemia resulting in tissue lactate levels less than 16 mmol/kg produces selective neuronal damage in predictably vulnerable areas. Astrocytes and endothelial cells are spared, thus providing a protective effect by preventing widespread cerebral edema. Ischemia resulting in levels greater than 16 mmol/kg damages astrocytes and endothelium, as well as neurons, resulting in infarction and progressive cerebral edema.[142]

Further investigation has demonstrated that raising serum glucose levels prior to normothermic ischemia increases tissue lactate levels, thus further decreasing intracellular pH.[143, 158] Normoglycemic and hyperglycemic rats subjected to 15 minutes of normothermic, hemispheric ischemia experienced a substantial but similar decrease in phosphocreatine and adenosine triphosphate levels.[159] Lactate concentrations increased significantly in both groups; however, the hyperglycemic animals exhibited a notably greater rise in lactate levels. Recovery of energy metabolism was significantly poorer in the hyperglycemic group and this was associated with a marked, lingering acidosis.

During CPB, hypothermia is employed to reduce cellular metabolism and oxygen demand. During periods of ischemia, it is hoped that the reduced metabolic activity results in minimal anaerobic metabolism, lactate formation, and intracellular acidosis. As mentioned earlier, neural tissues can tolerate low levels of lactate accumulation.[142]

The role of hyperglycemia during hypothermic CPB has not been clearly defined. Nondiabetic patients often experience a temporary increase in blood glucose levels during CPB. In many centers, this is not treated and subsequently resolves without any apparent sequelae. Based on clinical and experimental data obtained using normothermic models, one could hypothesize that hyperglycemia, in the presence of focal or global ischemia occurring during CPB, could drive anaerobic glycolysis, resulting in increased lactate formation and cell damage. Alternatively, hypothermia and the resultant decrease in metabolism may protect against this.

Using serial measurements of creatine kinase BB as a marker for brain ischemia, Ekroth[160] found a positive correlation between hyperglycemia and increased creatine kinase BB levels during reperfusion following deep hypothermic circulatory arrest in infants.

In our laboratory, we presently are studying the role of hyperglycemia during CPB. Using phosphorus-31 nuclear magnetic resonance spectroscopy, we are attempting to determine the effects of hyperglycemia on high-energy phosphate metabolism and intracellular pH during ischemia and reperfusion in the sheep brain. Models of deep hypothermic circulatory arrest and low-flow CPB are being studied.

Interest in the use of pharmacologic agents for cerebral protection during CPB is relatively new. In 1986, Nussmeier and associates[161] reported on the effectiveness of thiopental to decrease neuropsychiatric complications following open ventricle procedures. The authors concluded that embolization was the most common cause of focal neurologic dysfunction following CPB, and that the administration of thiopental prior to cannulation reduced the clinical consequences of such embolic events. Barbiturate protection during global ischemia has not been demonstrated.

Cerebral vascular injury due to free radicals may be amenable to pharmacologic intervention. As previously described, both vitamin E[162] and deferoxamine[163] have been shown to reduce lipid peroxidation during CPB. Mannitol is a known hydroxyl radical scavenger; however, its effects on lipid peroxidation are unknown.[147]

Prostacyclin and its analogues have been used to prevent platelet aggregation and microembolism of small vessels. Radegran and associates[164] demonstrated that prostacyclin infused prior to and during extracorporeal circulation for coronary artery bypass preserved platelet numbers and reduced microaggregates. Clinical evidence that prostacyclin reduces postoperative neurologic deficit has not been convincing. Fish et al.[165] administered prostacyclin to patients prior to and during CPB. All patients underwent neuropsychologic testing and brain computed tomography preoperatively, and 1 week and 2 months postoperatively. No differences between the two groups were noted at 1 week or 2 months.

It has been suggested that increased intracellular calcium is the final common pathway for cell necrosis.[166] Recently, attention has been directed toward the role of calcium channel blockers in cerebral protection. Nimodipine is a lipid-soluble calcium channel blocker with potent vasodilating properties.[167, 168] Gelmers and associates[167] reported reduced mortality and improved neurologic outcome in patients with acute ischemic stroke who received nimodipine. Allen et al.[168] showed reduced arterial spasm in patients with subarachnoid hemorrhage treated with nimodipine. Steen[169] demonstrated that nimodipine administration after 17 minutes of complete cerebral ischemia in monkeys led to improved neurologic outcome. The role of nimodipine during CPB has not been defined.

Calcium entry into the cell is controlled by voltage-dependent calcium channels and agonist-operated conducting channels. Agonist-operated channels also may allow the uptake of sodium, chloride, and water into the nerve cells. The naturally occurring agonists controlling these channels appear to be glutamate and N-methyl D-aspartate, both of which are known to cause neuronal excitation.[147] Cerebral ischemia results in greatly increased levels of extracellular glutamate.[170, 171] If glutamate receptors are blocked with an N-methyl D-aspartate antagonist, neuronal ischemic damage is decreased.[172, 173] Studies examining the protective effects of N-methyl D-aspartate antagonists during CPB presently are under way.

Cerebroplegia

A novel attempt to protect the brain from ischemia involves the use of "cerebroplegia." In our laboratory, Robbins and Swain[174] used phosphorus-31 nuclear magnetic resonance spectroscopy to study the protective effect of "intermittent hypothermic asanguinous cerebral perfusion" during hypothermic circulatory arrest in sheep. Phosphocreatine and adenosine triphosphate remained at significantly higher levels throughout the 2-hour arrest period in animals receiving cerebroplegia. The adenosine triphosphate level was maintained at $63\% \pm 6\%$ of prearrest values, and phosphocreatine levels were $21\% \pm 2\%$ of prearrest levels after 2 hours of circulatory arrest at $12°$ C ($P < .0001$). In control animals, both phosphocreatine and adenosine triphosphate were depleted totally after 60 minutes of arrest. Animals receiving cerebroplegia maintained significantly higher intracellular pH values throughout the arrest period and during up to 2 hours of reperfusion (Fig 2). Electroencephalographic activity returned to baseline after 36 ± 6 minutes of reperfusion for the cerebroplegia group. Activity in the control animals did not return until 117 ± 23 minutes ($P < .05$).

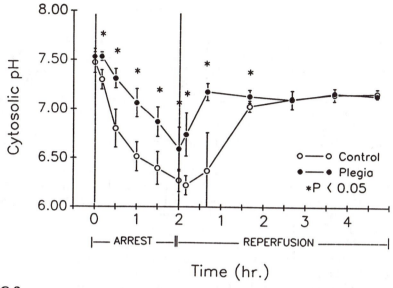

FIG 2.
Intracellular pH in control and cerebroplegia groups during circulatory arrest and reperfusion. (Courtesy of J Swain.)

Using the same model, Crittenden and Swain[175] demonstrated that sheep receiving antegrade cerebroplegia (i.e., carotid perfusion) had a better neurologic outcome than did animals cooled by surface cooling, core cooling, or retrograde cerebroplegia (i.e., internal jugular perfusion).

Whether or not cerebroplegia becomes a clinically useful adjunct for cerebral protection remains to be seen. However, this concept should generate much interest and future investigation.

Low Flow vs. No Flow

Potential neurologic insult limits the duration of hypothermic circulatory arrest. Continuous hypothermic low-flow perfusion has been advocated as an alternative to circulatory arrest, thereby allowing more time to complete complex procedures. Using creatine kinase BB as a marker for cerebral ischemia, Rossi and coworkers[176] compared deep hypothermic circulatory arrest with hypothermic low-flow CPB. Twenty-seven children undergoing repair of complex congenital heart defects were assigned to one of two groups. Patients in the low-flow group underwent perfusion at a rate calculated to be 25% of normal. Both the low-flow and the arrest group were cooled to 15° C. Arterial blood samples for the quantification of creatine kinase BB were obtained after induction and when the body temperature reached 15° C. Samples were taken also at the completion of the low-flow/ arrest periods and at 2 minutes, 30 minutes, and 1, 2, 3, 4, 5, 6, 7, and 8 hours. The period of low flow was 35 ± 6 minutes. The period of arrest was 46 ± 5 minutes.

None of the children had detectable preoperative or postoperative neurologic deficits. Creatine kinase BB levels increased from 4.3 ± 0.9 ng/mL to 10.4 ± 1.8 ng/mL in the circulatory arrest group, and from 2.8 ± 0.7 ng/mL to 9.9 ± 1.9 ng/mL in the low-flow group (Fig 3). The difference between the groups was not statistically significant. The authors concluded that low-flow CPB did not result in superior cerebral protection when compared with similar periods of circulatory arrest. Whether or not the continued flow of blood hampered the operation in the low-flow group was not addressed.

Using phosphorus-31 nuclear magnetic resonance spectroscopy, Swain and associates[177] examined cerebral energy metabolism during periods of hypothermic circulatory arrest, low-flow CPB, and circulatory arrest interrupted by a period of systemic, full-flow perfusion in sheep. Two hours of circulatory arrest at 15° C resulted in a large decrease of adenosine triphosphate (12% ± 2% of prearrest levels) and phosphocreatine (4% ± 2% of prearrest levels). Intracellular pH decreased markedly from 7.52 ± 0.04 to 6.65 ± 0.12 during the arrest period (Fig 4). Sheep undergoing hypothermic (15° C) low-flow bypass at 5 mL/kg/min also demonstrated a significant decrease in adenosine triphosphate (27% to ± 6% of prearrest values), phosphocreatine (13% ± 4%), and intracellular pH (7.61 ± 0.05 to 6.82 ± 0.03). Those animals perfused at 10 mL/kg/min maintained baseline levels of adenosine triphosphate (100% ± 2%), phosphocreatine (96% ± 5%), and intracellular pH (7.57 ± 0.02 vs. 7.67 ± 0.03 at the end of 2 hours) (see Fig 4).

A fourth group of animals underwent 60 minutes of circulatory arrest, 30 minutes of full-flow (75 to 100 mL/kg/min) reperfusion at 15° C, and another 60 minutes of arrest. As expected, 1 hour of arrest resulted in marked reductions in adenosine triphosphate, phosphocreatine, and pH. Reperfusion partially restored high-energy phosphates and intracellular pH; however, at the end of the second hour of arrest, adenosine triphosphate, phosphocreatine, and pH values were similar to those following 2 hours of perfusion at 5 mL/kg/min (Fig 5).

Pulsatile Flow

The issue of the most efficacious mode of arterial blood flow during CPB remains controversial. Nonpulsatile flow has been used since the clinical inception of CPB, mainly due to the technical complexity of trying to create pulsatile pump systems. Technologic advances have developed reliable pulsatile pump systems that are being used routinely now at a number of centers.

Intuitively, it would seem that pulsatile flow, and the creation of such a physiologic perfusion, would be more desirable. The theoretic aspects of pulsatile arterial physiology include the concept of energy-equivalent pres-

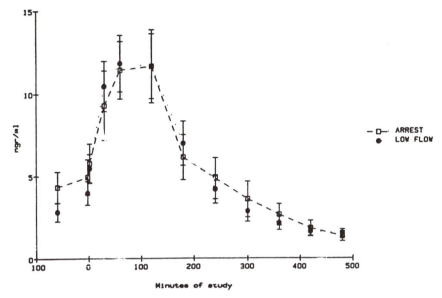

FIG 3.
Arterial creatine kinase BB (mean plus or minus standard error of the mean) of total circulatory arrest group and low-flow group before and after arrest/low-flow period (represented by 0). (From Rossi R, van der Linden J, Ekroth R, et al: *J Thorac Cardiovasc Surg* 1989; 98:193–199. Used by permission.)

sure.[178] The total hemodynamic energy per millimeter of blood passing a given arterial cross section can be calculated from phasic flow and pressure measurements and expressed as energy-equivalent pressure in millimeters of mercury. The difference between energy equivalent and mean pressures may represent energy contributed directly to the maintenance of peripheral perfusion. On this basis, a pulsatile arterial wave dissipates more utilizable energy to tissues than does a nonpulsatile wave of the same mean pressure. A higher mean flow rate is seen with pulsatile flow compared to nonpulsatile flow at equal perfusion pressures, although this may be secondary to lower peripheral vascular resistance. A second concept is that of capillary critical closing pressure and microcirculatory patency. It has been shown that nonpulsatile perfusion results in decreased flow of lymph and interstitial fluid, with decreased capillary flow.[179] Microcirculatory shunting and capillary collapse result in decreased oxygen consumption, tissue acidosis, and diminished metabolic uptake rates of oxygen and glucose. A third factor is the neuroendocrine reflex mechanisms triggered by baroreceptor discharge. Nonpulsatile flow results in a marked increase in discharge frequency of carotid sinus baroreceptors. This may be contributory to the vasoconstriction induced by nonpulsatile flow.[180]

The hemodynamic effects of arterial flow patterns during CPB are related intimately to peripheral vascular resistance. Nonpulsatile flow has

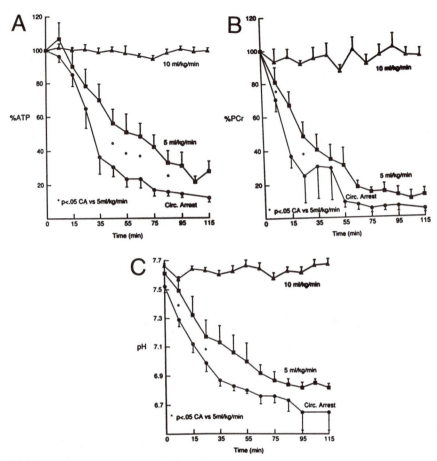

FIG 4.
Changes in cerebral adenosine triphosphate **(A)**, phosphocreatine **(B)**, and pH **(C)** during circulatory arrest and low-flow cardiopulmonary bypass. (From Swain J, McDonald T, Griffith P, et al: *J Thorac Cardiovasc Surg,* in press. Used by permission.)

been shown to result in elevated peripheral vascular resistance. A previous study demonstrated a marked increase in angiotensin II levels with nonpulsatile flow.[181] Furthermore, effective blockade of this effect has been demonstrated with angiotensin II inhibitors.[182] A more recent clinical study in patients requiring CPB for 60 minutes or more compared pulsatile and nonpulsatile flow in this regard. Pulsatile CPB resulted in less elevation of plasma angiotensin II and serum aldosterone levels.[183]

Earlier studies showed no correlation of catecholamine levels with the elevated peripheral vascular resistance of nonpulsatile perfusion. More recent clinical work has revealed a diminished catecholamine response to

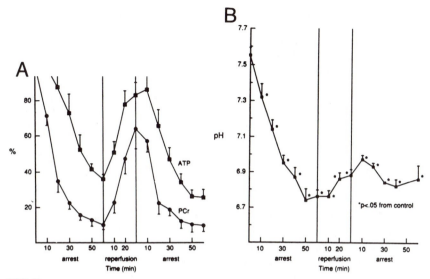

FIG 5.
Changes in cerebral adenosine triphosphate, phosphocreatine **(A)**, and pH **(B)** during circulatory arrest interrupted by 30 minutes of full-flow reperfusion. (From Swain J, McDonald T, Griffith P, et al: *J Thorac Cardiovasc Surg*, in press. Used by permission.)

pulsatile perfusion. This was associated with less fluid accumulation and improved recovery of patients during the postoperative phase, as evaluated by extubation time.[184] Additional clinical work has documented markedly reduced plasma norepinephrine levels with pulsatile perfusion.[185] Vasopressin also may play a contributory role in the hemodynamic effects.[186] Corroborating this, a recent study demonstrated that pulsatile perfusion resulted in decreased serum vasopressin levels as well as decreased urinary sodium and increased urine flow.[187] Increasing the flow rate and perfusion pressures of nonpulsatile flow has not been shown to prevent or ovecome increased peripheral vascular resistance and vasoconstriction. Recent studies with a canine model revealed that pulsatile perfusion was advantageous for both the kidney and systemic hemodynamics at flow rates of 80 and 100 mL/kg/min. Pulsatile and nonpulsatile perfusion seemed to be similar at lower and higher flow rates in terms of hemodynamics, renal circulation, and kidney metabolism.[188]

The metabolic effects of different arterial blood flow modes also have been studied extensively in the past. Pulsatile perfusion has been shown to result in higher oxygen consumption. Nonpulsatile perfusion has been associated with metabolic acidosis, reduced oxygen consumption, and reduced cellular glucose uptake.[189] Increased tissue water content with pulsatile flow may be a demonstration of cell membrane instability and sodium pump malfunction associated with impaired capillary perfusion.

However, recent clinical studies using pulsatile CPB for over 60 minutes of perfusion did not show a definite advantage for tissue metabolism, as assessed by serum lactate levels.[183]

Among the effects of nonpulsatile perfusion on the brain are decreased cerebral arteriolar and capillary diameter.[190] Additionally, during nonpulsatile perfusion, it has been demonstrated that the anterior pituitary failed to respond to a trophic stimulus from TRH.[191] Similarly, the secretion of adrenocorticotropic hormone and vasopressin was attenuated.[186, 187] Hence, the pituitary-adrenal axis shows evidence of switching off during nonpulsatile perfusion. These changes were prevented by the use of pulsatile perfusion. Elevated creatine kinase isoenzymes also were noted in the cerebrospinal fluid during nonpulsatile perfusion.[192] Canine experiments have shown that pulsatile flow is better than nonpulsatile flow in promoting cerebral perfusion. The differences between pulsatile and nonpulsatile flow seemed to be greater in the ischemic brain than in the nonischemic brain. Within ischemic regions, changing from nonpulsatile to pulsatile flow was associated with improvement in neuronal activity.[193] A recent study utilizing a pig model showed that pulsatile CPB resulted in cortical edema, possibly due to enhanced extravasation of serum proteins as a result of reduced cerebral blood flow during CPB. Pulsatile flow in this instance appeared to alter the permeability of the blood-brain barrier.[194] The results of a small clinical series have been reported recently.[195] In this study, neuropsychologic outcome was compared between pulsatile and nonpulsatile flow in 22 men undergoing aortocoronary bypass surgery. No difference was appreciated between the two groups with respect to neurologic outcome or the perioperative measurements of electrocardiogram, cerebral blood flow, and the cerebral metabolism of oxygen and glucose. To assess the degree of pulsatility of cerebral blood flow during CPB, transcranial Doppler ultrasound has been demonstrated to be a useful technique in clinical cases.[196] Using this technique, it was found that pulse frequency, pulse length, position of oxygenators within the circuit, and flow rate and CO_2 reactivity of the cerebral arteries were important factors influencing wave patterns in pulsatile CPB. This study also showed that minimal pulse levels are necessary to keep the microvasculature from undergoing collapse or shunting. It also was concluded that excessive systolic flow velocities may induce turbulence and vortices, especially in cases of cerebral artery stenoses. High pulse amplitude with low diastolic flow also should be avoided.

Observations of altered arterial flow patterns on the kidney are also noteworthy. Defects in renal excretory function have been shown during nonpulsatile perfusion. Tubular sodium excretion and increased secretion of renin have been seen also. Pulsatile perfusion has resulted in the preservation of cortical blood flow, renal venous return, and renal tubular histology.[197] Recent clinical studies have documented pulsatile perfusion to be advantageous in patients with preoperatively impaired renal function.[198] There was a greater elevation in postoperative serum creatinine, and a higher mortality in those who underwent nonpulsatile CPB. All patients in this series had a preoperative creatinine clearance below 30 mL/min. Canine experiments with CPB associated with profound hypothermia and total circulatory arrest have shown increased blood flow to the kidneys, liver, and pancreas, with pulsatile flow after reperfusion.[199] In addition to these beneficial effects of pulsatile perfusion, renal vascular autoregulation may provide protection to the kidneys.

The pancreas and liver have been seen to receive increased flow with pulsatile perfusion in the above-mentioned canine experiment. Clinical studies have revealed decreased serum amylase levels and a reduced incidence of elevated amylase-creatinine ratios with pulsatile flow.[200] Additional clinical studies have revealed that pulsatile flow is more effective in preserving pancreatic beta cell function and tissue metabolism during and early after open heart procedure.[201] This was assessed by measurement of immunoreactive insulin and C peptide, serum glucagon, glucose, and lactate levels. Nonpulsatile perfusion of the liver has resulted in vasoconstriction and decreased hepatic oxygen consumption.[202]

Current clinical use of pulsatile perfusion generally employs modified roller pump systems or intermittent occlusive systems, although several other systems are being developed also. Among the hematologic effects of the systems in common clinical use, significantly increased hemolysis or blood cell depletion have not been noted.[203] Clinical series have not demonstrated an increased requirement of homologous blood transfusion or need for postoperative reexploration for bleeding.[204] Additionally, a decreased need for intra-aortic balloon pump and inotropic drug support has been seen after pulsatile perfusion.[205] Pulsatile perfusion has resulted in improved core cooling and rewarming.[206] A clinical study incorporating 259 infants who underwent high-flow CPB with pulsatile flow showed benefits of this method of perfusion was in relation to operative techniques, water balance, and postoperative recovery.[207] Another recent clinical study in children did not show differences in plasma cortisol and adrenocorticotropic hormone concentrations during CPB with and without pulsatile flow.[208] Thus, there is a sound physiologic basis for the use of pulsatile flow, and good clinical results with this form of perfusion have been documented.

Percutaneous Cardiopulmonary Bypass

The application of CPB has extended beyond surgical management of cardiac disease to provide hemodynamic support in a number of clinical settings. Over the past 2 decades, emergent initiation of CPB for circulatory support has resulted in the salvage of patients with failing circulation. Catastrophic situations of impending death and cardiac arrest have been aborted using CPB for resuscitation.[209] It was through these endeavors that percutaneous and portable systems for CPB evolved.[210, 211] These systems now are gaining increasingly widespread use as a standby tool in the realm of interventional cardiology, during high-risk angioplasty and aortic valvuloplasty.[212–214]

The rationale for the use of percutaneous CPB support is based on the fact that 5% of patients undergoing angioplasty have acute arterial closure during the procedure, with subsequent risk of hemodynamic collapse.[215] Patients deemed to be at high risk for this occurrence are those in whom the target vessel supplies a large amount of the myocardium and those with severely reduced left ventricular function.[212] In addition, patients with left main coronary artery disease and those who have had several coronary artery bypass graft operations are at increased risk during catheterization.[216] Percutaneous CPB support also has been used in balloon valvuloplasty for aortic valvular stenosis in patients who are high operative risks or in whom surgery is contraindicated.[212]

Support of angioplasty with CPB is believed to reduce ischemia by lowering cardiac afterload and wall tension. Increased aortic diastolic pressure and reduced left ventricular pressures result in greater coronary artery perfusion gradients. Preload also is decreased during CPB.[217] During valvuloplasty, myocardial and cerebral ischemia are prevented while the balloon is inflated within the aortic valve. With prolonged balloon inflations during angioplasty or valvuloplasty, complete cardiopulmonary support is maintained. No chest pain or electrocardiographic changes have been observed, and symptomatic improvement has been reported in all surviving patients.[212] On-pump transfusion is often necessary, since priming volumes of about 1,400 mL generally are required in these circuits.[216] With nonreservoir centrifugal CPB, there is less need for α-agonists. Drops in blood pressure usually respond to volume infusion.[216] Significant complications of vessel and nerve injury have been incurred.

The results of percutaneous CPB have been assessed recently in the initial report on the National Registry of Elective CPB Supported Coronary Angioplasty, incorporating 105 patients in a multicenter study.[214] Patient criteria for inclusion in the study were those in whom the target vessel supplied more than 50% of the myocardium, those with an ejection fraction less than 25%, or both. The angioplasty success rate was 95%, with 1.7 dilatations per patient. A 39% morbidity of arterial, venous, or nerve injury associated with cannula insertion or removal was seen. Hospital mortality was 7.6%, with one half of these deaths in patients 75 years of age or older with left main coronary artery stenosis. Forty-three percent of patients required blood transfusion. None of the patients were CPB support–dependent after angioplasty. Thus, the majority of high-risk patients can undergo angioplasty with CPB support. However, there is an excessively high rate of associated vascular morbidity from the current method of percutaneous cannula insertion. It also was noted that a large number of patients did not have the anticipated hemodynamic collapse that would be prevented by CPB support. Hence, there is an unproven need for systemic circulatory support in all patients enrolled under the suggested inclusion criteria. On this basis, the current application of CPB probably should be made on a standby rather than routine basis in the cardiac catheterization laboratory. Improvements in cannula design and greater clinical experience may decrease the observed vascular complications. No randomized studies have been performed to compare high-risk angioplasty with and without CPB support.

Recent studies in a canine model have revealed significantly increased myocardial salvage and reduction in tension-time index utilizing percutaneous CPB with a synchronous pulsatile pump.[218] This may provide an effective means of providing seriously ill cardiac patients with temporary hemodynamic stability and myocardial protection before and during revascularization of fibrillating ischemic myocardium.

Extracorporeal Membrane Oxygenation

Extracorporeal membrane oxygenation (ECMO) continues to be the focus of much recent investigation in the management of acute respiratory insufficiency in infants and adults. Its efficacy is based on allowing pulmonary healing by providing gas exchange without damaging levels of inspired oxygen and by reducing barotrauma complications. Since long-term survival depends on the reversibility of the lung disease, applications of ECMO in the neonate have proved to be more diverse than in children or adults. It appears that pathologic conditions of more mature lung tissue heal by fibrosis, with little capacity for the regeneration of normal lung tissue. The ability of even the neonatal lung to recover is finite, so that ECMO yields best results when used within the first 5 to 7 days of life in term and near-term newborns weighing 2 kg or more.[219] Low–birth weight babies have a poor outcome with ECMO.[220]

Indications for ECMO in the neonate include reversible lung disease, failure of maximal medical therapy, and meeting the institution's criteria for 80% mortality or greater without ECMO. Indices of severity of lung disease include alveolar-arterial oxygen difference, a combination of alveolar-arterial oxygen difference and peak inspiratory pressure, oxygenation index, Pao_2/Pao_2, or just Pao_2. Serial alveolar-arterial oxygen difference determinations have been found to be particularly good indicators of severity, with a value of 600 or greater over a 12-hour period identifying a group with 94% mortality.[221] The acceptance criteria for neonates with congenital diaphragmatic hernia have been changed to include all of those in respiratory failure. Previously, in an attempt to exclude those with unsalvageable pulmonary hypoplasia, neonates were not considered for ECMO unless they had a "honeymoon period" with at least one preductal Pao_2 above 100 mm Hg or a postductal Pao_2 of 50 to 70. Contraindications to ECMO in neonates include weight less than 1,300 g, intracranial hemorrhage, neurologic deficit, multiple congenital anomalies, renal failure, and age greater than 7 days.

The overall results of ECMO therapy in adults and children have been disappointing.[222, 223] Irreversibility of acute pulmonary damage in this group of patients is the limiting factor. It has been shown that the pulmonary pathology is usually irreversible if the duration of the illness has been 5 days or more, the primary disease is infection or aspiration, or destruction of the lung architecture and fibrosis are found at biopsy. In children, however, irreversible damage seems to occur later, so that an ECMO trial may be indicated even after 5 days of respiratory failure.[224] Successful implementation of ECMO also has been demonstrated in the management of children with left ventricular or biventricular failure after CPB.[225] Left ventricular assist devices are not commonly available for the pediatric population. In adults, good results have been seen in conditions such as acute pulmonary embolism, pulmonary alveolar proteinosis, and iatrogenic venous gas embolism.[223] When improvement of pulmonary function is seen in adults, it generally begins to occur within 48 hours.[222] Contraindications to ECMO in adults include recent head trauma and hepatic or renal failure.

There are two types of ECMO in common use: venoarterial bypass and venovenous bypass. Venoarterial bypass is the most commonly used method in neonates, providing gas exchange and circulatory support. Venous cannulation is through the internal jugular vein, and arterial cannulation is via the carotid artery to the aortic arch. A possible disadvantage is the necessity of ligating the carotid artery, with uncertain long-term sequelae. Venovenous bypass provides gas exchange, with the left ventricle remaining as the pump for circulation to the arterial tree. Due to the recirculation of mixed venous blood, higher flow rates are required for adequate oxygenation. High mixed-venous saturation may help relax constricted pulmonary vessels. There also may be a benefit from maintaining pulmonary blood flow by this method. Venovenous perfusion may be best for adults in respiratory failure without cardiac failure. Recently, to-and-fro venovenous extracorporeal lung assist has been described as an alternative method.[226] This technique requires the cannulation of a single internal jugular vein and provides adequate gas exchange with alternating blood withdrawal and perfusion through the same catheter. Possible benefits with this method include unimpaired pulmonary blood flow and sparing of the carotid arteries. Other recent work has introduced the application of extracorporeal carbon dioxide removal, as opposed to extracorporeal oxygenation. Clinical trials in adults with this technique resulted in a 47% survival rate in a population with an expected mortality rate higher than 90%.[227] A recent canine study investigated respiratory support by means of arteriovenous extracorporeal membrane oxygenation driven by systemic arterial pressure, without the use of an external pump. It was found that achieving adequate flow rates with this technique adversely altered pulmonary and systemic hemodynamics. However, these effects could be modulated beneficially with moderate doses of inotropic medication.[228] A new intravascular blood gas exchange device is being developed. This intravenous mechanical blood oxygen/carbon dioxide exchange device is introduced into the vena cava through a jugular or femoral venotomy.[229] In an awake sheep model, this device has shown the capability of transferring more than 100 mL/min of oxygen and carbon dioxide to and from the venous blood. No adverse hemodynamic or hematologic sequelae were noted. This device employs multiple microporous hollow fibers, with 2,000 to 6,000 cm^2 of gas transfer surface area.

Complications of ECMO include bleeding, intracranial hemorrhage, technical problems, renal failure, sepsis, seizures, and vascular complications. Bleeding may occur at virtually any site, with systemic heparinization usually being the major contributory factor. Intracranial hemorrhage occurs in as many as 38% of neonates who undergo ECMO, and is the major cause of death.[224, 229] Neonates found to be at higher risk for intracranial hemorrhage are those born at less than 34 weeks of gestation and those weighing less than 2 kg at birth.[224] Neonates undergoing ECMO while in septic shock also have been found to be at higher risk for intracranial hemorrhage.[230] Technical problems include oxygenator leak or failure, heat exchanger leak, pump failure, tubing rupture, thromboemboli, and air emboli. Vascular complications include deep venous thrombosis and pseudoaneurysms with femoral vein cannulations.

ECMO in the neonate has resulted in an overall survival of 83%, as shown by the National ECMO Registry (July 1989). Neurologic follow-up has found that 72% to 75% of ECMO babies are normal, with non–ECMO-treated patients not doing as well.[224, 231] An adverse neurologic outcome is predicted by the occurrence of clinical seizures or cerebral infarction while on ECMO. Twenty-three percent of patients undergoing ECMO were found to have some degree of sensorineural hearing loss.[231] It has been found that individual outcomes cannot be predicted with neuroimaging; however, it can be a useful adjunct in assigning patients who survive with ECMO treatment to risk categories for developmental outcome.[232] Color Doppler imaging studies have demonstrated changing patterns of collateral cerebral circulation and adequacy of the collateral circulation following ligation of the right common carotid artery in ECMO patients.[233] Other transcranial Doppler studies have shown that there is no consistent correlation between lateralized cerebral hemodynamic abnormalities and lateralized neurologic sequelae in ECMO survivors.[234]

The incidence of chronic lung disease in ECMO survivors is 10% to 15%. Those at high risk are infants with sepsis and those placed on ECMO after 7 to 8 days.[224] Thus, overall ECMO has improved survival and decreased the incidence of intracranial hemorrhage and bronchopulmonary dysplasia as compared to conventional therapy.[229] These results have been obtained without increasing hospital utilization, cost, or morbidity compared to non-ECMO treatment.[235, 236]

References

1. Hanjuda M, Morimoto M, Sugenoya A, et al: Suppressive effect of ulinastatin on plasma fibronectin depression after cardiac surgery. *Ann Thorac Surg* 1988; 45:171–217.
2. Anderson LW, Baek L, Degn H, et al: Absence of circulating endotoxins during cardiac operations. *J Thorac Cardiovasc Surg* 1987; 93:115–119.
3. Faymonville ME, Deby-Dupont G, Larbuisson R, et al: Prostaglandin E$_2$, prostacyclin, and thromboxane changes during nonpulsatile cardiopulmonary bypass in humans. *J Thorac Cardiovasc Surg* 1986; 91:858–866.

4. Greeley WJ, Bushman GA, Kong DL, et al: Effects of cardiopulmonary bypass on eicosanoid metabolism during pediatric cardiovascular surgery. *J Thorac Cardiovasc Surg* 1988; 95:842–849.
5. Kim YD, Foegh ML, Wallace R, et al: Effects of CGS-13080, a thromboxane inhibitor, on pulmonary vascular resistance in patients after mitral valve replacement surgery. *Circulation* 1988; 78:44–50.
6. Mehta JL, Nichols WW, Schofield R, et al: TxA_2 inhibition and ischemia-induced loss of myocardial function and reactive hyperemia. *Am J Physiol* 1990; 258:H1402–H1408.
7. Dewar ML, Walsh G, Chui CJ, et al: Atrial natriuretic factor: Response to cardiac operation. *J Thorac Cardiovasc Surg* 1988; 96:266–270.
8. Schaff H, Mashburn JP, McCarthy PM, et al: Natriuresis during and early after cardiopulmonary bypass: Relationship to atrial natriuretic factor, aldosterone, and antidiuretic hormone. *J Thorac Cardiovasc Surg* 1989; 98:979–986.
9. Weinstein GS, Zabetakis PM, Clavel A, et al: The renin-angiotensin system is not responsible for hypertension following coronary artery bypass grafting. *Ann Thorac Surg* 1987; 43:74–77.
10. Gorin AB, Liebler J: Changes in serum angiotensin-converting enzyme during cardiopulmonary bypass in humans. *Am Rev Respir Dis* 1986; 134:79–84.
11. Robuschi G, Medici D, Fesani F, et al: Cardiopulmonary bypass: Low T_4 and T_3 syndrome with blunted thyrotropin (TSH) response to thyrotropin-releasing hormone (TRH). *Horm Res* 1986; 23:151–158.
12. Novitsky D, Cooper DKC, Zuhdi N: Triiodothyronine therapy in the cardiac transplant recipient. *Transplant Proc* 1988; 20:65–68.
13. Novitsky D, Human PA, Cooper DKC: Effect of triiodothyronine (T_3) on myocardial high energy phosphates and lactate after ischemia and cardiopulmonary bypass. *J Thorac Cardiovasc Surg* 1988; 96:600–607.
14. Novitsky D, Cooper DKC, Swanepoel A: Inotropic effect of triiodothyronine (T_3) in low cardiac output following cardioplegic arrest and cardiopulmonary bypass: An initial experience in patients undergoing open heart surgery. *Eur J Cardio-Thorac Surg* 1989; 3:140–145.
15. Novitsky D, Cooper DKC, Barton CI, et al: Triiodothyronine as an inotropic agent after open heart surgery. *J Thorac Cardiovasc Surg* 1989; 98:972–978.
16. Kangir CB, Madsen T, Peterson PH, et al: Calcium, magnesium, and phosphate during and after hypothermic cardiopulmonary bypass without temperature correction of acid base status. *Acta Anaesthesiol Scand* 1988; 32:676–680.
17. Fuhrer G, Heller W, Hoffmeister HE, et al: Levels of trace elements during and after cardiopulmonary bypass operations. *Acta Pharmacol Toxicol* (Copenh) 1986; 7: 352–357.
18. Sjogern A, Luhrs C, Abdulla M: Changed distribution of zinc and copper in body fluids in patients undergoing open heart surgery. *Acta Pharmacol Toxicol* (Copenh) 1986; 7: 348–351.
19. Del Canale S, Fiacadori E, Medici D, et al: Effects of low flux-low pressure cardiopulmonary bypass on intracellular acid-base and water metabolism. *Scand J Thorac Cardiovasc Surg* 1986; 20:167–170.
20. Del Canale S, Ficaccadori E, Vezzani A, et al: Cell metabolism response to cardiopulmonary bypass in patients undergoing aorto-coronary grafting. *Scand J Thorac Cardiovasc Surg* 1988; 22:159–164.

21. Addonizio VP: Platelet function in cardiopulmonary bypass and artificial organs. *Hematol Oncol Clin North Am* 1990; 4:145–155.
22. Copeland JG, Harker LA, Joist JG, et al: Bleeding and anticoagulation. *Ann Thorac Surg* 1989; 47:88–95.
23. Holloway DS, Summaria L, Sandesara J, et al: Decreased platelet number and function and increased fibrinolysis contribute to postoperative bleeding in cardiopulmonary bypass patients. *Thromb Haemost* 1988; 59:62–67.
24. Czer LS, Bateman TM, Gray RJ, et al: Treatment of severe platelet dysfunction and hemorrhage after cardiopulmonary bypass: Reduction in blood product usage with desmopressin. *J Am Coll Cardiol* 1987; 9:1139–1147.
25. Salzman EW, Weinstein MJ, Weintraub RM, et al: Treatment with desmopressin acetate to reduce blood loss after cardiac surgery. *N Engl J Med* 1986; 314:1402–1406.
26. Kucuk O, Kwaan HC, Frederickson J, et al: Increased fibrinolytic activity in patients undergoing cardiopulmonary bypass operation. *Am J Hematol* 1986; 23:223–229.
27. Kongsgaard UE, Smith-Erichsen N, Geiran O, et al: Changes in the coagulation and fibrinolytic systems during and after cardiopulmonary bypass surgery. *Thorac Cardiovasc Surg* 1989; 37:158–162.
28. Colman RW: Platelet and neutrophil activation in cardiopulmonary bypass. *Ann Thorac Surg* 1990; 49:32–34.
29. Wenger RK, Lukasiewicz H, Mikuta BS, et al: Loss of platelet fibrinogen receptors during clinical cardiopulmonary bypass. *J Thorac Cardiovasc Surg* 1989; 97:235–239.
30. Gluszko P, Rucinski B, Musial J, et al: Fibrinogen receptors in platelet adhesion to surfaces of extracorporeal circuit. *Am J Physiol* 1987; 252:H615–H621.
31. Mohr R, Martinowitz U, Golan M, et al: Platelet size and mass as an indicator for platelet transfusion after cardiopulmonary bypass. *Circulation* 1986; 74(suppl III):153–158.
32. Addonizio VP, Smith JB, Guiod LR, et al: The relationship between thromboxane synthesis and platelet protein release during simulated extracorporeal circulation. *Blood* 1979; 54:371–376.
33. Teoh KH, Christakis GT, Weisel RD, et al: Prevention of myocardial platelet deposition and thromboxane release with dipyridamole. *Circulation* 1986; 74(suppl III):145–152.
34. Addonizo VP, Macarak EJ, Nicolaou KC, et al: Effects of prostacyclin and albumin on platelet loss during in vitro simulation of extracorporeal circulation. *Blood* 1979; 53:1033–1042.
35. von Segesser LK, Turina M: Cardiopulmonary bypass without systemic heparinization. *J Thorac Cardiovasc Surg* 1989; 98:386–396.
36. Weinstein M, Ware JA, Troll J, et al: Changes in von Willebrand factor during cardiac surgery: Effect of desmopressin acetate. *Blood* 1988; 71:1648–1655.
37. Chard RB, Kam CA, Nunn GR, et al: Use of desmopressin in the management of aspirin-related and intractable haemorrhage after cardiopulmonary bypass. *Aust N Z J Surg* 1990; 60:125–128.
38. Hackmann T, Gascoyne RE, Naiman SC, et al: A trial of desmopressin (1-desamino-8-D-arginine vasopressin) to reduce blood loss in uncomplicated cardiac surgery. *N Engl J Med* 1989; 321:1437–1443.
39. Sear MD, Wadsworth LD, Rogers PC, et al: The effect of desmopressin acetate (DDAVP) on postoperative blood loss after cardiac operations in children. *J Thorac Cardiovasc Surg* 1988; 98:217–219.

40. D'Alauro FS, Johns RA: Hypotension related to desmopressin administration following cardiopulmonary bypass. *Anesthesiology* 1988; 69:962–963.
41. LoCicero J: Any value for desmopressin acetate (DDAVP) in cardiopulmonary bypass operations (letter)? *J Thorac Cardiovasc Surg* 1990; 99:945.
42. Van Oeveren W, Harder MP, Roozendaal KJ, et al: Aprotinin protects against the initial effect of cardiopulmonary bypass. *J Thorac Cardiovasc Surg* 1990; 99:788–797.
43. Bidstrup BP, Royston D, Sapsford RN, et al: Reduction in blood loss and blood use after cardiopulmonary bypass with high dose aprotinin (Trasylol). *J Thorac Cardiovasc Surg* 1989; 97:364–372.
44. Teoh KH, Christakis GT, Weisel RD, et al: Dipyridamole preserved platelets and reduced blood loss after cardiopulmonary bypass. *J Thorac Cardiovasc Surg* 1988; 96:332–341.
45. Fish KJ, Sarnquist FH, Van Steennis C, et al: A prospective, randomized study of the effects of prostacyclin on platelets and blood loss during coronary bypass operations. *J Thorac Cardiovasc Surg* 1986; 91:436–442.
46. Jestice KH, Humphreys JE, English TA, et al: A comparative study of prostacyclin infusion given before and during cardiopulmonary bypass to assess the first pass effect of the circuit on platelet number and function. *Eur J Cardiothorac Surg* 1990; 4:40–44.
47. Addonizio VP, Fisher CA, Jeffrey AB: Prevention of heparin-induced thrombocytopenia during open heart surgery with iloprost (ZK36374). *Surgery* 1987; 102:796–807.
48. Makhoul RG, McCann RL, Austin EH: Management of patients with heparin-associated thrombocytopenia and thrombosis requiring cardiac surgery. *Ann Thorac Surg* 1987; 43:617–621.
49. Teasdale SJ, Zulys VJ, Mycyk T, et al: Ancrod anticoagulation for cardiopulmonary bypass in heparin-induced thrombocytopenia and thrombosis. *Ann Thorac Surg* 1989; 48:712–713.
50. Kesteven J, Pasaoglu I, Williams T, et al: Significance of the whole blood activated clotting time in cardiopulmonary bypass. *J Cardiovasc Surg* 1986; 27:85–89.
51. Metz S, Keats AS: Low activated coagulation time during cardiopulmonary bypass does not increase postoperative bleeding. *Ann Thorac Surg* 1990; 49:440–444.
52. Tuman KJ, Spiess BD, McCarthy RJ, et al: Comparison of viscoelastic measures of coagulation after cardiopulmonary bypass. *Anesth Analg* 1989; 69:69–75.
53. Mohr R, Martinowitz U, Lavee J, et al: The hemostatic effect of transfusing fresh whole blood versus platelet concentrates after cardiac operations. *J Thorac Cardiovasc Surg* 1988; 96:530–534.
54. Lavee J, Martinowitz U, Mohr R, et al: The effect of transfusion of fresh whole blood versus platelet concentrates after cardiac operations. *J Thorac Cardiovasc Surg* 1989; 97:204–212.
55. McCarthy PM, Popovsky MA, Schaff HV, et al: Effect of blood conservation efforts in cardiac operations at the Mayo Clinic. *Mayo Clin Proc* 1988; 63:225–229.
56. Roy RC, Stafford MA, Hudspeth AS, et al: Failure of prophylaxis with fresh frozen plasma after cardiopulmonary bypass. *Anesthesiology* 1988; 69:254–257.
57. *Physicians Desk Reference 1989*. Oradell, New Jersey, Medical Economics Company Inc, 1989, pp 1197–1198.

58. Lee CN, Goh BL, Chin LG, et al: The role of protamine dose assay on reversal of heparin following extracorporeal circulation for open heart surgery. *Ann Acad Med Singapore* 1990; 19:41–44.

59. Gundry SR, Drongowski RA, Coran AG, et al: Failure of automated protamine titration to determine the protamine reversal dose of systemic heparin: Comparison with other methods. *Curr Surg* 1986; 43:110–112.

60. Shipton EA, Scanes TE, Fiessinger JN: Prototype of a new protamine sulphate titration kit for use in cardiopulmonary bypass surgery. *S Afr Med J* 1986; 70:809–811.

61. Stead SW: Comparison of two methods for heparin monitoring: A semi-automated heparin monitoring device and activated clotting time during extracorporeal circulation. *Int J Clin Monit Comput* 1989; 6:247–254.

62. Velders AJ, Wildevuur RH: Platelet damage by protamine and the protective effect of prostacyclin: An experimental study in dogs. *Ann Thorac Surg* 1986; 42:168–171.

63. Kresowik TF, Wakefield TW, Fessler RD II, et al: Anticoagulant effects of protamine sulfate in a canine model. *J Surg Res* 1988; 45:8–14.

64. Yang VC: A simple method for rapid and precise estimation of the protamine dose required for clinical heparin reversal. *ASAIO Trans* 1989; 274–277.

65. Teng CLC, Yang VC: A facile colorimetric protamine titration method. *J Lab Clin Med* 1989; 113:498–504.

66. Aren C, Feddersen K, Radegran K: Comparison of two protocols for heparin neutralization by protamine after cardiopulmonary bypass. *J Thorac Cardiovasc Surg* 1987; 94:539–541.

67. Kesteven PJ, Ahmed A, Aps C, et al: Protamine sulphate and heparin rebound following open-heart surgery. *J Cardiovasc Surg* 1986; 27:600–603.

68. Shanberge JN, Murato M, Quattrociocchi-Longe T, et al: Heparin-protamine complexes in the production of heparin rebound and other complications of extracorporeal bypass procedures. *Am J Clin Pathol* 1987; 87:210–217.

69. Horrow JC: Protamine: A review of its toxicity. *Anesth Analg* 1985; 64:348–361.

70. Alvarez J, Alvarez L, Escudero C, et al: Hemodynamics and morphologic alterations after experimental administration of protamine sulfate. *Am J Surg* 1988; 155:735–740.

71. Wakefield TW, Bouffard JA, Spaulding SA, et al: Sequestration of platelets in the pulmonary circulation as a consequence of protamine reversal of the anticoagulant effects of heparin. *J Vasc Surg* 1987; 5:187–192.

72. Morel DR, Zapol WM, Thomas SJ, et al: C5a and thromboxane generation associated with pulmonary vaso- and broncho-constriction during protamine reversal of heparin. *Anesthesiology* 1987; 66:597–604.

73. Conzen PF, Habazettl H, Gutmann R, et al: Thromboxane mediation of pulmonary hemodynamic responses after neutralization of heparin by protamine in pigs. *Anesth Analg* 1989; 68:25–31.

74. Hobbhahn J, Conzen PF, Zenker B, et al: Beneficial effects of cyclooxygenase inhibition on adverse hemodynamic responses after protamine. *Anesth Analg* 1988; 67:253–260.

75. Morel DR, Lowenstein E, Nguyenduy T, et al: Acute pulmonary vasoconstriction and thromboxane release during protamine reversal of heparin anticoagulation in awake sheep. *Circ Res* 1988; 62:905–915.

76. Kirklin JK, Chenoweth DE, Naftel DC, et al: Effects of protamine administration after cardiopulmonary bypass on complement, blood elements, and the hemodynamic state. *Ann Thorac Surg* 1986; 41:193–199.

77. Wakefield TW, Till GO, Lindblad B, et al: Complement depletion and persistent hemodynamic-hematologic responses in protamine heparin reactions. J Surg Res 1988; 45:320–326.
78. Hendry PJ, Taichman GC, Keon WJ: The myocardial contractile responses to protamine sulfate and heparin. Ann Thorac Surg 1987; 44:263–268.
79. Colman RW: Humoral mediators of catastrophic reactions associated with protamine neutralization (editorial). Anesthesiology 1987; 66:595–596.
80. Tan F, Jackman H, Skidgel RA, et al: Protamine inhibits plasma carboxypeptidase N, the inactivator of anaphylatoxins and kinins. Anesthesiology 1989; 70:267–275.
81. Weiler JM, Gelhaus MA, Carter JG, et al: A prospective study of the risk of an immediate adverse reaction to protamine sulfate during cardiopulmonary bypass surgery. J Allergy Clin Immunol 1990; 85:713–719.
82. Sharath MD, Metzger WJ, Richerson HB, et al: Protamine-induced fatal anaphylaxis. J Thorac Cardiovasc Surg 1985; 90:86–90.
83. Gupta SK, Veith FJ, Ascer E, et al: Anaphylactoid reactions to protamine: An often lethal complication in insulin-dependent diabetic patients undergoing vascular surgery. J Vasc Surg 1989; 9:342–350.
84. Depaulis R, Mohammad SY, Chiariello L, et al: A pulmonary mock circulation model for a better understanding of protamine reversal of heparin. ASAIO Trans 1988; 34:367–370.
85. Taylor RL, Little WC, Freeman GL, et al: Comparison of the cardiovascular effects of intravenous and intraaortic protamine in the conscious and anesthetized dog. Ann Thorac Surg 1986; 42:22–26.
86. Katz NM, Kim YD, Siegelman R, et al: Hemodynamics of protamine administration. J Thorac Cardiovasc Surg 1987; 94:881–886.
87. Mendeloff EN, Liang IYS, Swain JA, et al: Thromboxane A2 receptor specific blockade prevents the heparin-protamine reaction after cardiopulmonary bypass. Surg Forum 1990; 41:286–289.
88. Kreil E, Montalescot G, Greene E, et al: Nafamstat mesilate attenuates pulmonary hypertension in heparin-protamine reactions. J Appl Physiol 1989; 67:1463–1471.
89. Montalescot G, Kreil E, Lynch K, et al: Effect of platelet depletion on lung vasoconstriction in heparin-protamine reactions. J Appl Physiol 1989; 66:2344–2350.
90. Kim JS, Vincent C, Teng CLC, et al: A novel approach to anticoagulation control. ASAIO Trans 1989; 35:644–646.
91. Teng CLC, Kim JS, Port FK, et al: A protamine filter for extracorporeal blood heparin removal. ASAIO Trans 1988; 34:743–746.
92. Wakefield TW, Lindblad B, Whitehouse WM Jr, et al: Attenuation of hemodynamic and hematologic effects of heparin-protamine sulfate interaction after aortic reconstruction in a canine model. Surgery 1986; 100:45–50.
93. Wakefield TW, Hantler CB, Lindblad B, et al: Protamine pretreatment attenuation of hemodynamic and hematologic effects of heparin-protamine interaction. J Vasc Surg 1986; 3:885–889.
94. Protamine uses, hazards, and benefits in hemotec update. 1989; 4:1–4.
95. Teasdale SJ, Zulys VJ, Mycyk T, et al: Ancrod anticoagulation for cardiopulmonary bypass in heparin-induced thrombocytopenia and thrombosis. Ann Thorac Surg 1989; 48:712–713.
96. Zulys VJ, Teasdale SJ, Michel ER, et al: Ancrod (Arvin) as an alternative to heparin anticoagulation for cardiopulmonary bypass. Anesthesiology 1989; 71:870–877.

97. Doherty DC, Ortel TL, De Bruijn N, et al: "Heparin-free" cardiopulmonary bypass: First reported use of heparinoid (Org 10172) to provide anticoagulation for cardiopulmonary bypass. *Anesthesiology* 1990; 73:562–565.
98. Reigel W, Spillner G, Schlosser V, et al: Plasma levels of main granulocyte components during cardiopulmonary bypass. *J Thorac Cardiovasc Surg* 1988; 95:1014–1019.
99. Colman RW: Platelet and neutrophil activation in cardiopulmonary bypass. *Ann Thorac Surg* 1990; 49:32–34.
100. Nilsson L, Brunnkvist S, Nilsson U, et al: Activation of inflammatory systems during cardiopulmonary bypass. *Scand J Thorac Cardiovasc Surg* 1988; 22:51–53.
101. Hind CRK, Griffin JF, Pack S, et al: Effect of cardiopulmonary bypass on circulating concentrations of leucocyte elastase and free radical activity. *Cardiovasc Res* 1988; 22:37–41.
102. Wachtfogel YT, Kucich U, Greenplate J, et al: Human neutrophil degranulation during extracorporeal circulation. *Blood* 1987; 69:324–330.
103. Wachtfogel YT, Harpel PC, Edmunds LH, et al: Formation of C1s–C1 inhibitor, kallikrein-C1-inhibitor, and plasmin-alpha$_2$-plasmin-inhibitor complexes during cardiopulmonary bypass. *Blood* 1989; 73:468–471.
104. Moore FD, Warner KG, Assousa S, et al: The effect of complement activation during cardiopulmonary bypass. *Ann Surg* 1988; 208:95–103.
105. Kirklin JK: The postperfusion syndrome: Inflammation and the damaging effects of cardiopulmonary bypass, in Tinker JH (ed): *Cardiopulmonary Bypass: Current Concepts and Controversies.* Philadelphia, WB Saunders Company, 1989, pp 137–139.
106. Howard RJ, Crain C, Franzini DA, et al: Effects of cardiopulmonary bypass on pulmonary leukostasis and complement activation. *Arch Surg* 1988; 123:1496–1501.
107. Braude S, Nolop KB, Fleming JS, et al: Increased pulmonary transvascular protein flux after canine cardiopulmonary bypass. *Am Rev Respir Dis* 1986; 134:867–872.
108. Bando K, Pillai R, Cameron DE, et al: Leukocyte depletion ameliorates free radical-mediated lung injury after cardiopulmonary bypass. *J Thorac Cardiovasc Surg* 1990; 99:873–877.
109. Tennenberg SD, Bailey WW, Cotta LA, et al: The effects of methylprednisolone on complement-mediated neutrophil activation during cardiopulmonary bypass. *Surgery* 1986; 100:134–141.
110. Ide H, Kakiuchi T, Furuta N, et al: The effect of cardiopulmonary bypass on T cells and their subpopulations. *Ann Thorac Surg* 1987; 44:227–282.
111. Ryhanen P, Ilonen J, Helja-Marja S, et al: Characterization of in vivo activated lymphocytes found in the peripheral blood of patients undergoing cardiac operation. *J Thorac Cardiovasc Surg* 1987; 93:109–114.
112. Pollock R, Ames F, Rubio P, et al: Protracted severe immune dysregulation induced by cardiopulmonary bypass: A predisposing etiologic factor in blood transfusion-related aids. *J Clin Lab Immunol* 1987; 22:1–5.
113. Salama A, Hugo F, Heinrich D, et al: Deposition of terminal C5b-9 complement complexes on erythrocytes and leukocytes during cardiopulmonary bypass. *N Engl J Med* 1988; 318:408–414.
114. Haeffner-Cavaillon N, Roussellier N, Ponzio O, et al: Induction of interleukin-1 production in patients undergoing cardiopulmonary bypass. *J Thorac Cardiovasc Surg* 1989; 98:1100–1106.
115. Cavarocchi NC, Pluth JR, Schaff HV, et al: Complement activation during

cardiopulmonary bypass. *J Thorac Cardiovasc Surg* 1986; 91:252–258.

116. Tatsuo T, Yamasaki M, Maeo Y, et al: Complement activation in cardiopulmonary bypass, with special reference to anaphylatoxin production in membrane and bubble oxygenators. *Ann Thorac Surg* 1988; 46:47–57.

117. Nilsson L, Storm KE, Thelin S, et al: Heparin-coated equipment reduces complement activation during cardiopulmonary bypass in the pig. *Artif Organs* 1989; 14:46–48.

118. Melbye OJ, Froland SS, Lilleaasen P, et al: Complement activation during cardiopulmonary bypass: Comparison between the use of large volumes of plasma and dextran 70. *Eur Surg Res* 1988; 20:101–109.

119. Mann WK, Steger AC, Hosking SW, et al: Histamine release during cardiopulmonary bypass. *Perfusion* 1990; 5:107–116.

120. Marath A, Man W, Taylor KM, et al: Plasma histamine profiles in paediatric cardiopulmonary bypass. *Agents Actions* 1988; 23:339–342.

121. Marath A, Man W, Taylor KM: Histamine release in paediatric cardiopulmonary bypass—a possible role in the capillary leak syndrome. *Agents Actions* 1987; 20:299–302.

122. Menasche P, Pasquier C, Bellucci S, et al: Deferoxamine reduces neutrophil-mediated free radical production during cardiopulmonary bypass in man. *J Thorac Cardiovasc Surg* 1988; 96:582–589.

123. England MD, Cavarocchi NC, O'Brien JF, et al: Influence of antioxidants (mannitol and allopurinol) on oxygen free radical generation during and after cardiopulmonary bypass. *Circulation* 1986; 74:134–137.

124. Royston D, Fleming JS, Desai JB, et al: Increased production of peroxidation products associated with cardiac operations. *J Thorac Cardiovasc Surg* 1986; 91:759–766.

125. Cavarocchi NC, England MD, Schaff HV, et al: Oxygen free radical generation during cardiopulmonary bypass: Correlation with complement activation. *Circulation* 1986; 74(suppl III):130–133.

126. Cavarocchi NC, England MD, O'Brien JF, et al: Superoxide generation during cardiopulmonary bypass: Is there a role for vitamin E. *J Surg Res* 1986; 40:519–527.

127. Shumaker HB: Memoir for John H. Gibbon. *ASAIO Trans* 1973; 91:41.

128. Bigelow WG: *Cold Hearts. The Story of Hypothermia and the Pacemaker in Heart Surgery.* Toronto, McClelland & Stewart Ltd, 1984.

129. Gollan F: *Physiology and Cardiac Surgery. Hypothermia, Extracorporeal Circulation, and Extracorporeal Cooling.* Springfield, Illinois, Charles C Thomas, 1959.

130. Young W, Sealy W, Brown I, et al: Metabolic and physiologic observations on patients undergoing extracorporeal circulation in conjunction with hypothermia. *Surgery* 1959; 46:175–184.

131. Shaw PJ: The incidence and nature of neurological morbidity following cardiac surgery: A review. *Perfusion* 1989; 4:83–91.

132. Sotaniemi KA: Cerebral outcome after extracorporeal circulation: Comparison between prospective and retrospective evaluations. *Arch Neurol* 1983; 40:75–77.

133. Nussmeier NA, McDermott JP: Macroembolization: Prevention and outcome modification, in Hilberman M (ed): *Brain Injury and Protection During Heart Surgery.* Boston, Martinus Nijhoff Publishing, 1988, pp 85–107.

134. Blauth C, Arnold J, Kohoner E, et al: Retinal microembolism during cardiopulmonary bypass demonstrated by fluorescein angiography. *Lancet* 1986; 2:837–839.

135. Blauth C, Arnold J, Schulenberg W, et al: Cerebral microembolism during cardiopulmonary bypass. Retinal microvascular studies in vivo with fluorescein angiography. J Thorac Cardiovasc Surg 1988; 95:668–676.
136. Blauth C, Smith P, Newman S, et al: Retinal microembolism and neuropsychological deficit following clinical cardiopulmonary bypass: Comparison of a membrane and a bubble oxygenator. A preliminary communication. Eur J Cardio-thorac Surg 1989; 3:135–139.
137. Blauth C: Assessment of cerebrovascular microembolism by retinal fluorescein angiography. Perfusion 1989; 4:123–129.
138. Blauth C, Smith P, Arnold J, et al: Influence of oxygenator type on the prevalence and extent of microembolic retinal ischemia during cardiopulmonary bypass. Assessment by digital image analysis. J Thorac Cardiovasc Surg 1990; 99:61–69.
139. Treasure T: Interventions to reduce cerebral injury during cardiac surgery—the effect of arterial line filtration. Perfusion 1989; 4:147–152.
140. Pugsley W: The use of Doppler ultrasound in the assessment of microemboli during cardiac surgery. Perfusion 1989; 4:115–122.
141. Padayachee TS, Parsons S, Theobold R, et al: The effect of arterial filtration on reduction of gaseous microemboli in the middle cerebral artery during cardiopulmonary bypass. Ann Thorac Surg 1988; 45:647–649.
142. Lowery OH, Passonneau JV, Hasselberger FX, et al: Effect of ischemia on known substrates and cofactors of the glycolytic pathway in brain. J Biol Chem 1964; 239:18–30.
143. Siesjo BK, Wieloch T: Cerebral metabolism in ischemia: Neurochemical basis for therapy. Br J Anaesth 1985; 57:47–62.
144. Cheung JT, Bonventure JV, Malis CD, et al: Mechanisms of disease: Calcium and ischaemic injury. N Engl J Med 1986; 314:1670–1676.
145. Weiss SJ: Oxygen, ischaemia and inflammation. Acta Physiol Scand Suppl 1986; 548:9–37.
146. Roysten D: Free radicals, formation, function, and potential relevance in anaesthesia. Anaesthesia 1988; 43:315–320.
147. Roysten D: Interventions to reduce cerebral injury during cardiac surgery—the effect of physical and pharmacologic agents. Perfusion 1989; 4:153–161.
148. Murkin JM: Cerebral hyperfusion during cardiopulmonary bypass: The influence of PaCO$_2$, in Hilberman M (ed): Brain Injury and Protection During Heart Surgery. Boston, Martinus Nijhoff Publishing, 1988, pp 47–66.
149. Henriksen L, Hjelms E, Lindeburg T: Brain hyperperfusion during cardiac operations. J Thorac Cardiovasc Surg 1983; 86:202–208.
150. Govier A, Reves J, McKay R, et al: Factors and their influence on regional cerebral blood flow during nonpulsatile cardiopulmonary bypass. Ann Thorac Surg 1984; 38:592–600.
151. Swan H: The importance of acid-base management for cardiac and cerebral preservation during open heart operations. Surg Gynecol Obstet 1984; 158:391–414.
152. Lundar T, Lindegaard K, Froysaker T, et al: Dissociation between cerebral autoregulation and carbon dioxide reactivity during nonpulsatile cardiopulmonary bypass. Ann Thorac Surg 1985; 40:582–587.
153. Prough DS, Stump DA, Roy RC, et al: Response of cerebral blood flow to changes in carbon dioxide tension during hypothermic cardiopulmonary bypass. Anesthesiology 1986; 64:576–581.
154. Murkin JM, Farrar JK, Tweed WA, et al: Cerebral autoregulation and flow/me-

tabolism coupling during cardiopulmonary bypass: The influence of $PaCO_2$. *Anesth Analg* 1987; 66:665–672.

155. Prough DS, Stump DA, Troost BT: $PaCO_2$ management during cardiopulmonary bypass: Intriguing physiologic rationale, convincing clinical data, evolving hypothesis? *Anesthesiology* 1990; 72:3–6.

156. Bashein G, Townes B, Nessly M, et al: A randomized study of carbon dioxide management during hypothermic cardiopulmonary bypass. *Anesthesiology* 1990; 72:7–15.

157. Gravlee G, Roy R, Stump D, et al: Regional cerebrovascular reactivity to carbon dioxide during cardiopulmonary bypass in patients with cerebrovascular disease. *J Thorac Cardiovasc Surg* 1990; 99:1022–1029.

158. Ibayashi S, Fujishima M, Sadoshima S, et al: Cerebral blood flow and tissue metabolism in experimental cerebral ischemia of spontaneously hypertensive rats with hyper-, normo-, and hypoglycemia. *Stroke* 1986; 17:261–266.

159. Gardiner M, Smith M, Kagstrom E, et al: Influence of blood glucose concentration on brain lactate accumulation during severe hypoxia and subsequent recovery of brain energy metabolism. *J Cereb Blood Flow Metab* 1982; 2:429–438.

160. Ekroth R, Thompson R, Lincoln C, et al: Elective deep hypothermia with circulatory arrest: Changes in plasma creatine kinase BB, blood glucose, and clinical variables. *J Thorac Cardiovasc Surg* 1989; 97:30–35.

161. Nussmeier N, Arlund C, Slogoff S: Neuropsychiatric complications after cardiopulmonary bypass: Cerebral protection by a barbiturate. *Anesthesiology* 1986; 64:165–170.

162. Nicholas C, Cavarocchi M, Michael D, et al: Superoxide generation during cardiopulmonary bypass: Is there a role for vitamin E? *J Surg Res* 1986; 40:519–527.

163. Menasche P, Pasquier C, Bellucci S, et al: Deferoxamine reduces neutrophil mediated free radical production during cardiopulmonary bypass in man. *J Thorac Cardiovasc Surg* 1988; 96:582–589.

164. Radegran K, Ahren C, Teger-Nilsson A: Prostacyclin infusion during extracorporeal circulation for coronary bypass. *J Thorac Cardiovasc Surg* 1982; 83:205–211.

165. Fish K, Helms K, Sarnquist F, et al: A prospective, randomized study of the effects of prostacyclin on neuropsychologic dysfunction after coronary artery operation. *J Thorac Cardiovasc Surg* 1987; 93:609–615.

166. Wrogemann K, Pena S: Mitochondrial calcium overload. A general mechanism for cell necrosis in muscle disease. *Lancet* 1977; 1:672–673.

167. Gelmers H, Gorter K, de Weerdt C, et al: A controlled trial of nimodipine in acute ischemic stroke. *N Engl J Med* 1988; 318:203–207.

168. Allen GS, Ahn HS, Prezoisi TJ, et al: Cerebral arterial spasm—a controlled trial of nimodipine in patients with subarachnoid hemorrhage. *N Engl J Med* 1983; 308:619–624.

169. Steen PA, Grisvold SE, Milde JM, et al: Nimodipine improves outcome when given after complete cerebral ischemia in primates. *Anesthesiology* 1985; 62:406–414.

170. Benveniste H, Drejer J, Schousboe A, et al: Elevation of the extracellular concentrations of glutamate and aspartate in rat hippocampus during transient cerebral ischaemia monitored by intracerebral microdialysis. *J Neurochem* 1984; 43:1369–1374.

171. Rothman SM, Olney JW: Glutamate and the pathophysiology of hypoxic-ischemic brain damage. *Ann Neurol* 1986; 19:105–111.

172. Ozyurt E, Graham D, Woodruff G, et al: Protective effect on the glutamate antagonist, MK-801 in focal cerebral ischemia in the cat. *J Cereb Blood Flow Metab* 1988; 8:138–143.
173. Kochar A, Zivin J, Lyden P, et al: Glutamate antagonist therapy reduces neurologic deficits produced by focal central nervous system ischemia. *Arch Neurol* 1988; 45:148–153.
174. Robbins R, Balaban R, Swain J: Intermittent hypothermic asanguinous cerebral perfusion (cerebroplegia) protects the brain during prolonged circulatory arrest: A phosphorous-31 nuclear magnetic resonance study. *J Thorac Cardiovasc Surg* 1990; 99:878–884.
175. Crittenden M, Roberts C, Rosa L, et al: Neurologic outcome after prolonged circulatory arrest using hypothermic asanguinous cerebral perfusion (cerebroplegia) to protect the brain. *Ann Thorac Surg,* in press.
176. Rossi R, van der Linden J, Ekroth R, et al: No flow or low flow? A study of the ischemic marker creatine kinase BB after deep hypothermic procedures. *J Thorac Cardiovasc Surg* 1989; 98:193–199.
177. Swain J, McDonald T, Griffith P, et al: Low flow cardiopulmonary bypass protects the brain. *J Thorac Cardiovasc Surg,* in press.
178. Shepard RB, Simpson DC, Sharp J: Energy equivalent pressure. *Arch Surg* 1966; 93:70.
179. Parsons RJ, McMaster PD: The effect of the pulse upon the formation and flow of lymph. *J Exp Med* 1938; 68:353.
180. Angell-James JE, de Burgh-Daly M: Effects of graded pulsatile pressure on the reflex vasomotor responses elicited by changes of mean pressure in the perfused carotid sinus-aortic arch regions of the dog. *J Physiol* 1971; 214:51.
181. Taylor KM, Bain WH, Morton JJ: The role of angiotensin II in the development of peripheral vasoconstriction during open-heart surgery. *Am Heart J* 1980; 100:935–937.
182. Taylor KM, Casals J, Morton JJ, et al: The hemodynamic effects of angiotensin blockade after cardiopulmonary bypass. *Br Heart J* 1978; 41:380.
183. Nagaoka H, Innami R, Arai H: Effects of pulsatile cardiopulmonary bypass on the renin-angiotensin-aldosterone system following open heart surgery. *Jpn J Surg* 1988; 18:390–396.
184. Minami K, Korner MM, Vyska K, et al: Effects of pulsatile perfusion on plasma catecholamine levels and hemodynamics during and after cardiac operations with cardiopulmonary bypass. *J Thorac Cardiovasc Surg* 1990; 99:82–91.
185. Mori A, Tabata R, Nakamura Y, et al: Effects of pulsatile cardiopulmonary bypass on carbohydrate and lipid metabolism. *J Cardiovasc Surg (Torino)* 1987; 28:621–626.
186. Philbin DM, Levine FH, Emerson CW, et al: Plasma vasopressin levels and urinary flow during cardiopulmonary bypass. *J Thorac Cardiovasc Surg* 1979; 78:779.
187. Levine FH, Philbin DM, Coggins CH, et al: Plasma vasopressin levels and urinary sodium excretion during cardiopulmonary bypass: A comparison of pulsatile and nonpulsatile flow. *Surg Forum* 1978; 29:320–322.
188. Nakamura K, Koga Y, Sekiya R, et al: The effects of pulsatile and non-pulsatile cardiopulmonary bypass on renal blood flow and function. *Jpn J Surg* 1989; 19:334–345.
189. Shepard RB, Kirklin JW: Relation of pulsatile flow flow to oxygen consumption and other variables during cardiopulmonary bypass. *J Thorac Cardiovasc Surg* 1969; 58:694.

190. De Paepe J, Pomerantzeff PA, Nakiri K, et al: Observation of the microcirculation of the cerebral cortex of dogs subjected to pulsatile and non-pulsatile flow during extracorporeal circulation, in *A Propos du Debit Pulse*. Belgium, Cobe Laboratories Inc, 1979, pp

191. Taylor KM, Wright GS, Bain WH, et al: Comparative studies of pulsatile and non-pulsatile flow during cardiopulmonary bypass. III. Anterior pituitary response to thyrotropin-releasing hormone. *J Thorac Cardiovasc Surg* 1978; 75:579.

192. Taylor KM, Devlin BJ, Mittra SM, et al: Assessment of cerebral damage during open-heart surgery. A new experimental model. *Scand J Thorac Cardiovasc Surg* 1980; 14:197–203.

193. Tranmer BI, Gross CE, Kindt GW, et al: Pulsatile versus nonpulsatile blood flow in the treatment of acute cerebral ischemia. *Neurosurgery* 1986; 19:724–731.

194. Laursen H, Bodker A, Andersen K, et al: Brain oedema and blood-brain barrier permeability in pulsatile and nonpulsatile cardiopulmonary bypass. *Scand J Thorac Cardiovasc Surg* 1986; 20:161–166.

195. Henze T, Stephan H, Sonntag H: Cerebral dysfunction following extracorporeal circulation for aortocoronary bypass surgery: No differences in neuropsychological outcome after pulsatile versus nonpulsatile flow. *J Thorac Cardiovasc Surg* 1990; 38:65–68.

196. Kaps M, Haase A, Mulch J, et al: Pulsatile flow pattern in cerebral arteries during cardiopulmonary bypass. An evaluation based on transcranial Doppler ultrasound. *J Cardiovasc Surg (Torino)* 1989; 30:16–19.

197. Many M, Soroff HS, Birtwell WC, et al: The physiologic role of pulsatile and non-pulsatile blood flow: II. Effects on renal function. *Arch Surg* 1967; 95:762.

198. Matsuda H, Hirose H, Nakano S, et al: Results of open heart surgery in patients with impaired renal function as creatinine clearance below 30 ml/min. The effects of pulsatile perfusion. *J Cardiovasc Surg (Torino)* 1986; 27:595–599.

199. Mori A, Watanabe K, Onoe M, et al: Regional blood flow in the liver, pancreas and kidney during pulsatile and nonpulsatile perfusion under profound hypothermia. *Jpn Circ J* 1988; 52:219–227.

200. Murray WR, Mittra S, Mittra D, et al: The amylase creatinine clearance ratio following cardiopulmonary bypass. *J Thorac Cardiovasc Surg* 1982; 82:248–253.

201. Nagaoka H, Innami R, Watanabe M, et al: Preservation of pancreatic beta cell function with pulsatile cardiopulmonary bypass. *Ann Thorac Surg* 1989; 48:798–802.

202. Mathie R, Desai J, Taylor KM: Hepatic blood flow and metabolism during pulsatile and non-pulsatile cardiopulmonary bypass. *Life Support Systems* 1984; 2:303–305.

203. Taylor KM: Pulsatile cardiopulmonary bypass. A review. *J Cardiovasc Surg (Torino)* 1981; 22:561–568.

204. Taylor KM: Why pulsatile flow during cardiopulmonary bypass?, in Longmore DB (ed): *Towards Safer Cardiac Surgery*. Lancaster, MTP, 1981, pp 481–500.

205. Taylor KM, Bain WH, Davidson KG, et al: A comparative study of pulsatile and non-pulsatile cardiopulmonary bypass in 325 patients. *Proc Eur Soc Artif Organs* 1979; 6:238.

206. Williams GD, Seifen AB, Lawson NW, et al: Pulsatile perfusion versus conventional high-flow nonpulsatile perfusion for rapid core cooling and rewarming of infants for circulatory arrest in cardiac operation. *J Thorac Cardiovasc Surg* 1979; 78:667–677.
207. Yasui H, Yonenaga K, Kado H, et al: Open-heart surgery in infants using pulsatile high-flow cardiopulmonary bypass. *J Cardiovasc Surg (Torino)* 1989; 30:661–668.
208. Pollock EM, Pollock JC, Jamieson MP, et al: Adrenocortical hormone concentrations in children during cardiopulmonary bypass with and without pulsatile flow. *Br J Anaesth* 1988; 60:536–541.
209. Overlie PA: Emergency use of portable cardiopulmonary bypass. *Cathet Cardiovasc Diagn* 1990; 20:27–31.
210. Phillips SJ: Percutaneous initiation of cardiopulmonary bypass. *Ann Thorac Surg* 1983; 36:2.
211. Litzie AK, Roberts CP: Emergency femoro-femoral cardiopulmonary bypass. *Proc Am Acad Perfusionists* 1987; 8:60–65.
212. Vogel RA, Shawl F, Tommaso C, et al: Initial report of the National Registry of Elective Cardiopulmonary Bypass Supported Coronary Angioplasty. *J Am Coll Cardiol* 1990; 15:23–29.
213. Shawl FA: Percutaneous cardiopulmonary support in high-risk angioplasty. *Cardiol Clin* 1989; 7:865–875.
214. Vogel RA, Tomasso CL: Elective supported angioplasty: Initial report of the national registry. *Cathet Cardiovasc Diagn* 1990; 20:22–26.
215. Cowley MJ, Dorros G, Kelsey SF, et al: Acute coronary events associated with percutaneous transluminal coronary angioplasty. *Am J Cardiol* 1984; 53:12C–16C.
216. Gundry SR, Brinkley J, Wolk M, et al: Percutaneous cardiopulmonary bypass to support angioplasty and valvuloplasty; technical considerations. *ASAIO Trans* 1989; 35:725–727.
217. Tomasso CL: Use of percutaneously inserted cardiopulmonary bypass in the cardiac catheterization laboratory. *Cathet Cardiovasc Diagn* 1990; 20: 32–38.
218. Axelrod HI, Murphy MS, Galloway AC, et al: Percutaneous cardiopulmonary bypass limits myocardial injury from ischemic fibrillation and reperfusion. *Circulation* 1988; 78(suppl III):148–152.
219. Krummel TM, Greenfield LJ, Kirkpatrick BV, et al: Extracorporeal membrane oxygenation in neonatal pulmonary failure. *Pediatr Ann* 1982; 11:905–908.
220. Revenis M, Glass P, Sanchez L, et al: Outcome of low birth weight (LBW) babies on extracorporeal membrane oxygenation (ECMO). *Pediatr Res* 1990; 27:254A.
221. Krummel TM, Greenfield LJ, Kirkpatrick BV, et al: Alveolar-arterial oxygen gradients versus the neonatal pulmonary insufficiency index for prediction of mortality in ECMO candidates. *J Pediatr Surg* 1984; 19:380–384.
222. Egan TM, Duffin J, Glynn MF, et al: Ten-year experience with extracorporeal membrane oxygenation for severe respiratory failure. *Chest* 1988; 94:681–687.
223. Zapol WM: ECMO: A view from the east, in Stanley TH, Sperry RJ (eds): *Anesthesia and the Lung.* Dordrecht, Netherlands, Kluwer Academic Publishers, 1989, pp 295–301.
224. Wetmore N, McEwen D, O'Connor M, et al: Defining indications for artificial organ support in respiratory failure. *ASAIO Trans* 1979; 25:459–461.

225. Trento A, Thompson A, Siewers R, et al: Extracorporeal membrane oxygenation in children. New trends. *J Thorac Cardiovasc Surg* 1988; 96:542–547.
226. Tsuno K, Terasaki H, Tsutsumi R, et al: To-and-fro veno-venous extracorporeal lung assist for newborns with severe respiratory distress. *Intensive Care Med* 1989; 15:269–271.
227. Pesenti A, Gattinoni L, Kolobow T, et al: Extracorporeal circulation in adult respiratory failure. *ASAIO Trans* 1988; 34:43–47.
228. Chapman J, Adams M, Geha A: Hemodynamic response to pumpless extracorporeal membrane oxygenation. *J Thorac Cardiovasc Surg* 1990; 99:741–750.
229. Mortensen JD, Berry G: Conceptual and design features of a practical, clinically effective intravenous mechanical blood oxygen/carbon dioxide exchange device (IVOX). *Int J Artif Organs* 1989; 12:384–389.
230. Bartlett RH, Andrews AF, Toomasian JM, et al: Extracorporeal membrane oxygenation for newborn respiratory failure: Forty-five cases. *Surgery* 1982; 92:425–433.
231. McCune S, Short BL, Miller MK, et al: Extracorporeal membrane oxygenation therapy in neonates with septic shock. *J Pediatr Surg* 1990; 25:479–482.
232. Hofkosh D, Clouse H, Smith-Jones J, et al: Ten years of ECMO: Neurodevelopmental outcome among survivors. *Pediatr Res* 1990; 27:245A.
233. Taylor GA, Glass P, Fitz C, et al: Neurologic status in infants treated with extracorporeal membrane oxygenation: Correlation of imaging findings with developmental outcome. *Radiology* 1987; 165:679–682.
234. Desai HJ, Mitchell D, Wolfson P, et al: Color Doppler imaging of brain blood flow pattern following right common carotid artery ligation for ECMO in neonates. *Pediatr Res* 1990; 27:343A.
235. Fenton GA, Gomez CR, Kotagal S, et al: Evaluation of cerebral circulation by transcranial Doppler in patients having undergone extracorporeal membrane oxygenation. *Neurology* 1990; 40(suppl 1):558.
236. Roloff DW, Bartlett RH, Schumacher RE, et al: Does neonatal ECMO increase treatment cost or late morbidity? *Pediatr Res* 1990; 27:315A.

Coronary Revascularization for Acute Myocardial Infarction

Gary S. Benton, M.D.

Senior Fellow in Cardiothoracic Surgery, Medical College of Virginia, Richmond, Virginia

Andrew S. Wechsler, M.D.

Stuart McGuire, Professor of Surgery, Chairman, Department of Surgery, Professor of Physiology, Medical College of Virginia, Virginia Commonwealth University, Richmond, Virginia

Acute myocardial infarction (AMI) is the leading cause of death in America today. Although coronary revascularization plays a major role in treating the symptoms and complications of coronary atherosclerosis, its role in the treatment of AMI is less clear. General surgeons are taught that the more proximate an operation is to a myocardial infarction, the greater the risk of reinfarction. Indeed, multiple reports have defined the perils of general anesthesia and operation in the first 6 months following myocardial infarction.[1–4] The mortality for reinfarction is reported to be as great as 50% in this patient population. With this bias formed early in their general surgical training, it was little wonder that cardiac surgeons were hesitant to operate on patients with AMI. However, in 1979, Phillips et al. reported a series of 75 patients with AMI who underwent emergency revascularization with saphenous vein grafts and had an overall mortality of 4%.[5] In that same year, DeWood et al. reported improved survival in patients with AMI treated with early surgical revascularization as opposed to those managed medically.[6] They reported their extended experience of 701 patients with AMI managed with surgical revascularization with an operative mortality of 4.4% in 1983.[7] These reports opened the debate over the appropriate place for emergency surgical coronary revascularization (ESCR) in reperfusion following AMI.

Background

Most investigators studying animal models conclude that, in order to salvage myocardium, reperfusion must occur within 6 hours after acute coronary occlusion.[8-10] However, these studies are open to criticism, because they were performed in animals with normal coronary circulation that does not mimic the collateralization seen in patients with coronary atherosclerosis. Recently, Beyersdorf et al. have reported that myocardial salvage may occur after 6 hours of regional ischemia.[11] Additionally, there is evidence that surgical reperfusion is superior to medical reperfusion in the chronic dog model.[12]

Prior to the thrombolytic era, medical management of AMI consisted of oxygen, pain control, hemodynamic monitoring and support, coronary vasodilators, and anticoagulation. This is the "historic" control against which reperfusion strategies are measured. In 1967, Killip et al. reported a series of 250 patients with AMI who were treated with conservative management in a coronary care unit initially. In-hospital mortality in this study was 27%.[13] Reduction of this number has consumed the efforts of cardiologists and cardiothoracic surgeons.

Reperfusion Strategy

In any current reperfusion strategy, one begins with thrombolytic therapy, since it is the modality most readily available to the population at risk. The first thrombolytic agent to be tested widely in clinical trials was streptokinase. It is reported to be approximately 50% effective in achieving thrombolysis in myocardial infarction when given within 6 hours of the onset of chest pain at the high dose of 1.5 million units intravenously.[14] Intracoronary administration of streptokinase is reported to be 73% to 79% effective in the recanalization of thrombosed coronary arteries after AMI.[15-17]

Although streptokinase's efficacy as a thrombolytic was proven quickly, it was not until the Western Washington trial that reported in 1983 that its ability to reperfuse was equated with improved patient survival.[18] In this study, a 98% 1-year survival was demonstrated for the 80 patients who had complete reperfusion vs. an 85% survival for the 13 patients with partial reperfusion. Forty-one patients with no reperfusion had a reported 1-year survival of 77%. This conclusion was supported further by the Gruppo-Italiano per lo Studio della Streptocninasi nell' Infarto Miocardico (GISSI) study, which involved over 11,000 patients had validated streptokinase's efficacy in reducing mortality from AMI.[19]

Streptokinase proteolytically converts plasminogen to its active form, plasmin, which is fibrinolytic, but not thrombus-specific. It is obtained from a bacterial source and allergic reactions, including hypotension, have been reported. In addition, resistance to its thrombolytic properties can occur through an antibody-mediated response. Its effectiveness is considerably better with recent thrombi (<3 hours) than with more organized thrombi.[14, 20]

Recombinant tissue-type plasminogen activator (t-PA) has been tested widely clinically and is reported to be clot-specific, yielding it the theoretic advantage of being fibrin-sparing.[21] However, as doses of t-PA were increased to improve thrombolysis and, therefore, reperfusion rates, a dose-dependent decline in circulating fibrinogen was observed.[21, 22] In fact, it may be that greater care must be taken when using t-PA because of its more direct action and the potential for dissolving more organized clots. In the Thrombolysis in Myocardial Infarction (TIMI) study, the incidence of periaccess hematoma and transfusion requirements following emergency coronary catheterization or percutaneous transluminal coronary angioplasty (PTCA) in patients who had received t-PA was similar to that seen with streptokinase.[23]

The first conclusive study using t-PA in AMI was reported by Collen et al. and involved 45 patients with transmural infarction secondary to complete coronary occlusion.[24] Seventy-five percent (33 of 45) of the patients recanalized after 90 minutes using intravenous doses of t-PA at 0.5 to 0.75 mg/kg. The average time to recanalization in this study was 46 minutes. The 13 patients who received placebo initially later received t-PA, and 9 of them (69%) recanalized with an average of 23 minutes of intracoronary t-PA therapy. With the dose range of t-PA used in this study, a plasma fibrinogen level decline of only 8% was observed.

The excellent results of initial clinical trials using t-PA prompted further randomized prospective trials comparing its efficacy to that of streptokinase in AMI. The TIMI study group reported its phase I findings, which included 214 patients with AMI.[23] These patients were randomized to two treatment groups. The first group was treated with 80 mg of t-PA over 3 hours and the second group received 1.5 million IU of streptokinase intravenously over 1 hour. Fifty-nine of 99 patients, or 60% of the patients randomized to t-PA therapy, reperfused the infarcted artery. This was in contrast to 40 of 115 patients (35%) treated with streptokinase. In the European multicenter clinical trial, the efficacy of intravenous t-PA (0.75 mg/kg over 90 minutes) was compared to that of intravenous streptokinase (1.5 million IU over 60 minutes).[14] The infarct-related coronary arteries were reperfused in 70% of 61 patients in the t-PA group and in 55% of 62 patients in the streptokinase treatment limb. This study also reported fewer bleeding-related complications in the t-PA group compared to the streptokinase group (21 vs. 39 events).

The long-term drawback of thrombolytic therapy is rethrombosis. This is logical, since the coronary anatomy that predisposed a given patient to coronary thrombosis is not altered with thrombolytic therapy. Reports of in-hospital rethrombosis rates after streptokinase have ranged between 5% and 29%.[25, 31] Similar rates of reocclusion have been reported with t-PA.[32] Rethrombosis requires invasive intervention if viable myocardium is at risk. Currently, there are two modalities to achieve recanalization after rethrombosis:

PTCA and ESCR. The modality chosen is based upon coronary anatomy and may be used sequentially in a given patient. An article addressing this problem in 1985 by Braunwald has detailed an algorithm for reperfusion after AMI.[33]

Emergency PTCA without previous thrombolysis may be performed by passage of a guide wire through the thrombus followed immediately by PTCA. This offers the advantage of a recanalization rate of 85% to 95% without the risks of thrombolytic therapy.[34-36] In addition, the risk of rethrombosis may be lower, probably due to decrease in the residual stenosis. However, there are potential disadvantages to emergency PTCA. It is estimated that only 10% to 15% of patients with AMI could reach a well-staffed and equipped catheterization laboratory within 4 hours of their infarction.[33] PTCA is operator-dependent and requires additional skill in the face of AMI. A 24-hours-a-day, 7-days-a-week dedicated catheterization laboratory is necessary, including available personnel. It takes more time to perform PTCA than it does to administer an intravenous thrombolytic. Finally, it requires the availability of a cardiac surgical team and an operating room on a 24-hour basis to perform ESCR in case the procedure fails. More recently, TPCA has been used as an adjunct to thrombolytic therapy in the event of failure or high-grade stenosis.

There have been three recent randomized studies attempting to measure the benefit of coronary angioplasty as an adjunct to thrombolytic therapy. The thrombolysis and angioplasty in myocardial infarction (TAMI) study involved 386 patients who were given 150 mg of t-PA intravenously; those who were reperfused successfully were randomized to either immediate or delayed (7 days) angioplasty.[32] The European Cooperative Study Group reported 367 patients who were given 100 mg of t-PA, and those who were eligible were randomized to immediate or no angioplasty.[37] Finally, TIMI-IIA involved 389 patients who received 100 to 150 mg of t-PA and those who were eligible were randomized to immediate vs. delayed (18 to 48 hours) angioplasty.[38] The results of these studies were similar, although their experimental protocols were somewhat different. Bleeding complications were seen more commonly in the immediate vs. the delayed angioplasty group. This is evidenced by a 10% vs. 4% bleeding complication rate in the European Cooperative Study Group trial and a 19.5% vs. 7.2% rate reported by the TIMI-IIA group. Additionally, the rate of emergency coronary surgery was higher in the immediate vs. the delayed group, as witnessed by 6% vs. 2% in the TIMI-IIA trial and 7% vs. 2% in the TAMI trial. No improvement was seen in predischarge left ventricular ejection fraction in either group. Finally, the mortality of the immediate angioplasty group was higher in all studies than that of the delayed group (4%, 7%, and 8% vs. 1%, 3%, and 5% for TAMI, the European Cooperative Study Group, and TIMI-IIA, respectively). Therefore, these studies concluded that there probably was no short-term benefit to immediate angioplasty in patients with successful thrombolytic therapy.

ESCR for AMI has been reported since the early 1970s, and now there are collective series of over 2,000 patients with a mortality of 6% or less.[5-7, 39-61] This compares favorably to the 11.7% to 27% mortality reported in similar patients managed medically.[6, 13, 59] This is particularly interesting, since ESCR usually is the modality of last resort and therefore the most delayed.

Emergency Surgical Coronary Revascularization

The widespread use of ESCR as primary therapy for AMI is limited logistically by estimates that only 10% of patients with AMI are within 4 hours of a referral center with a modern catheterization facility.[33] This limitation will diminish with quicker patterns of referral, faster methods of medical evacuation, and the proliferation of cardiac surgical facilities. For the present, the challenge is to determine the best therapeutic modality for patients referred to centers with waiting catheterization laboratories and the ready availability of PTCA and ESCR. This question has yet to be answered with randomized clinical trials; however, there are some results in the literature that seem to warrant such trials.

In most centers, ESCR is not the procedure of choice for AMI. However, it is the procedure of second choice for selected patients following coronary angiography, thrombolytic therapy, PTCA, or a combination of these. Certainly, ESCR has been shown to be effective in maintaining coronary reperfusion established by thrombolytic or catheter techniques.[55, 57] The possible indications for ESCR are summarized in Table 1. Patients should be considered for ESCR if they have left main coronary disease or left main equivalent disease (high-grade proximal left anterior descending and

TABLE 1.
Possible Indications for Emergency Surgical Coronary Revascularization

Pharmacologically reperfused patients with high-risk coronary artery anatomy
  Significant stenosis of left main coronary artery
  Left main equivalent disease (significant stenosis in both the left anterior
    descending and circumflex coronary arteries)
  Multivessel coronary disease not amenable to percutaneous transluminal
    coronary angioplasty or with ongoing ischemia and regions of "stunned"
    myocardium in noninfarct zones
Failure to reperfuse myocardium at risk with pharmacologic or mechanical means
  with evidence of ongoing ischemia (ongoing chest pain and/or
  electrocardiographic
  evidence of ongoing ischemia)
Rethrombosis after percutaneous transluminal coronary angioplasty from residual
  stenosis or coronary dissection with viable myocardium at risk.

circumflex stenosis) after AMI, especially if large areas of viable myocardium are at risk for reinfarction. Timely ESCR is particularly important, since the extension of myocardial infarction has been associated with an increased mortality of 15% to 43%.[62-64] Another subset of patients in whom the use of early ESCR should be considered includes those who have been recanalized by thrombolytic therapy and have multivessel coronary disease not amenable to PTCA. This anatomy places patients at high risk for reocclusion. A third group of patients who might benefit from ESCR are those with failed PTCA in whom rethrombosis or failure to recanalize results in recurrent or persistent chest pain and/or electrocardiographic evidence of continued myocardial ischemia. The remaining group of patients who may benefit from ESCR are those in whom reperfusion is unsuccessful using existing thrombolytic and/or catheter techniques. Some have suggested that the interval of 6 hours or less should be used in the indications for ESCR. However, there is an evolving body of evidence suggesting that this interval should be extended.[11] Certainly, the clinical trials have not agreed clearly upon the ideal "window" for revascularization. A more complete discussion of interval and ESCR occurs later in this chapter. One further difficulty with the aforementioned indications involves using recurrent or ongoing chest pain as an indication for ESCR. Califf et al.[65] reported that 20% of patients in whom chest pain was unchanged with thrombolytic therapy had a 60% chance of infarct artery patency. In contrast, patients with partially resolved chest pain had a 71% likelihood of infarct artery patency, and those with complete resolution of chest pain had only an 84% chance of infarct artery patency. This discrepancy between clinical impression and infarct artery patency underlines the difficulty in deciding when to employ ESCR.

Many clinical studies have reported prognostic indicators of operative outcome, but there is no clear consensus on absolute indicators.* Age, left ventricular end diastolic pressure, preoperative cardiogenic shock, extent/ location of coronary artery disease, left ventricular ejection fraction, interval of revascularization, presence/absence of collaterals, and presence/absence of transmural myocardial infarction all have been identified as important variables. The difficulty in analyzing the variables for ESCR in AMI rests with the variability of clinical design of the studies and the subsets of patients studied.

Advanced age recently has been reported by Floten et al.[1] as a negative prognostic factor for long-term survival. They reported 5- and 10-year survival rates of 89% ± 2% and 80% ± 4% for patients under 65 years of age as opposed to survival rates of only 75% ± 3% and 58% ± 9% for patients over 65 years of age. Similarly, Athanasuleas et al. in 1987 reported a series of 83 patients in whom the mortality for ESCR in those under 65 years of age was 8.8% vs. 30.7% for those over 65 years of age.[50] Naunheim et al.[58] further support advanced age as a prognostic indicator for poor survival, with survivors in their series averaging 58.6 ± 10.1 years of age vs. 66.9 ± 7.6 years of age for nonsurvivors.

*References 7, 48, 50, 52, 53, 56–58, 61, 66–68.

Left ventricular end diastolic pressure has been reported to be a significant predictor of postoperative survival in a recent clinical series.[61] The 5- and 10-year survival rates were reported as 89% ± 2% and 75% ± 6% for patients with a left ventricular end diastolic pressure of less than 15 mm Hg. Survival rates for patients with left ventricular end diastolic pressures over 15 mm Hg were 77% ± 5% and 67% ± 7%, respectively. Others have reported reductions of 40% in left ventricular end diastolic pressure after ESCR, but no further clinical studies were found.[5]

Preoperative cardiogenic shock is a significant predictor of mortality in many clinical series.* These studies comprise 300 patients with preoperative cardiogenic shock and an overall mortality of less than 31%. The mortality of cardiogenic shock managed medically is 80%. There is a wide range of reported mortality for this problem (23% to 61.5%) in the surgical series that may reflect differences in operative technique or the interval between onset of cardiogenic shock and ESCR. Allen et al.[66] reported a mortality of 7% in patients with preoperative cardiogenic shock revascularized in 18 hours or less vs. 31% in those delayed after 18 hours.

Preoperative ejection fraction is one of the most debated predictors of surgical mortality, particularly since many of the recent series report improved survival in patients with poor ventricular function managed surgically vs. medically.[16, 69-71] These series demonstrated significantly improved survival in 598 surgically managed patients with impaired left ventricular function when compared with 897 medically managed patients. In general, patients with more left ventricular impairment benefited most from surgical intervention. This approach is not supported as clearly in series of patients undergoing ESCR. Only one series comments directly on ESCR and ejection fraction. This study, reported by Hochberg et al., compared 124 patients undergoing ESCR with ejection fractions greater than 50%. The former group had a hospital mortality of 22% vs. no deaths in the latter group. The authors concluded that patients with an ejection fraction of 50% or greater could be operated on at any point in their hospital course and, therefore, probably warranted early operation. However, they recommended that those with ejection fractions less than 50% have operation delayed 4 weeks. Athanasuleas et al.[50] reported a hospital mortality of 42.8% for patients undergoing ESCR with ejection fractions of 30% or less vs. 10% for patients with ejection fractions of greater than 30%. Although obviously it is not clear from the above discussion, patients with AMI and impaired left ventricular function may benefit from early ESCR.

The optimal interval between the onset of AMI and surgical revascularization has been thought to be 6 hours or less.[72] This was based on animal studies that suggested that myocardial salvage beyond this point was not possible with coronary reperfusion. Roberts et al. reported a series of 20 patients with postinfarction angina who underwent intensive medical stabilization for a mean of 10 days prior to coronary bypass surgery with no mortality. Based on this experience, they urged attempted medical stabilization prior to coronary revascularization. However, more recent clinical

*References 7, 48, 50, 53, 57, 58, 61, 66, 67.

series have suggested exactly the opposite, i.e., that early revascularization is the key.[7, 61] DeWood et al. reported their series of 440 patients with transmural infarction. Patients undergoing early surgical reperfusion (<6 hours) had a mortality of 3.8% vs. 8.0% for patients undergoing late reperfusion (>6 hours). Floten et al.,[61] in their series of 832 patients, divided the mortality based upon these reperfused before or after 24 hours of the onset of AMI. They reported a mortality of 7.6% in the "early" group as opposed to a mortality of 4.1% in the late group. However, the differences in mortality were not statistically significant. Both Naunheim et al.[58] and Athanasuleas et al.[50] reported no difference in mortality based upon interval to reperfusion, and concluded that surgical reperfusion could be performed at any time in the course of a stable patient with the same mortality. Thus, the optimal interval between onset of AMI and ESCR is not defined. However, the trend is to earlier surgical reperfusion, and perhaps the 6-hour limitation can be extended with similar results.

Technique

Standard cardiopulmonary bypass should be established in patients undergoing ESCR as soon as possible. Left ventricular decompression is advisable; it is mandatory if there is any tendency to distention. The cardioplegia system should be organized so that both the aortic root and the subsequent vein grafts may be perfused, or a retrograde (coronary sinus) system should be used. It may be of some advantage to arrest the heart with warm, nutrient-enriched, blood cardioplegic solution while the saphenous vein is dissected. Systemic cooling should be used and hypothermic blood cardioplegic solution should be instituted. In patients with severe proximal coronary artery disease or multivessel coronary disease, retrograde cardioplegic perfusion through the coronary sinus may be required to attain rapid arrest and adequate hypothermia. Topical hypothermia should be added. The order of grafting should follow from the largest, most viable region of myocardium in jeopardy to the area of infarct last. It may be beneficial to infuse warm-blood, nutrient-enriched cardioplegia prior to removing the aortic cross-clamp. After completing the proximal anastomoses, warm-blood perfusion should be allowed, with the mean arterial systolic pressure maintained at 60 to 80 mm Hg while systemic warming is occurring. Aggressive use of intra-aortic balloon support should be instituted early and inotropic support should be minimized. Placement of a femoral arterial line prior to beginning cardiopulmonary bypass will facilitate aortic balloon placement should it be required to wean the patient from bypass.

Results

The overall mortality of over 2,000 patients undergoing ESCR is less than 6% and is summarized in Table 2. Some series have reported mortalities in low-risk patients comparable to those reported for elective coronary artery revascularization.[5-7, 52, 56, 58, 59, 73] Unfortunately, the differences in clinical trial design make it difficult to draw valid conclusions with respect to

TABLE 2.
Mortality in Emergency Surgical Coronary Revascularization Series

Series	Number of Patients	Mortality (%)
Phillips[5] 1979	75	1.3
DeWood[6] 1979	169	1.2
Mathey[55] 1981	48	0
Nunley[48] 1982	80	5.0
Krebber[47] 1982	20	0
DeWood[7] 1983	701	4.4
Walker[54] 1984	53	2.0
Vanhaecke[60] 1985	13	0
Kirklin[52] 1985	35	2.9
Phillips[53] 1986	261	5.7
Athanasuleas[50] 1986	51	5.9
Sutton[49] 1986	99	4.0
Koshal[59] 1988	34	2.9
Naunheim[58] 1988	313	4.7
Kereiakes[57] 1989	82	6.0
Messmer[56] 1989	70	1.4
Floten[61] 1989	832	4.7

patient selection, operative technique, interval, and operative mortality.

Several recent studies have reviewed patient survival after ESCR and found it to be comparable to elective coronary revascularization.[5, 6, 50, 61] In these series, patients with less extensive coronary artery disease or shorter intervals between the onset of symptoms and ESCR seemed to have improved survival. The reported postdischarge mortality of 2% to 3% in surgical patients compares favorably to that of similar patients managed medically. In addition, surgical patients have less postinfarction angina and improved functional capacity.

Left ventricular ejection fraction has been shown to improve in most of the clinical trials that evaluated this parameter in patients undergoing ESCR.[5, 6, 47, 50, 55, 60] It may be that the shorter the interval between the onset of symptoms and surgical coronary revascularization, the more improvement seen in the postoperative left ventricular ejection fraction. The relationship between improved ejection fraction and improved patient survival has yet to be defined in the surgical series. However, ejection fraction at hospital discharge after AMI has been shown to be an important predictor of 1-year survival. It may be that the improved ejection fraction seen after surgical reperfusion is related to reduced ischemic damage secondary to left ventricular decompression and improved cardioplegic solutions used during the procedure.[74, 75]

Unlike medical reperfusion, as compared with thrombolysis or PTCA, surgical reperfusion is controlled and the conditions of reperfusion may be modified. Specific reperfusion options may be beneficial in decreasing myocardial necrosis and accelerating recovery from "stunning." These modifications include "gentle" reperfusion at decreased pressures that may minimize cellular swelling, hypocalcemic reperfusion that diminishes cellular calcium overload, hyperosmotic reperfusion that may facilitate restoration of cellular volume regulation, reperfusion under conditions of cellular arrest that may allow selective utilization of cellular energy stores for reparative processes, and specific metabolic interventions such as free radical "traps" that may be introduced, thereby minimizing oxidant injury.

There are theoretic concerns regarding hemorrhage when ESCR is used in patients who have had thrombolytic therapy. However, these proved unfounded in over 600 patients who underwent ESCR after streptokinase therapy.[72] These individuals had a reported in-hospital mortality of 4% and a rate of reexploration for hemorrhage of less than 5%. Kereiakes et al.[57] reported a similarly low rate of clinically significant hemorrhage in 5 of 82 patients who underwent ESCR following thrombolytic therapy with t-PA. Therefore, it seems that postoperative hemorrhage following thrombolytic therapy is not as major a concern as once was feared. However, many of the clinical series reporting these results include patients operated on further than 24 hours from the cessation of thrombolytic therapy, and the true risk of hemorrhage immediately after thrombolytic therapy is not well defined.

Summary

The cardiologist and/or cardiac surgeon facing a patient with AMI has multiple potential therapeutic modalities from which to choose. ESCR frequently has been seen as the procedure of last resort because of logistic problems. Its use is reserved for those patients who cannot be reperfused by thrombolytics and/or PTCA. In addition, certain subsets of patients who are reperfused but have high-risk coronary anatomy for rethrombosis are offered ESCR. Certainly, any center that performs emergency catheterizations for AMI should have ESCR readily available.

The real debate concerns the best technique for the reperfusion of patients who reach a major referral center and, therefore, have all modalities available to them. This has not been defined in a prospectively randomized clinical study. In addition, the effects of age, ejection fraction, and interval between onset of AMI and ESCR have not been determined. Randomized, multicenter, clinical trials with uniform study design will be necessary to define these parameters. Until then, patients with multivessel coronary disease and AMI can be revascularized safely within 6 hours. There is evolving clinical and basic science data indicating that this interval may be extended successfully as a consequence of improved cardioplegic solutions. In general, the sicker the patient with AMI, the more the potential benefit of early ESCR.

Experimental and clinical studies support the powerful efficacy of operative reperfusion in AMI, particularly in the setting of multivessel coronary disease and major infarction. Such an approach may be ideal for an individual patient, but it currently has cost and logistic implications that limit its widespread application. It is unlikely that large-scale, prospectively randomized studies will be initiated. Given that ESCR is not likely to become the standard of care for the nation, the goal and compromise position is to make medical reperfusion resemble operative reperfusion as closely as possible.

References

1. Manney FM Jr, Ebert PA, Sabiston DC Jr: Postoperative myocardial infarction: A study of predisposing factors, diagnosis, and mortality in a high risk group of surgical patients. *Ann Surg* 1970; 172:497–502.
2. Baer S, Nakhjavan F, Kajani M: Postoperative myocardial infarction. *Surg Gynecol Obstet* 1965; 120:315–322.
3. Tarhan S, Emerson A, Moffitt EA, et al: Myocardial infarction after general anesthesia. *JAMA* 1972; 220:1451–1454.
4. Arkins R, Gmessaert AA, Hicks RG: Mortality and morbidity in surgical patients with coronary artery Disease. *JAMA* 1964; 190:425–428.
5. Phillips SJ, Kowgtahwonn C, Zeff R, et al: Emergency coronary artery revascularization: A possible therapy for acute myocardial infarction. *Circulation* 1979; 2:241–246.
6. DeWood MA, Spores J, Notske RW, et al: Medical and surgical management of myocardial infarction. *Am J Cardiol* 1979; 44:1356–1364.
7. DeWood MA, Spores J, Berg R, et al: Acute myocardial infarction: A decade of experience with surgical reperfusion in 701 patients. *Circulation* 1983; 68:(suppl II):8–16.
8. Reimer KA, Jennings RB: The "wavefront phenomenon" of myocardial ischemic cell death: II. Transmural progression of necrosis within the framework of ischemic bed size (myocardium at risk) and collateral flow. *Lab Invest* 1979; 40:633–644.
9. Cerra FB, Lajos TZ, Montes M, et al: Structural functional correlates of reversible myocardial anoxia. *J Surg Res* 1974; 10:140.
10. Jennings RB, Reimer KA: Savage of ischemic myocardium. *Mod Concepts Cardiovasc Dis* 1974; 43:125.
11. Beyersdorf F, Allen B, Buckberg GD, et al: Studies on prolonged acute ischemia. *J Thorac Cardiovasc Surg* 1989; 98:112–126.
12. Cheung EH, Arcid JM Jr, Dorsey LMA, et al: Reperfusion of infarcting myocardium: Benefit of surgical reperfusion in alcoholic model. *Ann Thorac Surg* 1989; 48:331B.
13. Killip III T, Kimball JT: Treatment of myocardial infarction in a coronary care unit. *Am J Cardiol* 1967; 20:457–464.
14. Verstrate M, Bory M, Brower RW, et al: Randomized trial of intravenous recombinant tissue-type plasminogen activator versus intravenous streptokinase in acute myocardial infarction. *Lancet* 1985; 1:842–847.
15. Cowley MJ, Hastillo A, Vetrovec GW, et al: Effects of intracoronary streptokinase in acute myocardial infarction. *Am Heart J* 1981; 6:1149–1150.

16. Rogers WJ, Mantle JA, Hood WP Jr, et al: Prospective randomized trial of intravenous and intracoronary streptokinase in acute myocardial infarction. *Circulation* 1983; 68:1051–1061.
17. Serruys PW, Suryapranata H, Simoons ML, et al: Intracoronary thrombolysis in patients with acute myocardial infarctions: The Netherlands randomized trial and current status. *Circulation* 1987; 76(suppl II): II-63–II-67.
18. Kennedy JW, Ritchie JL, Davis KB, et al: Western Washington randomized trial of intracoronary streptokinase in acute myocardial infarction. *N Engl J Med* 1983; 309:1477–1482.
19. Gissi-Gruppo Italiano per lo Studio della Streptocninasi nell' Infarto Miocardico: Effectiveness of intravenous thrombolytic treatment of acute myocardial infarction. *Lancet* 1986; 1:397.
20. Chesebro JH, Knatterud G, Roberts R, et al: Thrombolysis in Myocardial Infarction (TIMI) trial, phase 1: A comparison between intravenous plasminogen activator and intravenous streptokinase. *Circulation* 1987; 76:(suppl I):I–142.
21. Collen D: Human tissue type plasminogen activator: From the laboratory to the bedside. *Circulation* 1986; 72:18–20.
22. Gold HK, Leinbach RL, Garabedian SM, et al: Acute coronary reocclusion after thrombolysis with recombinant tissue type plasminogen activator: Prevention by a maintenance infusion. *Circulation* 1986; 2:347–352.
23. TIMI Study Group: The Thrombolysis in Myocardial Infarction (TIMI) trial. *N Engl J Med* 1985; 312:932–936.
24. Collen D, Topol EJ, Tiefenbrunn AJ, et al: Coronary thrombolysis with recombinant human tissue type plasminogen activator: A prospective randomized placebo controlled trial. *Circulation* 1984; 70:1012–1017.
25. Rentrop P, Bianke H, Karsch KR, et al: Changes in left ventricular function after intracoronary streptokinase infusion in clinically evolving myocardial infarction. *Am Heart J* 1981; 102:1193.
26. Cribier A, Berland J, Champoud O, et al: Intracoronary thrombolysis in evolving myocardial infarction: Sequential angiographic analysis of left ventricular performance. *Br Heart J* 1983; 50:410.
27. Ganz W, Geft I, Maddahi J, et al: Nonsurgical reperfusion in evolving myocardial infarction. *N Am Coll Cardiol* 1983; 1:1253.
28. Schwarz F, Schuler G, Katus H, et al: Intracoronary thrombolysis in acute myocardial infarction: Duration of ischemia as a major determinant of late results after recanalization. *Am J Cardiol* 1982; 50:937.
29. Rogers WJ, Mantle SA, Hood WP, et al: Prospective randomized trial of intravenous and intracoronary streptokinase in acute myocardial infarction. *Circulation* 1983; 68:1051–1061.
30. Schroder R, Biamino G, Enz-Rudineger L, et al: Intravenous short-term infusion of streptokinase in acute myocardial infarction. *Circulation* 1983; 67:536–548.
31. Serruys PW, Wijns W, Van Denbrand M, et al: Is transluminal coronary angioplasty mandatory after successful thrombolysis? Quantitative coronary angiography study. *Br Heart J* 1983; 50:257–265.
32. Topol EJ, Califf RM, George BS, et al: A randomized trial of immediate versus delayed elective angioplasty after intravenous tissue plasminogen activator in acute myocardial infarction. *N Engl J Med* 1987; 317:501–588.
33. Braunwald E: The aggressive treatment of acute myocardial infarction. *Circulation* 1985; 71:1087–1092.
34. Stack RS, O'Connor CM, Mark KDB, et al: Coronary reperfusion during acute

myocardial infarction with a combined therapy of coronary angioplasty and high-dose intravenous streptokinase. *Circulation* 1988; 77:151–161.

35. Rothaum DA, Linne Meier TJ, Landin RJ, et al: Emergency percutaneous transluminal coronary angioplasty in acute myocardial infarction: A three year study experience. *J Am Coll Cardiol* 1987; 10:204–272.

36. Pepine CJ, Prida X, Hill JA, et al: Percutaneous transluminal coronary angioplasty in acute myocardial infarction. *Am Heart J* 1984; 107:820–822.

37. Simoons ML, Betriu A, Col J, et al: Thrombolysis with tissue plasminogen activator in acute myocardial infarction: No additional benefit from immediate percutaneous angioplasty. *Lancet* 1900; 1:197–202.

38. The TIMI Research Group: Immediate versus delayed catheterization following thrombolytic therapy for acute myocardial infarction. *JAMA* 1988; 260:2849–2850.

39. Fanaloro RG, Effler DB, Cheanvechai C, et al: Acute coronary insufficiency (impending myocardial infarction and myocardial infarction). Surgical treatment by the saphenous vein graft technique. *Am J Cardiol* 1971; 28:598–607.

40. Cohn LH, Fogarty TJ, Daily PO, et al: Emergency coronary artery bypass: *Surgery* 1971; 70:821–829.

41. Scanlon PJ, Nemickas R, Tobin JR, et al: Pifarrer: Myocardial revascularization during acute phase of myocardial infarction. *JAMA* 1971; 218:207–212.

42. Cohn LH, Gorlin R, Herman MV, et al: Aortocoronary bypass for acute coronary occlusion. *J Thorac Cardiovasc Surg* 1972; 64:503–513.

43. Keon WJ, Bedard P, Shankar RK, et al: Experience with emergency aortocoronary bypass grafts in the presence of acute myocardial infarction. *Circulation* 1973; 57/58(suppl III):111–151.

44. Cheanvechai C, Effler DB, Loop FD, et al: Emergency myocardial revascularization. *Am J Cardiol* 1973; 32:901–908.

45. Bolooki H, Kotler MD, Lottenberg L, et al: Myocardial revascularization after acute infarction. *Am J Cardiol* 1975; 36:395–406.

46. Berg R, Kendall RW, Duvoisin GE, et al: Acute myocardial infarction: A surgical emergency. *J Thorac Cardiovasc Surg* 1975; 70:432–439.

47. Krebber HJ, Mathey D, Kuck KJ, et al: Management of evolving myocardial infarction by intracoronary thrombolysis and subsequent aorta coronary bypass. *J Thorac Cardiovasc Surg* 1982; 83:186–193.

48. Nunley DL, Grunkemeiber GL, Teply JF, et al: Coronary bypass operation following acute complicated myocardial infarction. *J Thorac Cardiovasc Surg* 1983; 85:485–491.

49. Sutton JM, Taylor GL, Mikell FL, et al: Thrombolytic therapy followed by early revascularization for acute myocardial infarction. *Am J Cardiol* 1986; 57:1227–1231.

50. Athanasuleas CL, Geer DA, Arciniegas JG, et al: A reappraisal of surgical intervention for acute myocardial infarction. *J Thorac Cardiovasc Surg* 1987; 93:405–414.

51. Berg R Jr, Selinger SL, Leonard JJ, et la: Immediate coronary artery bypass for evolving myocardial infarction. *J Thorac Cardiovasc Surg* 1981; 81:493–497.

52. Kirklin JK, Blackstone EH, Zorn GL, et al: Intermediate-term results of coronary artery bypass grafting for acute myocardial infarction. *Circulation* 1985; 72(suppl II):II-175–II-178.

53. Phillips SJ, Zeff RH, Skinner JR, et al: Reperfusion protocol and results in 738

patients with evolving myocardial infarction. *Ann Thorac Surg* 1986; 41:119–125.

54. Walker WE, Smalling RW, Fuentes F, et al: Role of coronary artery bypass surgery after intra-coronary streptokinase for myocardial infarction. *Am Heart J* 1984; 107:826–829.

55. Mathey DG, Rodeward G, Rentrop P, et al: Intracoronary streptokinase thrombolytic recanalization and subsequent surgical bypass of remaining atherosclerotic stenosis in acute myocardial infarction: Complementary combined approach effecting reduced infarct size, preventing reinfarction and improving left ventricular function. *Am Heart J* 1981; 102:1194–1201.

56. Messmer BJ, Uebis R, Rieger C, et al: Late results after intracoronary thrombolysis and early bypass grafting for acute myocardial infarction. *J Thorac Cardiovasc Surg* 1989; 97:10–18.

57. Kereiakes DJ, Topol EJ, and the TAMI Study Group: Favorable early and long-term prognosis following coronary bypass surgery therapy for myocardial infarction. Results of a multicenter trial: *Am Heart J* 1989; 118:199–206.

58. Naunheim KS, Kesler KA, Kanter KR, et al: Coronary artery bypass for recurrent myocardial infarction. Predictors of mortality. *Circulation* 1988; 78:(suppl K):I-122–I-128.

59. Koshal A, Beanlands DS, Davies RA, et al: Urgent surgical reperfusion in acute revolving myocardial infarction. *Circulation* 1988; 78:(suppl I):I-171–178.

60. Vanhaecke J, Flameng W, Sergeant P, et al: Emergency bypass surgery: Late effects on size of infarct and ventricular function. *Circulation* 1985; 72:(suppl II):179–184.

61. Floten HS, Ahmad A, Swanson JS, et al: Long-term survival after post infarction bypass operation: Early versus late operation. *Ann Thorac Surg* 1989; 48:757–763.

62. Fraker TD Jr, Wagner GS, Rosati RA: Extension of myocardial infarction: Incidence and prognosis. *Circulation* 1979; 60:1126–1129.

63. Maisel AS, Ahnve S, Gilpin E, et al: Prognosis after extension of myocardial infarct: The role of Q wave or non Q wave infarction. *Circulation* 1985; 71:211–216.

64. Buda AJ, MacDonald IL, Dubbin JD, et al: Myocardial infarct extension: Prevalence clinical significance and problems in diagnosis. *Am Heart J* 1983; 105:744–749.

65. Califf RM, O'Neil WW, Stack RS, et al: Failure of simple clinical measure to predict perfusion status after intravenous thrombolysis. *Ann Intern Med* 1988; 108:658–662.

66. Allen BS, Rosenkranz E, Buckberg GD, et al: Studies on prolonged acute regional ischemia VI. Myocardial infarction with left ventricular power failure: A medical surgical emergency requiring urgent revascularization with maximal protection of remote muscle. *J Thorac Cardiovasc Surg* 1989; 98:691–703.

67. Stuart RS, Baumgartner WA, Soule L, et al: Predictors of perioperative mortality in patients with unstable post-infarction angina. *Circulation* 1988; 78(suppl I):I-163–165.

68. Roberts AJ, Sanders JH Jr, Moran JH, et al: The efficacy of medical stabilization prior to myocardial revascularization in early refractory post infarction angina. *Ann Surg* 1983; 197:91–98.

69. Alderman EL, Fisher LD, Litwin P, et al: Results of coronary artery surgery in patients with poor ventricular function. *Circulation* 1983; 68:785–795.

70. Scott SM, Luchi RJ, and the Veterans Unstable Angina Cooperative Study Group: Veterans Administration cooperative study for treatment of patients

with abnormal left ventricular function. *Circulation* 1988; 78(suppl I):I-113–I-121.

71. Bounous EP, Mark DB, Pollock BG, et al: Surgical survival for coronary disease patients with left ventricular dysfunction. *Circulation* 1988; (suppl I):I151–I157.

72. Kereiakes DJ: The role of emergency surgical revascularization in AMI. Topol EJ (ed): Acute Coronary Intervention. New York, AR Liss, Wiley 1987.

73. Hochberg MS, Parsonnet V, Gielchnsky I, et al: Timing of coronary revascularization after acute myocardial infarction. *J Thorac Cardiovasc Surg* 1984; 88:914–921.

74. Laschinger JC, Gross EA, Cunningham JN Jr, et al: Adjunctive left ventricular unloading during myocardial reperfusion plays a major role in minimizing myocardial infarct size. *J Thorac Cardiovasc Surg* 1985; 90:80–85.

75. Rosenkranz ER, Okamoto F, Buckberg GD, et al: Safety of prolonged aortic cross clamping with blood cardioplegia. III. Aspartate enrichment of glutamate—blood cardioplegia in energy depleted hearts after ischemia and reperfusion injury. *J Thorac Cardiovasc Surg* 1986; 91:428–435.

Myocardial Protection in Cardiac Surgery: Subcellular Basis for Myocardial Injury and Protection

Anwar S. Abd-Elfattah Ph.D.

Associate Professor of Surgery and Pharmacology and Toxicology, Division of Cardiothoracic Surgery, Department of Surgery, Medical College of Virginia, Virginia Commonwealth University, Richmond, Virginia

Andrew S. Wechsler, M.D.

Stuart McGuire Professor of Surgery, Chairman, Department of Surgery, Professor of Physiology, Medical College of Virginia, Virginia Commonwealth University, Richmond, Virginia

Although the morbidity and mortality associated with coronary artery bypass graft (CABG) surgery in uncomplicated cases are low, recent studies suggest that they are increasing as the demographic profile of the operative population changes. Patients presenting for CABG surgery now are older and sicker. Most of them are being sustained on multiple medical therapies, such as β- and calcium channel blockers, and have undergone one or more angioplasties. Recent estimates conclude that the number of angioplasties performed each year exceeds the number of CABG operations. However, frequent coronary artery restenosis occurs in a large number of patients. The development of myocardial ischemia before cardiopulmonary bypass surgery has been shown to have a strong causal relationship to the outcome of surgery. Ischemia occurring prior to bypass doubles or triples the risk of subsequent myocardial infarction. Indicators of perioperative ischemia include (1) electrocardiographic determination of ST segment depression, (2) increases in left ventricular end-diastolic pressure, and (3) segmental wall motion and wall thickening abnormalities. Both segmental shortening and wall thickening abnormalities provide the most sensitive clinical measure of ischemia. Reduction in perioperative cardiac morbidity requires new approaches to the management of cardiac surgery patients and high-risk noncardiac surgery patients.

The role of basic science investigations in elucidating subcellular and

*Supported in part by National Institutes of Health grant HL#26302.

molecular mechanisms of myocardial injury and protection is greatly appreciated when clinically applied for patient management. It would be unrealistic to cover all aspects of myocardial injury and protection in this review. However, our discussion will deal with old (but controversial) as well as new mechanisms of myocardial protection in different events of ischemic syndromes. Due to well-documented age-related differences, a comparison will be made, whenever appropriate, between strategies of myocardial protection in adult and pediatric cardiac surgery.

When Should Myocardial Protection Be Applied?

Four phases of myocardial protection against ischemic and reperfusion injury in association with cardiac surgery should be considered: (1) preoperative interventions, including pharmacologic management with β-blockers and calcium channel blockers, vasodilator drugs that relieve vasospasm, percutaneous transluminal coronary angioplasty, and thrombolytic therapy; (2) intraoperative interventions managed by the anesthesiologist, providing adequate oxygen supply and minimizing intraoperative hypotension and tachycardia, and by the surgeon, providing adequate cooling; (3) postoperative intervention that prevent short-term reperfusion-mediated injury, low cardiac output, and hypotension especially in high-risk patients in the intensive care unit; and (4) interventions that prevent postoperative low cardiac output and other cardiac morbidity mediated by long-term reperfusion injury before or after hospital discharge. Since perioperative ischemic disease and intraoperative and postoperative pathophysiologic changes contribute to cardiac morbidity and patient mortality following open heart surgery, the relationship between intraoperative ischemia and the outcome of cardiac surgery should be reemphasized. Deleterious effects of the extracorporeal circuit, including platelet and neutrophil activation and adhesion to incompatible materials, may occur during the initiation of cardiopulmonary bypass.[1, 2] Release of active substances from activated platelets and neutrophils may produce additional vascular damage, including thrombus formation, free radical production, and the adhesion of these cells to coronary artery endothelium, which may cause vascular plugging in addition to preexisting myocardial ischemia and anticipated reperfusion injury. It is well established that a dramatic reduction of platelet and neutrophil counts (60% to 70%) occurs with the initiation of cardiopulmonary bypass.[3] Hypothermia and alkalinity shift hemoglobin/oxygen association and dissociation curves and induce changes in the shape of platelets from discoid to flat,[4, 5] similar to the changes that precede pharmacologic platelet activation.

Myocardial Ischemic and Reperfusion Injury

In order to discuss the rationale behind the evolution of myocardial protective techniques, it is important to emphasize certain physiologic facts and subcellular mechanisms of myocardial ischemic injury and possible strategies for myocardial protection that may be employed during elective cardiac surgery. Biochemical and physiologic principles, and experimental laboratory observations, therefore, are valuable to the surgeon for better management of patients' safety. Disruption of coronary blood flow and lack of oxygen with the onset of ischemia induce acute subcellular biochemical changes in the myocardium.[6, 7] First, lack of molecular oxygen uncouples the respiratory chain from oxidative phosphorylation, resulting in the cessation of adenosine triphosphate (ATP) synthesis, while the demand for energy utilization is increased concomitantly in an attempt to maintain mechanical function and regulate ionic homeostasis.[8] In addition, uncouplers are known to convert mitochondrial ATP synthetase complex (Factor 1/Factor 0 complex) to ATP phosphatase (Fig 1). Therefore, with the onset of ischemia, the critical balance between energy production and utilization is impaired, allowing the transient accumulation of intramyocardial adenosine diphosphate (ADP) and adenosine monophosphate (AMP).

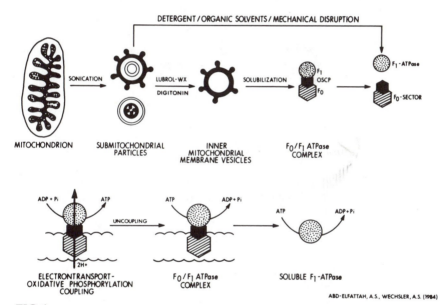

FIG 1.
Intact mitochondria can synthesize adenosine triphosphate *(ATP)* in the presence of appropriate substrates and oxygen and when oxidative phosphorylation is coupled to the electron transport. The resolution of mitochondrial adenosine triphosphatase *(ATPase)* by solubilization or mechanical distribution results in the separation of F_1-ATPase from the F_0-sector and oligomycin-sensitive conferring protein *(OSCP)*, the loss of ATP synthesis activity, and the dramatic stimulation of ATPase activity. Ischemia and uncouplers produce similar effects in vivo and in isolated heart models. Rapid reduction in myocardial ATP during ischemia is related partially to the stimulation of mitochondrial ATPase activity. *ADP* = adenosine diphosphate.

The turnover of ATP is minimized and will be dependent solely on inefficient anaerobic glycolysis. In normal hearts, subcellular levels of myocardial ATP regulate the activity of key enzymes involved in the degradative pathway of adenine nucleotides.[9, 10] Upon ATP depletion, a cascade of enzymes is stimulated, converting adenine nucleotides (ADP, AMP) to diffusible nucleosides (adenosine and inosine) (Fig 2). In addition to the loss of ATP as an energy source, the myocardial cell membrane becomes permeable to NA^+ and Ca^{2+}, and the sarcoplasmic reticulum becomes inefficient in sequestering cytosolic calcium, which leads to the development of a "stone heart."[11] Proteolytic enzymes and phospholipases subsequently are activated upon availability of cytosolic calcium during myocardial ischemia.[12, 13] It also is believed that Ca^{2+} stimulates complement formation, which is necessary for neutrophil activation, i.e., production of superoxide radicals and adhesion to endothelial cells during postischemic reperfusion.[14] Also, Ca^{2+} may be involved in arachidonic acid production[15] and the intraconversion of xanthine dehydrogenase into xanthine oxidase.[16] During ischemia, catecholamine levels increase, while β-adrenergic receptors and their responsiveness are compromised.[17]

The early diagnosis of acute or chronic myocardial ischemic syndromes is extremely crucial for myocardial salvage and patient survival. In most clinical instances, myocardial infarction and irreversible damage occur prior to any medical or surgical procedures. The success of myocardial salvage is measured by the extent of myocardial necrosis during the ischemic episode. Relieving coronary artery stenosis and restoring blood perfusion is critical in patients with acute myocardial infarction. Although reperfusion is a prerequisite for myocardial salvage, in addition to the injurious effects of ischemia, reperfusion may cause injury that contributes to postischemic ventricular dysfunction.[18-20] Ventricular arrhythmias, low cardiac output, and the "no-reflow" phenomenon are common events observed by surgeons following lengthy ischemia and reperfusion. Metabolic interventions capable of minimizing ischemic injury and shortening the period of vulnerability during reperfusion reduce postoperative ventricular dysfunction. Therefore, pharmacologic interventions that prevent reperfusion-mediated injury have assumed renewed clinical significance.

The forthcoming discussion is organized to follow the cascade of events triggered by myocardial ischemia (see Fig 2). ATP depletion is the first signal of ischemia, followed by increased calcium entry into the myocyte. Calcium stimulates calcium-dependent proteases and phospholipases that ac-

---

FIG 2.
The graph illustrates the tight linkage between oxidative metabolism, the production of reducing equivalents nicotinamide-adenine dinucleotide and flavin adenine dinucleotide$_2$ *(NADH and FADH$_2$),* and the coupling between respiratory chain and oxidative phosphorylation. During normoxia, adenosine triphosphate *(ATP)* turnover is fast. However, under hypoxic or ischemic stress, the critical balance between ATP supply and demand shifts toward ATP utilization, while ATP produc-

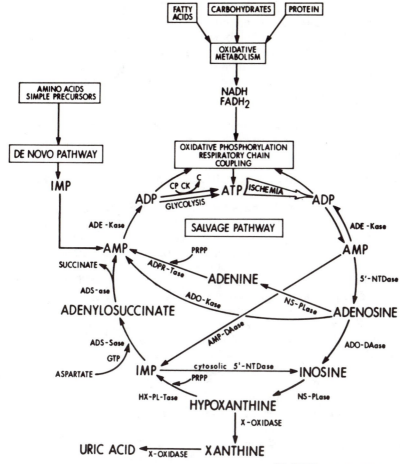

FATTY ACIDS   CARBOHYDRATES   PROTEIN

OXIDATIVE METABOLISM

NADH FADH$_2$

AMINO ACIDS SIMPLE PRECURSORS

DE NOVO PATHWAY

IMP

OXIDATIVE PHOSPHORYLATION RESPIRATORY CHAIN COUPLING

CP CK / C
ADP $\longleftarrow$ ATP ISCHEMIA $\longrightarrow$ ADP
GLYCOLYSIS

SALVAGE PATHWAY

ADE -Kase   ADE -Kase

AMP   AMP

SUCCINATE   PRPP
                    ADPR-Tase   5'-NTDase
ADS-ase   ADENINE
                         ADO-Kase   NS-PLase
ADENYLOSUCCINATE   ADENOSINE

                    AMP-DAase
ADS-Sase   ADO-DAase
GTP
ASPARTATE — IMP cytosolic 5'-NTDase → INOSINE
                    PRPP
HX-PL-Tase   NS-PLase
              HYPOXANTHINE

              X -OXIDASE

URIC ACID ←—— XANTHINE
        X-OXIDASE

ABD-ELFATTAH, A.S., WECHSLER, A.S. (1986)

tion is limited to anaerobic glycolysis. ATP depletion stimulates several degradative enzymes in order to prevent any significant accumulation of catabolites. The majority of ATP catabolites during ischemia are inosine. Nucleosides and purine bases are washed out of the myocardium during reperfusion. The salvage pathway of adenine nucleotides utilizes salvage precursors adenosine monophosphate *(AMP)*, adenosine, hypoxanthine, and inosine monophosphate *(IMP)* only when they are entrapped. Normally, postischemic recovery of adenine nucleotide is dependent on the slow de novo pathway rather than the salvage pathway. *ADE-Kase* = adenosine kinase; *5'-NTDase* = 5'-nucleotidase; *ADO-DAase* = adenosine deaminase; *NS-Plase* = nucleoside phosphorylase; *X-Oxidase* = xanthine oxidase; *AMP* = adenosine monophosphate; *ADP* = adenosine diphosphatase; *GTP* = guanosine triphosphate; *PRPP* = phosphoribosylpyrophosphate; *HX-PL-Tase* = hypoxanthine phosphorylatranferance; *ADS-Sase* = adenosylsuccinate synthesis; *ADS-ase* = adenosylsuccinase; *CP* = creatine phosphate; *CK* = creatine kinase; *ADO-Kase*=adenosine kinase; *ADP-ase*=adenosine-diphosphatase; *ADE*= adenylate kinase; *ADPR-Tase*=adenylphosphopyrophosphate transferase.

tivate complement and stimulate neutrophils. During postischemic reperfusion, several mechanisms may be involved in the alleged "reperfusion-mediated injury." The possible contribution of each mechanism to ventricular dysfunction during postischemic reperfusion will be discussed. The dual role of myocardial ATP in ischemia/reperfusion injury and functional and metabolic recovery also will be reviewed, along with other possible mechanisms of myocardial injury.

Role of Adenine Nucleotide Pool in Myocardial Ischemic Injury

It is well established that approximately 95% of the chemical energy produced by mitochondrial oxidative metabolism is stored in the form of high-energy phosphate bonds in the ATP molecule. Phosphocreatine, a high-energy phosphate, acts as an energy transfer buffer between ATP and ADP. The interconversion is catalyzed by creatine kinase. The myocardium needs ATP for the regulation of ionic homeostasis, basic metabolism, and ventricular mechanical function. Both ventricular systole and diastole are ATP-dependent biochemical processes. During systole, ATP is required also for troponin subunit phosphorylation, which allows interaction between actin and myosin in the presence of increased levels of systolic calcium released from the sarcoplasmic reticulum at the beginning of the cardiac cycle. Cardiac muscle relaxation during diastole and the sequestration of systolic calcium by the sarcoplasmic reticulum is also ATP-dependent. Therefore, it is apparent that the myocardial ATP level at the end of ischemia and during reperfusion is an important determinant for recovery of myocardial metabolism and cardiac function.[21, 22]

Interventions that prevent the depletion of myocardial ATP during ischemia also preserve myocardial function. For example, hypothermia and hyperkalemia provide adequate preservation of myocardial ATP metabolism as well as functional recovery.[23, 24] In models of brief coronary artery occlusion, persistent ventricular dysfunction ("myocardial stunning") is associated with the loss of myocardial ATP.[25, 26] Other investigators have reported that in unprotected, reversibly ischemic myocardium, functional recovery usually is not associated with complete ATP recovery.[27–29] These findings are consistent, despite the fact that complete repletion of phosphate or creatine occurs within a few minutes of reperfusion, even in hearts that perform poorly. Repletion of myocardial ATP normally lags as long as 1 to 7 days following brief ischemia,[30, 31] during which time ventricular function may be totally recovered. Factors affecting incomplete repletion of myocardial ATP following brief ischemia apparently are related to the loss of essential precursors such as adenosine and hypoxanthine during reperfusion.[9, 10, 32] Studies have demonstrated that the higher the ATP at the end of ischemia, the better the functional recovery.[33] More precise techniques are now available to assess ventricular function and measure levels of myocardial adenine nucleotide pool intermediates. Results from recent studies have shown that ventricular function may recover without concomitant recovery of myocardial ATP following brief ischemia.[34, 35] A short period (15 minutes) of regional ischemia produces ventricular dysfunction (myocardial stunning), while ATP is reduced only slightly ($\approx$30%).[34–36] These studies demonstrate dissociation between ATP levels and ventricular function. These discrepancies may be attributed to at least two factors that have been overlooked. First, the myocardium apparently contains more ATP than is needed to support ventricular function and basal cellular regulation.[37] Second, a lack of separation between ventricular dysfunction mediated by ischemia and that mediated by reperfusion hinders efforts to determine the correlation between myocardial ATP and function assessed only during reperfusion.[37, 38] We have separated ischemia and reperfusion components using the nucleoside transport blocker p-nitrobenzylthioinosine (NBMPR) and adenosine deaminase inhibitor erythro-9-(2-hydroxy-3-nonyl) adenine (EHNA).[37–40] In recent studies,[37, 38] myocardial ATP was depleted to less than 20% of normal levels by prolonging the period of normothermic global ischemia (to 30, 60, and 90 minutes). In the untreated control group, the relationship between myocardial ATP and function was biphasic. However, when reperfusion injury was prevented by specific metabolic and transport inhibitors, myocardial ATP did not correlate with function as long as ATP was above critical levels. From these studies, the critical myocardial ATP was estimated to be less than 20% of normal ATP (8 to 9 nmol/mg of protein). Below critical levels of ATP, ventricular function was impaired and the myocardium developed either ischemic contracture or cardiogenic shock during reperfusion. These results demonstrate the dual role of myocardial ATP: (1) as an essential element for ventricular function when myocardial ATP is reduced to critical levels, and (2) as an important source of free-radical substrates. As mentioned, the myocardium apparently contains more ATP than is required for contraction-relaxation coupling and other basic biochemical and physiologic functions. Therefore, the loss of myocardial ATP (by 80%) still allows adequate ventricular performance when reperfusion is managed.[37–40] The correlation between ATP and ventricular function exists at significantly reduced, but critical, levels of ATP, and when reperfusion injury is prevented.[40]

Role of Calcium in Myocardial Ischemic Injury

Calcium overload during ischemia and reperfusion is one of the major mechanisms of myocardial injury.[41, 42] The glycocalyx layer and sarcolemmic membranes also play an important role in calcium binding and entry into normal myocardial cells. Disruption of calcium binding sites of the glycocalyx is believed to facilitate calcium entry into the cardiomyocyte. The removal of sialic acid, an amino sugar, from the glycocalyx layer by neuraminidase increases sarcolemmic membrane permeability to calcium ions. Morphologic studies have demonstrated separation of the glycocalyx layer from the sarcolemmic membrane during ischemia.[43] Therefore, sarcolemmic membrane damage during myocardial ischemia promotes calicum entry during and presumably after ischemia. The loss of ATP and rise in intracellular calcium promotes the activation of calcium-dependent phospholipase, and proteolytic enzymes.[12, 13] Therefore, pharmacologic interventions that reduce ATP loss during ischemia, stabilize the sarcolemmic membrane glycocalyx complex, or specifically limit calcium ion entry would be effective in attenuating myocardial damage mediated by calcium overload during ischemia and also during reperfusion injury.[44]

Calcium channel blockers (verapamil, diltiazem, nifedipine, lidoflazine, and mioflazine) have extremely high affinity to membrane phospholipids and exert membrane-stabilizing effects. These molecules, due to their high affinity to phospholipids, block calcium ions, nucleosides, and many other molecules released or taken up by cardiomyocytes.[45, 46]

Role of Calcium in Postischemic Ventricular Arrhythmias

A common factor shared by clinical events following significant ischemia is a prolonged recovery period during which the heart is susceptible to ventricular arrhythmias and/or pump failure. This phenomenon of electrophysiologic disturbances is quite reproducible in experimental animal models following varying periods of ischemia and reperfusion.[47-49] The frequency of ventricular arrhythmias is species-dependent (Abd-Elfattah et al, unpublished data, 1990). For example, the pig is more susceptible to regional myocardial ischemia and reperfusion-induced arrhythmias than is the dog. These differences could be related to the lack of preexisting coronary collaterals, species-related differences in endothelial vasculature, conduction system differences, or ischemic heterogeneity.

Both oxygen-derived free radicals and calcium have been implicated in myocardial injury and ventricular arrhythmias.[49-53] It has been shown that cytosolic calcium rises during ischemia, which may set the stage for arrhythmias during reperfusion. Calcium overload during the first few minutes of reperfusion also plays a significant role in ventricular arrhythmias. Calcium entry during reperfusion may be provoked by endothelial cell membrane damage mediated by free radicals generated immediately with reperfusion. Hearse and coworkers reported that ventricular arrhythmias induced by free radicals could be attenuated by free-radical scavengers.[54-56] Recent reports dissociated the arrhythmogenic effects of free radicals produced during reperfusion.[57]

The hypothesis implicating oxygen-derived free radicals in ventricular arrhythmias and fibrillation has been challenged by other investigators. Pharmacologic interventions that reduce calcium entry during ischemia improve metabolic and functional recovery and prevent arrhythmias during reperfusion.[44] Therefore, calcium antagonists are more cardioprotective when administered prior to ischemia.[58] The administration of calcium antagonists during reperfusion is not as effective as administration prior to ischemia.[59]

A combination of calcium channel blockers and other drugs has been of interest in experimental and clinical settings of thrombolytic therapy.[60] Calcium antagonists alone or in combination have been used to reduce ischemia-mediated injury.[61, 62] Other strategies include the infusion of calcium channel blockers prior to thrombolytic therapy.[63] Delayed infusion of calcium antagonists following acute myocardial ischemia may have adverse effects when combined with thrombolytic therapy.[63] Pharmacologic interventions with β-blockers to reduce ischemic injury have been reported.[64] Adenosine also has been used experimentally in combination with verapamil to provide additional myocardial protection during ischemia and reperfusion.[65]

The Phenomenon of Reperfusion Injury: Mechanisms and Protection

The overall injury sustained by the heart during ischemia and reperfusion may be divided into two components (Fig 3). The first component of myocardial injury is that induced by biochemical changes mediated by ischemia. This process begins with ATP depletion and the build-up of ATP catabolites, acidosis, the influx of sodium and calcium, and the activation of phospholipases, proteolytic enzymes, and complement. The second component of injury is reperfusion phenomena. By definition, reperfusion injury is myocardial damage, in addition to that of ischemia, that occurs only with reperfusion. The separation of these two components of injury is thoroughly discussed by Bulkely.[66] Jennings' and Schaper's groups have urged against the phenomenon of reperfusion injury.[7, 67] Their argument, based on morphologic assessment, is that the injury sustained by the heart following ischemia and reperfusion is related solely to the ischemia, and that reperfusion does not cause additional trauma. During the last decade, numerous reports have implicated free radicals in postischemic reperfusion injury.[37-40, 68-70] This hypothesis has gained the acceptance of the majority of experimental and clinical investigators. However, the mechanisms by which oxygen-derived radicals are produced and exert their injurious effects remain controversial.[71-73] There are five major mechanisms for the production of oxygen free radicals during reperfusion: (1) ATP catabolism providing xanthine oxidase substrates, (2) neutrophil/complement activation, (3) phospholipase-arachidonic acid pathway intermediates, (4) mitochondria, and (5) auto-oxidation of catecholamines. Other mechanisms of free radicals may yet be identified.

Due to a lack of on-line direct measurement of free radical production during reperfusion, studies to demonstrate the mechanism of reperfusion-mediated injury have been indirect and limited to the use of free-radical scavengers. The efficacy of free-radical scavengers,[69, 74] iron chelators,[75] and neutrophil depletion[76] has been assessed by measuring myocardial infarct size. Limited numbers of studies have assessed ventricular function as a determinant of the success of pharmacologic intervention. Superoxide

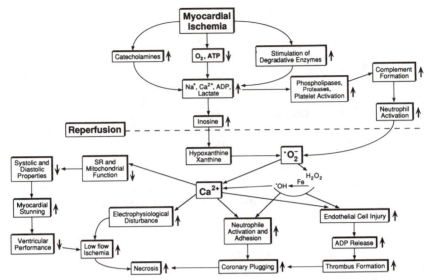

FIG 3.
Dramatic representation of the cascade events that takes place with the onset of ischemia. The sudden loss of oxygen supply due to interruption of the blood flow sends a signal of stress that leads to catecholamine release, increased contractility, and massive adenosine triphosphate *(ATP)* utilization. The loss of ATP triggers a cascade of degradative reactions of adenine nucleotides to nucleoside and disrupts ionic hemostasis across plasma membranes. The entry of extracellular calcium and inability to sequester cytosolic calcium results in the activation of calcium-dependent phospholipases, proteases, and platelets. The stimulation of phospholipid catabolism activates complements. The end product of ATP catabolism is inosine.

The introduction of oxygen during reperfusion allows the formation of free radicals via multiple mechanisms. Hydrogen peroxide and hydroxyl radicals, derived from superoxide radicals, may cause membrane phospholipid oxidation directly and stimulate calcium overflow. The lack of adequate high-energy stores, inflow of calcium, activation of platelets, and neutrophil adhesion may aggravate cellular damage upon reperfusion. Calcium overload and free radicals impair sarcoplasmic reticulum (SR) myofibril and mitochondrial function, resulting in contactile dysfunction and electrophysiologic disturbance. *ADP* = adenosine diphosphate.

dismutase, a natural enzyme that scavenges superoxide radicals to H_2O_2 has long been the strategy of choice in protecting the myocardium against reperfusion injury. Lack of agreement between different studies performed in various laboratories using superoxide dismutase has made it difficult to elucidate the role of free radicals in reperfusion injury.[73, 77-79] A short half-life and the lack of a simple transport mechanism of the native superoxide dismutase through membranes make it difficult to interpret study results, especially when infarct size is used as the sole determinant of the efficacy of myocardial protection. In contrast, Ambrosio et al.[29] have shown that superoxide dismutase decreased ATP depletion and improved functional recovery when administered during reperfusion using an isolated rabbit model. Conjugation between superoxide dismutase and the polyethylene glycol molecule increased the half-life of superoxide dismutase and improved its efficacy in vitro. Polyethylene glycol superoxide dismutase slightly reduced the infarct size[80, 81] and minimally improved ventricular function in vivo when administered 24 hours prior to surgery in pig[82] and isolated rabbit heart[83] models.

A variety of interventions have been introduced to protect the myocardium during ischemia and reperfusion (Table 1). Most of these agents, however, do not prevent reperfusion injury or dramatically reduce the

TABLE 1.
Pharmacologic Interventions for Myocardial Protection*

Additives	Adenosine Triphosphate Recovery	Functional Recovery	Reduced Infarct Size	Reference
Glucose, insulin	No	?	NR	84
Calcium antagonists	No	Yes	No	85
β-Blockers	No	Yes	?	86
Anesthetic agents	No	Yes	?	87
Membrane stabilizers	No	Yes	Yes	88
High-molecular-weight starch	No	Yes	?	89
Adenosine, adenosine deaminase inhibitors	?	Yes	NR	90
Adenine, ribose, hypoxanthine	No	Yes	NR	91
Glutamate aspartate	No	Yes	NR	92, 93
Xanthine oxidase inhibitors	No	?	?	94, 95
Free-radical scavengers, mannitol, SOD, CAT, PEG-SOD	No	?	?	74, 76, 77, 96

(Continued.)

TABLE 1 (cont.).
Pharmacologic Interventions for Myocardial Protection*

Additives	Adenosine Triphosphate Recovery	Functional Recovery	Reduced Infarct Size	Reference
Iron chelators	No	?	?	97
Inhibitors of arachidonic acid	No		?	98
Anti-inflammatory agents	No	?	?	99
Complement inactivators	No	?	?	100
University of Wisconsin solution	Six hours of myocardial preservation of rat hearts	Yes	NR	101, 102
AICAR	Partial recovery with 24 hours of continuous infusion	Yes	NR	103, 104
Calcium antagonists with nucleoside transport blocking actions	No	Yes	No	105, 106
Specific adenine nucleoside transport inhibitors	Full recovery within 30 minutes when drugs were infused before ischemia	Full recovery within 30 minutes when drugs were infused before or after ischemia	NR	37–40, 107

*NR = not reported; ? = controversial; SOD = superoxide dismutase; CAT = catalase; PEG-SOD = polyethylene glycol-SOD; AICAR = 5-amino-4-imidazole carboxamide riboside.

infarct size. Some of them provided modest protection and reduced myocardial infarct size. New pharmacologic strategies have been introduced and have attracted widespread attention. Therefore, a successful pharmacologic strategy for myocardial protection against oxygen free radical–mediated injury should fulfill the following requirements: (1) a simple chemical structure readily diffusible via plasma membranes, (2) an adequate half-life (90 to 180 minutes), (3) effectiveness at low concentrations, (4) an ability to prevent oxygen-derived free radical–mediated injury when the drug is administered before ischemia and/or during reperfusion, and (5) recovery of global or regional ventricular function assessed by highly sensitive indices of contractility.

Hypothermia and Hyperkalemia in Myocardial Protection

Interventions that prevent or slow biochemical changes induced by myocardial ischemia are effective means of myocardial protection. For example, preventing ATP depletion by using specific inhibitors of adenosine triphosphatases has been shown to protect against the progression of cellular injury due to ischemia.[108, 109] Unfortunately, most of these inhibitors are not reversible and may have other cardiovascular toxicity. Hypothermic arrest and myocardial cooling also prevent, or at least slow, ATP depletion during ischemia and improve functional recovery during reperfusion.[110–112] Melrose and his colleagues used potassium citrate to produce flaccid cardiac asystole.[113] Although it arrested the heart and provided a quiet operating field, potassium citrate proved to induce myocardial necrosis.[114,115] An increased potassium chloride concentration induces cardiac asystole by depolarizing the plasma membranes and dissociating actin and myosin. The concentration of potassium should be sufficient to produce rapid cardiac arrest following cross-clamping of the aorta, without damaging the myocardium or causing circulatory potassium overload. A high potassium concentration (> 20 milli equivalent) has been shown to be more injurious than a relatively lower concentration (<16 to 20 milli equivalent). Calcium concentration in the cardioplegic solution should be lowered to avoid calcium overload during cardiac arrest and reperfusion, but not totally omitted, to prevent calcium paradox during reperfusion. Magnesium is another potential constituent of cardioplegic solutions. Magnesium antagonizes calcium entry and protects the myocardium following ischemia. However, high concentrations of magnesium (16mM) have been reported to produce an atrioventricular nodal block. The potassium solution should be buffered to counteract the intramyocardial acidosis that is produced during myocardial ischemia. In addition, it is important to maintain normal, or slightly elevated, extracellular osmolality.

Several adjuvants have been added to potassium cardioplegic solutions. It has been thought that the presence of glucose, with or without insulin, in a cardioplegic solution enhances anaerobic metabolism during cardioplegic cardiac arrest. Theoretically, the benefits of glucose under hypothermic conditions (4° C to 18° C) are questionable, due to changes in the membrane permeability and limited diffusibility of any solute as a result of the phase transition of membrane phospholipids. Some surgeons do not employ potassium cardioplegic solution to arrest the heart. Basically, deep hypothermic cardiac arrest is used as a routine procedure for myocardial protection during surgery. The mortality rate is slightly higher using only hypothermia compared with adding potassium cardioplegia. Some surgeons employ intermittent aortic cross-clamping and reperfusion every 20 minutes during CABG. Others briefly occlude the coronary artery while performing anastomosis of the graft distal to the obstruction, without making any attempt to arrest the heart. These groups report excellent recovery and short surgical procedures.

The induction of a warm potassium cardioplegic solution enriched with dicarboxylic amino acids has been used in experimental and clinical settings of cardiac surgery during ischemic arrest and/or reperfusion.[92, 116–120] Buckberg and his colleagues report excellent results in patients and experimental models with warm cardioplegia enriched with glutamate and aspartate.[92, 120] Although their results are very convincing, only recently have a few surgeons followed this procedure and obtained an excellent outcome. The rational for using glutamate and aspartate has been based on triggering the Krebs cycle and producing reducing equivalents (reduced nicotinamide adenine dinucleotide and reduced flavin adenine dinucleotides) that enhance the respiratory chain-oxidative phosphorylation coupling, thereby enhancing ATP production. A prolonged normothermic ischemic period (45 to 60 minutes significantly depletes adenine nucleotides (ATP, ADP, and AMP and accumulates inosine, hypoxanthine, and xanthine. During reperfusion with glutamate-containing cardioplegia, precursors for adenine nucleotides usually have been washed from the myocardium within the first minute. Even if it is conceivable that reducing equivalents are elevated in glutamate-treated hearts, the lack of ADP and AMP should be limiting for ATP synthesis.

Despite numerous efforts, the perfect cardioplegic solution has not been designed. Cardioplegic solution recipes vary from one institution to another. The rationale and biochemical mechanisms of action of the main components of cardioplegic solutions should be defined clearly. The ideal solution theoretically should have excellent buffering capacity, be slightly hypertonic, and contain an arresting agent, a membrane-stabilizing agent, nutritious substrates, and agents that antagonize calcium overload and modify free radical–mediated injury. New strategies of myocardial protection also should focus on preventing reperfusion-mediated injury in addition to the protection afforded during cardioplegic arrest. Several investigators have added glucose and insulin,[84] calcium channel blockers,[85] mannitol,[96] free-radical scavengers,[74, 76, 77] iron chelators,[97] β-receptor antagonists,[86] and other agents as adjuvants to the basic potassium cardioplegic solutions (see Table 1). However, few of these "cardioprotective" agents have been introduced into the heart during reperfusion and proven to be effective and suitable for clinical application.

Route of Administration of Cardioplegic Solutions

Surgeons have debated whether continuous administration of cold cardioplegic solution is more efficacious than intermittent administration. The notion has been that continuous infusion washes out harmful metabolites.

Our experimental data demonstrated that cold cardioplegia causes a change in the phase transition of membrane phospholipids in such a way that they become rigid and possibly impermeable to diffusible metabolites.[121] Membrane permeability is regained with rewarming and reperfusion. In the clinical setting, myocardial temperature tends to rise to 10 to 15° C between each bolus of intermittent cardioplegia. A slight elevation of myocardial temperature increases the rate of metabolic drainage during cardiac surgery. Myocardial protection afforded by hypothermic cardioplegia is known to vary when administered antegrade into the aortic root distal to the cross-clamp or retrograde into the coronary sinus.[122] Therefore, retrograde coronary sinus reperfusion provides better cooling and rapid cardioplegic arrest in cases of coronary artery stenosis.[122, 123] Both routes provide excellent myocardial preservation in normal hearts.[124, 125] However, in cases of coronary artery stenosis, antegrade cardioplegia may not be adequate for myocardial protection distal to coronary artery obstruction. Recently, both techniques were used simultaneously. Shumway[126] and Menasche[127] have demonstrated that retrograde cardioplegia is a suitable technique for myocardial protection during aortic valve replacement.

The basic aim of cardioplegic solutions has been to depolarize the membrane, prevent the interaction of actin and myosin, and stop electrical activity and metabolic demand. When hypothermia is applied with potassium cardioplegia, it is believed that metabolic activities not affected by the extracellular rise in potassium concentration are slowed further. Several investigators have demonstrated that hypothermia alone may be adequate for myocardial protection. Other researchers and surgeons have obtained better results by combining chemically induced arrest of the myocardium with systemic and/or myocardial cooling. Despite well-recognized age-related differences, procedures of myocardial protection used in adult cardiac surgery have been applied also to pediatric cardiac surgery. Recent work from our laboratory demonstrated that profound rapid cooling produced necrosis and cell death in rabbit hearts.[128] In addition, we have demonstrated that hypothermic St. Thomas solution, when combined with systemic circulatory arrest, caused metabolic derangement and increased morbidity and mortality in newborn and infant patients.[129] Myocardial injury with St. Thomas solution was found to be related inversely to patient age. Similar injurious effects of St. Thomas solution in neonatal rabbit hearts have been reported.[130] Hypothermia alone was more effective in improving ventricular developed pressure than was hypothermic cardioplegia with St. Thomas solution in neontal rabbit hearts. These observations recently were supported by Hearse's group.[131] The mechanism(s) by which rapid cooling and/or St. Thomas solution exert myocardial damage remains to be elucidated. However, age-related differences have been demonstrated with respect to adenine nucleotide pool metabolism.[132–136] It is believed that immature myocardium is different from adult myocardium with respect to membranous glycocalyx, phospholipid composition, and Ca^{2+} regulation. Therefore, efforts should be directed toward the development of a special cardioplegic strategy for pediatric cardiac surgery.

This issue is especially crucial in myocardial preservation for pediatric heart transplantation.

It has been demonstrated that continuous retrograde cardioplegia is effective during surgery on ischemically injured hearts. Although successful myocardial protection during ischemia is essential, it may not prevent postischemic reperfusion injury.[137] The new strategy of myocardial protection, therefore, should take into account reperfusion injury as well as ischemic injury as determinants for overall postoperative ventricular functional recovery.

Mechanisms of Cellular Repair Following Myocardial Ischemic and Reperfusion Injury

Preventing ischemic and reperfusion injury and augmenting cardiac repair is the goal of cardiologists and cardiac surgeons. The process of myocardial repair involves the initiation of protein, phospholipid, and carbohydrate synthesis for healing in injured sarcolemmic membranes and contractile apparatuses. These myocardial reparative mechanisms require an adequate supply of high-energy phosphates (ATP) and essential building substrates. The signal(s) for genetic expression for compensatory mechanisms of repair represents a challenge for basic scientist. It would be logical to activate the repair mechanisms before allowing the heart to work and utilize energy for cardiac contraction-relaxation coupling during reperfusion. Rewarming the myocardium and supplying it with oxygen and essential precursors while the heart remains arrested may augment myocardial salvage. Accelerated myocardial metabolic recovery has been demonstrated with terminal warm blood cardioplegia.[138, 139] Clinical application of this procedure is promising. Preventing postischemic reperfusion injury is important in order to shorten the period of myocardial recovery during reperfusion. Oxygenation is believed to be responsible for oxygen-derived free radical–mediated reperfusion injury, and several studies have shown that lowering oxygen tension during reperfusion improves function and mediates recovery.

The metabolic and functional role of myocardial purine nucleotides is well recognized. Several enzymes are regulated by adenine nucleotides that are either inhibited or activated by normal ATP. These enzymes are normally involved in the synthetic pathway of ATP precursors. On the other hand, ATP depletion stimulates the salvage synthetic pathway of adenine nucleotides whenever intramyocardial precursors are entrapped. ATP is involved indirectly in the activation of protein kinases and is regulated by cyclic AMP–dependent protein phosphorylation. These mechanisms regulate calcium sequestration by the sarcoplasmic reticulum in the heart,[140] thereby affecting diastolic properties of the ventricle. ATP also is essential for the genetic expression and production of RNA and DNA, thus regulating protein synthesis and compensatory mechanisms for myocardial salvage. Adult cardiomyocytes continue to synthesize RNAs, while there is no evidence for DNA replication. Immature cells are able to produce both DNA and RNA. It is anticipated that in a severely ATP-depleted myocardium, protein synthesis for compensatory hypertrophy in noninfarcted myocardium also is compromised following acute mycoardial infarction.

Subcellular compartmentalization of adenine nucleotides is known to be important in cell regulation. ATP is produced mainly in the mitochondria when the respiratory chain is coupled to oxidative phosphorylation. However, ADP also could be phosphorylated in the presence of phosphocreatine and creatine kinase. The cytosolic level of myocardial ATP could reach 5mM in cardiomyocytes, and may be twice as much in endothelial cells. ATP levels in the smooth muscle cells may fall between those of the myocytes and the endothelial cells. Within the myocyte, ATP is distributed subcelluarly in the cytoplasm, mitochondrial sarcoplasmic reticulum, and nucleus. ATP and ADP also bind the myofibrillar proteins. Isolated cardiomyocyte preparations represent an excellent experimental model with which to investigate mechanism(s) of injury and protection in a system devoid of endothelial, smooth muscle, hormonal, or neural regulation. During myocardial ischemia, ATP is depleted rapidly in cardiomyocytes as well as in endothelial cells. Any intervention to modify ATP metabolism should consider cellular compartmentalization, i.e., myocytes vs. endothelial cells, metabolic flux of diffusible nucleosides, and purine bases. These metabolites have been implicated in reperfusion-mediated injury.[38-40]

ATP depletion in cardiomyocyte preparations normally leads to the release of adenosine and inosine. In vivo, adenosine is deanimated. Inosine has been shown to be the end product of ATP catabolism in isolated cardiomyocyte preparations.[141-142] Detection of uric acid in the coronary sinus or coronary flow with postischemic reperfusion is strong evidence for the presence of xanthine oxidase in the myocardium. These findings support the notion that adenosine and inosine are produced in the cytosol of cardiomyocytes in the absence of an interstitial space compartment or endothelial cell involvement. The success of pharmacologic intervention requires that any metabolic inhibitor reach the myocyte via the endothelial cell bed and interstitial space. In the intact heart, it is difficult to separate cellular and subcellular compartmentalization of adenine nucleotides, nucleosides, and purine bases. It is interesting to note that ATP depletion in isolated cardiomyocytes does not release hypoxanthine, xanthine, or uric acid,[141, 142] suggesting that cardiomyocytes are deficient of xanthine oxidase. Endothelial cells are known to have an active xanthine oxidase, especially in small coronaries and capillaries.[143, 144] These findings proved to be true in human, pig, and rabbit species, once thought to be deficient in xanthine oxidase.

In the last few decades, investigators have been interested in establishing the correlation between myocardial adenine nucleotides and ventricular function. Unfortunately, most studies reported only levels of ATP, ADP, and AMP. Previous work from our laboratory emphasized the importance of measuring all adenine nucleotide pool intermediates during ischemia-induced ATP depletion and assessing the activity of the salvage pathway during reperfusion.[136] Therefore, it is essential to characterize the key enzymes involved in either the degradative or the synthetic pathway of the ATP pool during ischemia and reperfusion. Several methods are used to assay for other enzyme activities, including spectrophotometric, fluorometric, radiometric, and histochemical localization. High-performance liquid chromatography analysis is superior over other methods in providing an accurate measurement of the levels of substrate, products, inhibitors, and possible other products produced by other enzymes copurified with the enzymes of concern.[136] The infusion of hypoxanthine to enhance myocardial ATP is limited by its ability to pass via endothelial and smooth muscle cells and interstitial spaces in intact form and be taken up by myocytes to be incorporated into the ATP salvage pathway. There is no experimental evidence demonstrating the presence of a transport system for hypoxanthine.

De Novo Synthesis Pathway of Adenine Nucleotides

ATP synthesis via the de novo pathway is energy-dependent. Four molecules of ATP are consumed to produce a single purine ring. The rate of ATP synthesis via the de novo pathway is slower than that of the salvage pathway to match metabolic demand for myocardial adenine nucleotide replenishment following an ischemic insult. 5-Amino imidazole-4-carboxamide riboside (AICAR) is an intermediate for the de novo synthesis pathway for inosine monophosphate (IMP) (Fig 4). Two more reactions are needed to produce AMP: (1) the formation of S-adenosylsuccinate, and (2) desuccinylation by adenosylsuccinase. The continuous perfusion of AICAR for 24 hours augments ATP recovery following brief acute ischemia.[103] AICAR is phosphorylated rapidly in the heart, utilizing one molecule of ATP, to the corresponding nucleotide (AICAR-P). The infusion of AICAR results in an increase in the level of myocardial IMP. The latter is catabolized rapidly into hypoxanthine and xanthine, and a small amount of it is incorporated into the ATP pool. Several reports have demonstrated the efficacy of AICAR in reperfusion-mediated injury.[116, 117] It is most likely that AICAR is involved in other activities in addition to enhancing the de novo synthesis pathway of nucleotides. Recent studies have shown the beneficial effects of AICAR in myocardial stunning by augmentation of the production of adenosine.[145, 146] It is known that the half-life of adenosine in vivo is very short (6 to 8 seconds) due to the presence of a large quantity of adenosine deaminase. Without an adenosine deaminase inhibitor, the adenosine generated from AICAR may not last very long. Other mechanisms may be involved in AICAR's cardioprotective action, which deserves further investigation.

Modulation of Enzyme Kinetics and Nucleoside Transport

Although ATP is a prerequisite for cardiac function, it is a major source of free-radical substrates. Therefore, metabolic interventions capable of mini-

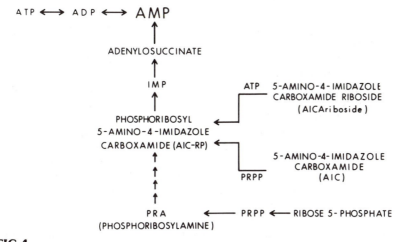

FIG 4.
Enhancement of the de novo pathway of adenosine triphosphate *(ATP)* synthesis by 5-amino imidazole-4-carboxamide riboside. The phosphorylation of this riboside consumes ATP. Riboside, phosphate, and pyrophosphate are incorporated to produce 5-amino imidazole-4-carboxamide riboside phosphate. The native pathways are relatively slower than the salvage pathways. *ADP* = adenosine diphosphate; *AMP* = adenosine monophosphate; *PRPP* = phosphoribosylpyrophosphate.

mizing ATP catabolism eventually would help in preventing metabolic energy drainage, increased acidosis, overflow of calcium, and free radical–mediated reperfusion injury. Strategies of myocardial protection using hypothermic hyperkalemic arrest remarkably reduce ATP catabolism during elective cardiac surgery, but do not totally prevent ATP depletion. Since cardiac muscle contains more ATP than it may need, our efforts should be directed toward preventing the degradation of ADP, AMP, and salvageable nucleoside (adenosine) and modulating their release from the myocardium into the vasculature bed. There are several possible means of metabolic intervention to augment ATP recovery and/or prevent reperfusion injury mediated by ATP catabolites: (1) inhibition of ATP utilization and catabolism and adenine nucleotides, (2) reversible inactivation of the degradative enzymes and stimulation of the enzymes involved in the salvage and de novo pathways of adenine nucleosides, (3) stimulation of salvage and de novo pathways by supplementation of the rate-limiting substrates needed for ATP synthesis, and (4) modulation of nucleoside and nucleotide transport to augment the recovery of high energy stores and prevent ATP catabolite–mediated reperfusion injury.

During the early phase of myocardial protection, the inhibition of ATP utilization immediately prior to myocardial planned global ischemia, either by specific inhibitors or by slowing down the rate of degradative metabolism with hypothermic potassium cardioplegic arrest, provides the ideal approach to the preservation of high-energy phosphate stores and manages the reperfusion injury mediated by ATP catabolites. In experimental settings, the infusion of mitochondrial adenosine triphosphatase inhibitors such as oligomycin has been shown to reduce the rate of myocardial ATP depletion significantly following ischemia in the isolated rat heart model. Metabolic intervention utilizing oligomycin and other mitochondrial adenosine triphosphatase inhibitors is not appropriate for clinical application due to irreversible inhibition and acute toxicity. Transport through the plasma membrane, mitochondrial uptake, and possible side effects are factors that may limit the use of well-known mitochondrial adenosine triphosphatase inhibitors before or during ischemic arrest. On the other hand, in clinical situations, ischemic insult usually occurs prior to any possible intervention for myocardial preservation during surgical or medical procedures. During the second phase of myocardial protection, myocardial ATP is depleted rapidly during ischemia, accompanied by the build-up of ADP and AMP.

AMP is the most important precursor of ATP production and is produced mainly via the de novo or salvage synthetic pathways during or following stress. The phosphorylation of intracellular AMP to ADP by adenylate kinase or myokinase and transport of ADP into the mitochondrial matrix via regulation by ADP/ATP translocase are essential and rate-limiting steps in ATP replenishment with reperfusion following reversible ischemia (Fig 5). The loss of ATP and accumulation of intracellular AMP during myocardial ischemia trigger kinetic enhancement of 5'-nucleotidase. This enzyme catalyzes the dephosphorylation of AMP, producing adenosine. Since adenine nucleotides (ATP, ADP, and AMP) are less permeable to the plasma membrane, while adenine nucleosides (adenosine and inosine) and purine bases (hypoxanthine and xanthine) are readily diffusible, the inhibition of 5'-nucleotidase during ischemia had been an attractive biochemical intervention to prevent or at least minimize AMP degradation and elevate intracellular AMP levels. We introduced, for the first time, the use of bromo-AMP as a novel inhibitor of 5'-nucleotidase activity to prevent AMP catabolism during normothermic global ischemia in an isolated rat heart model.[147] Significant myocardial functional and ATP recovery were demonstrated with pretreatment with bromo-AMP. Bromo-AMP has been shown to be effective when added as an adjuvant to cardioplegic solution.[148] Different isoenzymes of 5'-nucleotidase have been detected and partially characterized in the liver[149] and cardiac muscle. The enzyme activity has been determined in various subcellular fractions (plasma membrane, sarcoplasmic reticulum, Golgi membranes, mitochondria, and the cytosolic soluble fraction). The roles of cytosolic and membrane-bound isoenzymes of 5'-nucleotidase in AMP depletion and adenosine production during normoxia, hypoxia, and ischemia are not clearly characterized.[148, 150, 151] Several studies have demonstrated that both isoenzymes are kinetically distinct. While the soluble 5'-nucleotidase is stimulated by ATP and ADP, the membrane-bound enzyme is regulated by both nucleotides.[152] In addition, substrate specificity studies have shown that the Michaelis-Menten constant (K_m) value of cytosolic 5'-nucleotidase for IMP

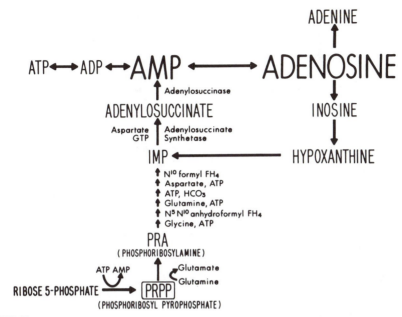

FIG 5.
The incorporation of glutamate into the de novo pathway of adenine nucleotide is depicted. The rate-limiting reaction in this pathway is the incorporation of glutamine into phosphoribosylpyrophosphate *(PRPP)*. Several other steps are involved to promote the production of inosine monophosphate *(IMP)*. It seems possible to enhance the salvage pathway rather than the de novo pathway. *ATP* = adenosine triphosphate; *ADP* = adenosine diphosphate; *AMP* = *adenosine monophosphate; GTP* = guanosine triphosphate. (From Pasque MK, Spray TL, Pellon GL, et al: *J Thorac Cardiovasc Surg* 1982; 83:390. Used by permission.)

is significantly lower than that for AMP (more specific), while the membrane-bound enzyme favors AMP over IMP.

Several analogues of adenine nucleotides have been introduced as specific potent inhibitors of 5'-nucleotides. α, β-Methylene-5'-adenosine diphosphate (α, β-MeADP) is the most widely used inhibitor for 5'-nucleotidase activity during myocardial hypoxia and ischemia. Theoretically, the inhibition of 5'-nucleotidase during ischemic arrest should enhance intracellular AMP, which can be phosphorylated readily to ADP. It has been demonstrated that the infusion of inhibitors of 5'-nucleotidase (i.e., α, β-MeADP or Conconavlin A [ConA]) alone does not increase myocardial AMP levels significantly.[153] Similar results were obtained in our laboratory, where α, β-MeADP was infused into the cardiopulmonary bypass reservoir prior to global normothermic ischemia and reperfusion.[153] However, when adenine or adenosine supplementation was used in combination with α, β-MeADP or ConA, reduced ATP depletion and improved metabolic recovery, in terms of myocardial ATP level, were noted during reperfusion in dogs.[154] Work from our laboratory demonstrated that α, β-MeADP strongly inhibited 5'-nucleotidase activity in isolated microsomal and cytosolic fractions. Results from these studies indicate that ConA inhibits 5'-nucleotidase activity in vitro and in vivo, but does not inhibit the enzyme in isolated rat cardiac myocytes separated by collagenase/hyaluronidase treatment.[134] These results suggest that ConA does not interact directly with the catalytic site of 5'-nucleotidase, but rather that it binds to the glycocalyx, which leads to masking of the catalytic binding site of AMP on the enzyme.

Substrate Enhancement for Myocardial Salvage

It is possible that kinetic modulation of the degradation enzymes of adenine nucleotides and their important precursors using hypothermic potassium arrest and specific inhibitors may not be adequate for myocardial protection of severely injured hearts. The provision of essential precursors bypassing the rate-limiting enzymes or steps has attracted widespread attention recently in attempts to augment cardiac repair mechanisms following ischemia/reperfusion.

Carbohydrates

During anaerobiosis induced by ischemia or hypoxia, the only source of ATP is anaerobic glycolysis. The idea of substrate enhancement of glycogen and glucose during ischemia and hypoxia was introduced in the 1960s. Improved functional and metabolic recovery of isolated hearts infused with glucose and insulin was reported.[155] Myocardial protection using glycogen/glucose, glucose and insulin, and fructose-1,6-diphosphate invariably yielded mixed results. These interventions have little, if any, effect on AMP synthesis via either de novo or salvage pathways. Increasing the availability of glycogen or glucose prior to hypoxia increases myocardial tolerance to hypoxia during sustained perfusion.[156] These results may be different in myocardial ischemia. A few reports have concluded that the administration of glucose and insulin may cause myocardial damage.[157] Moreover, the phosphorylation of one molecule of glucose requires two ATP molecules, while anaerobic glycolysis produces only two ATP molecules. The infusion of fructose-1,6-diphosphate during ischemia may enhance the turnover of ATP. A lack of direct metabolic effects of fructose-1,6-diphosphate on ischemic myocardium has been demonstrated in relation to the replenishment of adenine nucleotides.

Krebs Cycle Intermediate Precursors

In well-oxygenated, perfused hearts, about 95% of the ATP produced is synthesized in the mitochondria. Reducing equivalents in the form of reduced nicotinamide-adenine dinucleotide and reduced flavin adenine dinucleotide$_2$ are produced in each cycle, driving the electron transport chain, which then is coupled tightly to oxidative phosphorylation, where three or two molecules of ATP are produced, respectively. The availability of an adequate supply of ADP is a prerequisite for ATP synthesis, even if the rate of the Krebs cycle has been stimulated by substrate enhancement.

Interesting results from Buckberg's group[92, 117, 118, 120] have demonstrated excellent myocardial functional recovery following severe ischemia with glutamate cardioplegia before and after ischemia and prior to reperfusion. In a recent report, complete reversal of severe ischemic injury (45 minutes at 37° C) occurred when glutamate and aspartate were included in normothermic postischemic cardioplegia for 5 minutes. This "hot shot" following cold ischemic arrest resulted in complete functional and metabolic (i.e., O_2 consumption) recovery.[92, 120] The authors suggested that the infusion of glutamate and aspartate cardioplegia for 5 minutes enhanced the level of Krebs cycle intermediates α_1-ketoglutarate and oxaloacetate, respectively, thus increasing O_2 consumption and ATP production by the Krebs cycle. In these particular studies, adenine nucleotide measurements were not made. Studies from our laboratory have demonstrated that glutamate did not provide either metabolic or functional advantages in the isolated rat heart model, with or without potassium cardioplegia infused after ischemic insult.[158]

Since mitochondrial O_2 consumption is coupled very tightly with the oxidative phosphorylation of ADP, the ADP/O ratio represents an important determinant for both O_2 consumption and ATP synthesis. It is reasonable to speculate that substrate enhancement of the Krebs cycle will increase reduced nicotinamide-adenine dinucleotide and reduced flavin adenine dinucleotide$_2$. However, the massive depletion of adenine nucleotides associated with 45 minutes of warm ischemia results in a very low level of ADP available for oxidative phosphorylation. In this respect, alternative mechanism(s) should be investigated to explain the observed functional and metabolic recovery following glutamate provision. In the salvage pathway of the adenine nucleotide pool, both aspartate and guanosine triphosphate are required for the formation of adenosylsuccinate catalyzed by adenylosuccinate synthase from IMP. Desuccinylation of adenylosuccinate catalyzed by adenosuccinase results in the production of AMP (see Figs 2 and 6). Since glutamate and aspartate are the only amino acids that mediate postischemic recovery, the mechanism of myocardial recovery may involve the enhancement of AMP production via the salvage synthetic pathway and, to a lesser extent, the de novo pathway. Employing radioactive tracers of glutamate and aspartate, one may provide more basic biochemical information on the mechanism of action of these dicarboxylic acids in overall adenine nucleotide metabolism. Another approach to elucidate the mechanism of action of glutamate and aspartate is to follow their transport and subcellular compartmentalization during ischemia and reperfusion. A dicarboxylic acid transporter has been identified. The role of this dicarboxylic acid carrier protein in glutamate and aspartate myocardial recovery needs further investigation, perhaps employing potent inhibitors of dicar-

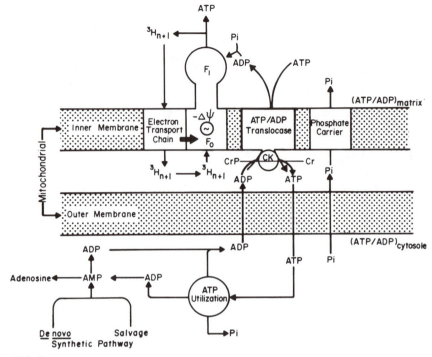

FIG 6.
The graph emphasizes the importance of adenosine triphosphate *(ATP)* precursor availability and active mitochondrial ATP adenosine diphosphate *(ADP)* translocase in the phosphorylation of ADP to ATP by inner mitochondrial adenosine triphosphatase complex (F_1/F_0). The stimulation of ATP/ADP translocase is believed to enhance ATP replenishment if ATP precursors are entrapped inside the cardiomyocyte. Mitochondrial coupling factor one is the catalytic site for ATP hydrolase in mitochondrial ATPase. Oligomycin-sensitivity conferring protein (OSCP) and mitochondrial coupling factor zero *(F₀)* are essential for conferring oligomycin-sensitivity and ATP synthase activity of mitochondrial ATPase *(F₁/F₀)* complex. The proton electron motive force $(^3H_{n+1} \rightarrow -\Delta)$ derives the required energy through ATPase complex for ADP phosphylation. ATP=adenosine-5'-triphosphate, *ADP*=adenosine-5'-diphosphate, *AMP*=adenosine-5'-monophosphate; *Cr*=creatine; *CrP*=creatine phosphate; *CK*=creatine kinase; Pi=inorganic phosphate.

boxylic acid transport. Utilizing these inhibitors, one may be able to determine the mechanisms of the cardioprotective effects of glutamate during cardiac surgery.

Replenishment of Myocardial Adenosine Triphosphate by Metabolic Intervention

High-energy phosphates have been administered prior to or following ischemia in attempts to improve the metabolic and functional status of the heart and shorten the period of recovery. Myocardial protective effects have been reported following reperfusion with ATP, ADP, or AMP. Chaudry and his associates have demonstrated significant improvement in cardiac output following myocardial ischemia when ATP-magnesium chloride (ATP-MgCl$_2$) was infused into both experimental animal models[159] and patients.[160] Robinson et al.[161] have reported the beneficial effects of creatine phosphate added to cardioplegic solutions in dogs. Due to permeability restrictions, adenine nucleotides are not easily diffusible through plasma membranes compared to adenine nucleosides and purine bases. Depolarization of cell membranes with moderately high concentrations of potassium (10mM to 26mM) may alter their permeability to high-energy phosphates and cause endothelial cell damage.[162] Mechanisms of myocardial protection with ATP-MgCl$_2$ deserve further investigation.

The repletion of AMP by substrate enhancement of salvageable precursors has been of great interest. Myocardial recovery following ischemia may be increased by replacing essential intermediates washed out upon reperfusion. Several investigators have administered adenine nucleoside before ischemia and during reperfusion. Recently, increased numbers of reports demonstrate the cardioprotective actions of exogenous adenosine in several models of ischemic syndromes.[163–165] It has been reported that the administration of adenosine to ischemically injured myocardium results in slightly improved myocardial energy stores (AMP and ATP) and functional recovery.[166] The mechanisms by which adenosine provides cardioprotective action are not well elucidated. Adenosine can be either phosphorylated directly to AMP or cleaved to adenine, then ribopyrophosphorylated to AMP (see Fig 2). Inhibiting adenosine deaminase (by EHNA or deoxycoformycin) and blocking adenosine transport by NBMPR redirects the salvage pathway toward adenosine conversion to AMP.[37–40] These data support the importance of AMP repletion in adenine nucleotide replenishment. Possible limitations of adenosine therapy following ischemia are related to its vasodilation and function as a potential source of the free-radical substrates hypoxanthine and xanthine and as a potent renal vasoconstrictor.[167] Adenine, the adenosine catabolite, also has been shown to cause renal dysfunction.[168]

To avoid adenosine vasoactivity, inosine has been used in experimental animal models during myocardial ischemia in an attempt to enhance the rate of the salvage pathway for high-energy phosphate repletion.[169–171] The hypothesis was that providing inosine might allow the formation of salvageable hypoxanthine. Improved myocardial function and the repletion of adenine nucleotide have been demonstrated following the infusion of inosine to ischemic myocardium.[171] The conversion of inosine to hypoxanthine is necessary for its use in the salvage pathway inside the myocyte. The stimulation of nucleoside phosphorylase and inhibition of xanthine oxidase could be desirable biochemical maneuvers to make the salvage pathway more efficient (see Fig 2). Several reports have demonstrated, by unknown mechanisms, that the infusion of inosine enhances myocardial contractility in normal and injured hearts. The inotropic effect of inosine does not appear to be mediated by adrenergic stimulation. Administration of adenine as an intermediate of the salvage pathway also has been demonstrated to improve myocardial function and the total adenine nucleotide pool in ischemic myocardium in the presence of ribose,[172] adenine and a specific inhibitor of 5'-nucleotidase (α,β-methylene-ADP)[154]. Adenine administration, however, has been limited, possibly because of its known nephrotoxicity.[168]

The de novo synthetic pathway of AMP is based on the incorporation of simple amino acids (glycine, etc.) and phosphoribosylpyrophosphate (PRPP) to produce IMP, which in turn is converted to AMP, as shown in Figure 6. The availability of PRPP is a rate-limiting step of the de novo pathway for AMP synthesis. Several studies have focused on increasing the rate of the de novo pathway by elevating myocardial PRPP or administering precursors that enter the pathway at a step distal to rate-limiting synthetic steps for PRPP. Metabolic manipulations that enhance PRPP availability in the myocardium predicted augmentation AMP synthesis.[173, 174] The administration of ribose results in its immediate transport into the cell, where it is phosphorylated to ribose-5-phosphate, an essential precursor of PRPP. Several experiments have demonstrated the enhancement of PRPP and an increased rate of adenine nucleotide synthesis following ribose administration to ischemic and hypoxic myocardium. Zimmer and his associates have shown that ribose administration to rats treated with isoproterenol resulted in the recovery of myocardial ATP and prevented cardiac cell necrosis.[175] Myocardial functional and ATP recovery have been reported in ribose-treated rats following 15 minutes of warm ischemia.[176] Since the rate of the de novo pathway is slower than that of the salvage pathway, it is suggested that the primary involvement of ribose is in the salvage pathway of adenine nucleotide synthesis.

Enhancing the rate of the de novo pathway distal to the rate-limiting precursor (PRPP) can be achieved by AICAR. This precursor is taken up readily by the cell and phosphorylated by ATP to form phosphoribosyl-5-amino-4-imidazole carboxamide ribonucleotide (AICRP), which enters the de novo pathway of adenine nucleotide synthesis. The infusion of AICA-riboside for 24 hours following 12 minutes of coronary artery occlusion in dogs significantly improved ATP and guanosine triphosphate recovery of the injured myocardium.[103, 104] This again emphasizes that the de novo pathway is slow, and that prolonged infusion of AICA-riboside may be required.

The manipulation of hormonal regulation for kinetic enhancement of enzymes involved in the adenine nucleotide pool has not been investigated in relation to myocardial preservation, protection, and postischemic recovery. The regulation of enzyme activities and the role of membrane properties in the control of metabolic flux can be of great importance for myocardial protection. The activity of important enzymes can be modulated by (1) enhancing substrates or their precursors; (2) increasing their uptake and diffusion; (3) simulators, inhibitors, or specific covalent modifiers, such as phosphorylation/dephosphorylation, methylation/demethylation; and (4) hormonal stimulation of enzyme synthesis or prevention of its down-regulation and internalization.

One of the most important biochemical aspects is regulation of the transport of substrates, precursors, and modulators through membranes. This process often has been ignored in studies reported in relation to biochemical interventions when hearts are infused with these solutions. Membrane properties are modulated by low temperature and depolarization with potassium cardioplegia.

Role of Mitochondria in Adenosine Triphosphate Replenishment

The oxidative phosphorylation of ADP is very much restricted by its availability in the mitochondrial matrix. The transport of ADP from the cytoplasm through the outer mitochondrial membrane is not well defined. However, ADP transport is regulated by ATP/ADP translocase localized in the inner mitochondrial membrane.[177] This carrier protein transports ADP into the mitochondria in exchange for ATP (see Fig 6). Factors that reduce the rate of ADP transport via adenine nucleotide translocase may include (1) a low level of cytoplasmic ADP, (2) the inhibition of translocase activity, and (3) the inhibition of oxidative phosphorylation. The machinery of production for high-energy phosphates in the mitochondrion is intact following reversible myocardial ischemia, as demonstrated by the recovery of phosphocreatine during postischemic reperfusion. Nevertheless, prolonged delay in ATP repletion is observed with reperfusion, and this has been related to the unavailability of washed-out salvageable precursors. Biochemical manipulations that enhance de novo and salvage synthesis of AMP enhance the availability of ADP in the cytoplasm. It has been suggested that the phosphorylation potential of ATP/ (ADP × pi) regulates adenine nucleotide translocase activity.[177] The role of adenine nucleotide translocase in the postischemic recovery of myocardial ATP is of great interest and deserves investigation. Kinetic enhancement of this carrier protein activity increases the turnover of ATP and, subsequently, myocardial metabolic recovery. Investigations with biochemical interventions that cause favorable allosteric stimulation of adenine nucleotide translocase activity are needed. It would be of interest to assess the role of ATP/ADP translocase in normoxic hearts perfused with specific inhibitors of mitochondrial/ADP transporter activity in relation to adenine nucleotide metabolism and myocardial function and metabolism. Triiodothyronine has been shown to have an inotropic effect and to enhance ATP/ADP translocase ATP synthesis and utilization.

Since the phosphorylation of adenosine is catalyzed by adenosine kinase, to AMP, the hypothesis that adenosine level can be raised by either blocking its degradation to inosine or enhancing its substrate is an attractive approach to increasing the rate of metabolic recovery during ischemia and reperfusion. Adenosine deaminase catalyzes the deamination of adenosine to inosine. The enzyme is localized in the cytoplasm, interstitial space, and endothelial and smooth muscle cells in the coronary vessels.[178] Several specific inhibitors of adenosine deaminase have been used in experimental animal models. The infusion of EHNA, coformyocin, and deoxycoformyocin during myocardial ischemia and hypoxia reduced the rate of ATP depletion, especially when adenine or adenosine was infused simultaneously. The administration of an adenosine deaminase inhibitor and provision of adenosine to the myocardium during ischemia and reperfusion increased the probability of adenosine uptake by myocardial and endothelial cells and enhanced its phosphorylation to AMP.

Adenosine Triphosphate Contribution to Ventricular Dysfunction Mediated by Free Radicals During Reperfusion

Although ATP is the critical energy source required for ventricular function and myocardial metabolism, it is also a major source of free-radical substrate precursors.[40] About 90% to 95% of the ATP depleted during normothermic ischemia is retained inside the cardiomyocyte as inosine. Upon reperfusion, inosine is converted rapidly to hypoxanthine, xanthine, and uric acid. These are substrates that favor oxygen free radical formation under appropriate enzymatic conditions, with a single passage via the interstitial space and smooth muscle and endothelial cell layers. This was demonstrated by collecting the coronary sinus effluent during the first minutes of reperfusion during CABG surgery.[179] Similar data are available in rabbits, pigs, and dogs.[180] Since four superoxide radicals are produced for each ATP catabolized, a burst of free radicals is formed with the resumption of blood flow. These free radicals cause random damage in endothelial cell membranes, allowing calcium entry, cell swelling, and the infiltration of neutrophils.

We developed a strategy to modulate adenosine and inosine metabolism and transport in such a way as to limit the formation of free-radical substrates during reperfusion.[37–40] A combination of EHNA (adenosine deaminase inhibitor) and NBMPR (a specific nucleoside transport blocker) was used both to prevent adenosine deamination to inosine and to block adenosine and inosine release upon reperfusion. Reperfusion injury mediated by ATP catabolism was prevented with EHNA and NBMPR following 30[37] and 60 minutes[40] of normothermic global ischemia in vivo. Since adenosine has been shown to have cardioprotective actions, it has been thought that the entrapment of intramyocardial adenosine with EHNA and NBMPR was responsible for excellent ventricular functional recovery and the replenishment of ATP. To test this hypothesis, we administered EHNA and NBMPR only during reperfusion and not during ischemia. Results from these experiments demonstrated that functional recovery was associated with the entrapment of intramyocardial nucleosides, mainly inosine, while ATP was not recovered.[38] These data demonstrated that the entrapment of nucleosides generated during myocardial ischemia plays an important role in ventricular dysfunction mediated by reperfusion and emphasized the role of ATP as a source of damaging substrates.[40]

Biochemical intervention aimed at preventing hypoxanthine conversion to xanthine is important in two ways. First, the elevation of hypoxanthine levels increases the probability of its salvage for the formation of IMP (see Fig 2). Second, this elevation decreases the possibility of free radical formation upon reperfusion. These biochemical manipulations could be achieved either by inhibiting the transformation of xanthine-dehydrogenase into xanthine oxidase or by inactivating xanthine oxidase. The inhibition of xanthine oxidase has been demonstrated in vitro[181] and in vivo[182] using allopurinol or oxypurinol. Two reports from different laboratories found the beneficial effects[183] and failure[184] of allopurinol to provide myocardial protection against reperfusion injury. The modulation of xanthine dehydrogenase-xanthine oxidase intraconversion during ischemia and/or reperfusion may provide additional myocardial protection against observed reperfusion injury. The disadvantage of using xanthine oxidase inhibitors is that they are difficult to dissolve and may not reach the target site before oxidation of myocardial hypoxanthine and xanthine. Therefore, the entrapment of nucleoside during reperfusion by EHNA and NBMPR may provide an attractive and better pharmacologic intervention than inhibiting xanthine oxidase or scavenging free radicals after they have been formed.

Summary

Myocardial ischemic injury is initiated by the interruption of coronary blood flow. Lack of oxygen and depletion of ATP are the first recognized events that occur with the onset of ischemia. Although ATP is needed for myocardial function and metabolism, it represents a major source of catabolites that may produce oxygen-derived free radicals during postischemic reperfusion. Preventing reperfusion injury mediated by ATP catabolites could be achieved either by the inhibition of xanthine oxidase or the modulation of nucleoside transport.

Myocardial protection should involve preoperative, intraoperative, and postoperative phases of cardiac surgery. Long-term reperfusion injury may involve neutrophil activation and infiltration into damaged endothelial beds. The postoperative management of reperfusion injury may be as important as the intraoperative management in preventing the development of restenosis and necrosis. Therefore, basic research in cardiovascular surgery is not only important to provide a better understanding of the pathophysiology of myocardial injury and myocardial protection, but also to ensure improved patient management during widespread clinical events associated with ischemic syndromes.

References

1. Edmunds LH, Ellison N, Colman RW, et al: Platelet function during cardiac operation: Comparison of membrane and bubble oxygenator. *J Thorac Cardiovasc Surg* 1982; 83:805–812.
2. Lazenby WD, Ko W, Weksler BB, et al: Platelet function and hemostasis after cardiopulmonary bypass: A comparison of hypothermia and normothermic cardiopulmonary bypass. *Surg Forum* 1990; 41:307–309.
3. Wachtfogel YT, Kucich U, Greenplant J, et al: Human neutrophil degranulation during extracorporeal circulation. *Blood* 1987; 69:324–330.
4. White JG, Krivit W: An ultrastructural basis for the shape changes in platelets by chilling. *Blood* 1967; 39:625–634.
5. Valari CR, Cassidy G, Khuri SF, et al: Hypothermia induced reversible platelet dysfunction. *Ann Surg* 1987; 205:175–181.
6. Jennings RB, Ganote CE, Reimer KA: Ischemic tissue injury. *Am J Pathol* 1975; 81:179–198.
7. Jennings RB, Reimer KA, Steenbergen C: Complete global myocardial ischemia in dogs. *Crit Care Med* 1988; 16:988–996.
8. Schwerzmann K, Pedersen P: Regulation of the mitochondrial ATP synthesis/ATPase complex. *Arch Biochem Biophys* 1986; 250:1–18.
9. Maguire MH, Lukas MC, Rettie JF: Adenine nucleotide salvage synthesis in rat heart: Pathways of adenosine salvage. *Biochim Biophys Acta* 1972; 262:108–115.
10. Vary TC, Angelakos ET, Schaffer SW: Relationship between adenine nucleotide metabolism and irreversible ischemic tissue damage in isolated perfused rat heart. *Circ Res* 1979; 45:218–224.
11. Katz AM, Tada M: The "stone heart": A challenge to the biochemist. *Am J Cardiol* 1972; 29:578–580.
12. Chien KR, Han A, Sen A, et al: Accumulation of unesterified arachidonic acid in ischemic canine myocardium: Relationship to a phosphatidylcholine deacylation reacylation cycle and the depletion of membrane phospholipids. *Circ Res* 1984; 54:312–322.
13. Corr PB, Gross RW, Sobel BE: Amphipathic metabolites and membrane dysfunction in ischemic myocardium. *Circ Res* 1984; 55:135–154.
14. Cavarocchi NC, England MD, Schaff HV, et al: Oxygen free radical generation during cardiopulmonary bypass: Correlation with complement activation. *Circulation* 1986; 74(suppl III):III34.
15. Hagler HK, Buja LM: Subcellular calcium shifts in ischemia and reperfusion, in *Pathophysiology of Severe Ischemic Myocardial Injury*. Boston, Kluwer Academic Publishers, 1990, pp 283–296.
16. Battelli MG: Enzymic conversion of rat liver xanthine oxidase from dehydrogenase (D-form) to oxidase (O-form). *FEBS Lett* 1980; 113:47–51.
17. Penny WJ: The deleterious effects of myocardial catecholamines on cellular electrophysiology and arrhythmias during ischemia and reperfusion. *Eur Heart J* 1984; 5:960–973.
18. McCord JM: Oxygen-derived free radicals in postischemic tissue injury. *N Engl J Med* 1985; 312:159–163.
19. Peterson DA, Asinger RW, Elsperger KJ, et al: Reactive oxygen species may cause myocardial reperfusion injury. *Biochem Biophys Res Commun* 1985; 127:87–93.
20. Das DK, Engelman RM, Rouson JA, et al: Pathophysiology of superoxide

radical as potential mediator of reperfusion injury in pig heart. *Basic Res Cardiol* 1986; 81:155–166.

21. Hearse DJ, Garlick PB, Humphrey SM: Ischemic contracture of the myocardium: Mechanism and prevention. *Am J Cardiol* 1971; 39:986–993.

22. Deaton DW, Pasque MK, Pellom GL, et al: Comparative effects of calcium antagonists on ischemic contracture. *Surg Forum* 1982; 33:297–300.

23. Jones RN, Hill ML, Reimer KA, et al: Effect of hypothermia on the relationship between ATP depletion and membrane damage in total myocardial ischemia. *Surg Forum* 1981; 32:250–253.

24. Rosenfeldt FL, Hearse DJ, Cankovic-Darracott S, et al: The additive protective effects of hypothermia and chemical cardiac arrest in the dog. *J Thorac Cardiovasc Surg* 1980; 79:29.

25. Braunwald E, Kloner RA: The stunned myocardium: Prolonged, postischemic ventricular dysfunction. *Circulation* 1982; 66:1146–1149.

26. Glower DD, Spratt JA, Newton JR, et al: Disassociation between early recovery of regional function and purine nucleotide content in postischemic myocardium in conscious dogs. *Cardiovasc Res* 1987; 21:328–336.

27. Hoffmeister HM, Mauser M, Schaper W: Failure of postischemic ATP repletion by adenosine to improve regional myocardial function in coronary sinus, in Glogan D (ed): New York, Steinkopf-Verlag Darmstadt Springer-Verlag, 1984, pp 148–152.

28. Schaper W, Ito BR: The energetics of "stunned" myocardium, in De Jong JW (ed): *Myocardial Energy Metabolism.* Boston Martinus Nighoff Publishers, 1988, pp 203–213.

29. Ambrosio G, Jacobus WE, Bergman CA, et al: Preserved high energy phosphate metabolic reserve in globally "stunned" hearts despite reduction of basal ATP content and contractility. *J Mol Cell Cardiol* 1987; 19:953–964.

30. Swain JL, Sabina RL, McHale PA, et al: Prolonged myocardial nucleotide depletion after brief ischemia in the open-chest dog. *Am J Physiol* 1982; 242:H818–H826.

31. Reimer KA, Hill ML, Jennings RB: Prolonged depletion of ATP and the adenine nucleotides following reversible myocardial ischemic injury in dogs. *J Mol Cell Cardiol* 1981; 13:229–239.

32. Pasque MK, Wechsler AS: Metabolic intervention to affect myocardial recovery following ischemia. *Ann Surg* 1984; 200:1–12.

33. Goldstein JP, Salter DR, Murphy CE, et al: The efficacy of blood versus crystalloid coronary sinus cardioplegia during global myocardial ischemia. *Circulation* 1986; 74(suppl III):99–104.

34. Ambrosio G, Jacobus WE, Mitchell MC, et al: Effect of ATP precursor or ATP and free ADP content and functional recovery of post-ischemic hearts. *Am J Physiol* 1984; 256:H560–H566.

35. Murphy SM, Hallis DG, Seelye RN: Myocardial adenine pool depletion and recovery of mechanical function following ischemia. *Am J Physiol* 1985; 248:H644–H651.

36. Ambrosio G, Jacobus WE, Bergmon CA: Preserved high energy phosphate metabolic reserve in globally "stunned" hearts despite reduction of basal ATP content and contractility. *J Mol Cell Cardiol* 1987; 19:953–964.

37. Abd-Elfattah AS, Jessen ME, Hanan SA, et al: Is adenosine 5'-triphosphate derangement or free-radical-mediated injury the major cause of ventricular dysfunction during reperfusion? Role of adenine nucleotide transport in myocardial reperfusion injury. *Circulation* 1990; 82(suppl IV):341–350.

38. Abd-Elfattah AS, Wechsler AS: Differentiation between ischemic and reperfusion injury. (abstract) FASEB J 1991; 5:A705.
39. Abd-Elfattah AS, Jessen ME, Lekven J, et al: Myocardial reperfusion injury: Role of myocardial hypoxanthine and xanthine in free-radical mediated reperfusion injury. Circulation 1988; 78(suppl III):224–235.
40. Abd-Elfattah AS, Wechsler AS: Differentiation between ischemic and reperfusion injury: Role of adenine nucleotide transport. Jpn J Pharmacol 1990; 52(suppl III):86P.
41. Nayler WG, Panagiotopoulos S, Elz JS, et al: Calcium-mediated damage during post-ischemic reperfusion. J Mol Cell Cardiol 1988; 20(suppl II):41–54.
42. Opie LH, Coetzee WA: Role of calcium ions in reperfusion arrhythmias: Relevance to pharmacological intervention. Cardiovasc Drugs Ther 1988; 2:623–636.
43. Jennings RB, Reimer KA, Stenbergen C: Myocardial ischemia revisited: The osmolar load, membrane damage and reperfusion. J Mol Cell Cardiol 1986; 18:769–780.
44. Opie LH: Reperfusion injury and its pharmacologic modification. Circulation 1989; 80:1049–1062.
45. Belloni FL, Laing BC, Gerritsen ME: Effect of alkylxanthines and calcium antagonists on adenosine uptake by cultured rabbit coronary microvascular endothelium. Pharmacology 1987; 35:1–15.
46. Van Belle H, Goossens F, Wynants J: Normothermic global ischemia in the isolated working rabbit heart: The effect of different drugs on functional recovery and on the release of inorganic phosphated, lactic acid, nucleosides and norepinephrine. J Mol Cell Cardiol 1989; 21(suppl II):S-142.
47. Gulling W, Penny WJ, Lewis MJ, et al: Effect of myocardial catecholamine depletion on cellular electrophysiology and arrhythmias during ischemia and reperfusion. Cardiovasc Res 1984; 18:675–682.
48. Pogwizd SM, Corr PB: Electrophysiologic mechanisms underlying arrhythmias due to reperfusion of ischemic myocardium. Circulation 1987; 76:404–426.
49. Hearse DJ, Tosaki A: Free radical and calcium: Simultaneous interacting triggers as determinates of vulnerability to reperfusion-induced arrhythmias in the rat heart. J Mol Cell Cardiol 1983; 20:213–223.
50. Opie LH, Coetzee WA: Role of calcium ions in reperfusion arrhythmia: Relevance to pharmacological intervention. Cardiovasc Drug Ther 1988; 2:623–636.
51. Kusuoka H, Porterfield JK, Weisman HF, et al: Pathophysiology and pathogenesis of stunned myocardium: Depressed Ca^{2+} activation of contraction as a consequence of reperfusion-induced cellular calcium overload in ferret hearts. J Clin Invest 1987; 79:950–961.
52. Marban E, Lorestsune Y, Corretti M, et al: Calcium and its role in myocardial cell injury during ischemia and reperfusion. Circulation 1989; 80(suppl IV):IV-17–IV-22.
53. Hendricks GR, Millard RW, McRitchie RJ, et al: Regional myocardial functional and electrophysiological alterations after brief coronary occlusion in conscious dogs. J Clin Invest 1975; 56:978–985.
54. Manning AS, Hearse DJ: Reperfusion-induced arrhythmias: Mechanisms and prevention. J Mol Cell Cardiol 1984; 16:497–518.
55. Manning AS, Coltart DJ, Hearse DJ: Ischemia- and reperfusion-induced arrhythmias in the rat: Effects of xanthine oxidase inhibition with allopurinol. Circ Res 1984; 55:545–548.

56. Bernier M, Hearse DJ, Mannings AS: Reperfusion-induced arrhythmias and oxygen-derived free radicals: Studies with anti-free radical interventions and a free radical generating system in the isolated perfused rat heart. *Circ Res* 1986; 58:331–340.
57. Yamada M, Hearse DJ, Curtis MJ: Reperfusion and readministration of oxygen—pathophysiologic relevance of oxygen derived free radicals to arrhythmogenesis. *Circ Res* 1990; 67:1211–1224.
58. Fitzpatrick DB, Karmazyn M: Comparative effects of calcium channel blocking agents and varying extracellular calcium concentration on hypoxia/reoxygenation and ischemia/reperfusion-induced cardiac injury. *J Pharmacol Exp Ther* 1984; 228:761–768.
59. Lo HM, Kloner RA, Braunwald E: Effect of intracoronary verapamil on infarct size in the ischemic, reperfused canine heart: Critical importance of the timing of treatment. *Am J Cardiol* 1985; 56:672–677.
60. Lavie CJ, Murphy JG, Gersh BJ: The role of beta-receptor and calcium-entry-blocking agents in acute myocardial infarction in the thrombolytic era: Can the results of thrombolytic reperfusion be enhanced? *Cardiovasc Drugs Ther* 1988; 2:601–607.
61. Erbel R, Pop, T, et al: Combination of calcium channel blocker and thrombolytic therapy in acute myocardial infarction. *Am Heart J* 1988; 115:529–538.
62. Nayler WG, Ferrari R, William A: Protective effect of pre-treatment with verapamil, nifedipine and propranolol on nitrochondrial function in the ischemic and reperfused myocardium. *Am J Cardiol* 1980; 146:242–248.
63. Van de Werf F, Vanhaecke J, Jang I-K, et al: Reduction in infarct size and enhancement recovery of systolic function after coronary thrombolysis with tissue-type plasminogen activator combined with β-adrenergic blockade with metoprolol. *Circulation* 1987; 75:830–836.
64. Bush LR, Buja LM, Tilton G, et al: Effect of propranolol and diltiazem alone and in combination on the recovery of left ventricular segmental function after temporary coronary occlusion and long-term reperfusion in conscious dogs. *Circulation* 1985; 72:413–430.
65. Yanagida S, Ohsuzu F, Sakata N, et al: Protection of ATP depletion in the perfused heart by verapamil and adenosine (abstract). *Circulation* 1987; 76(suppl IV):IV-244.
66. Bulkely GB: Free radical-mediated reperfusion injury: A selective review. *Br J Cancer* 1987; 55(suppl I):66–73.
67. Schaper W, Schaper J: Problems associated with reperfusion of ischemic myocardium, in Piper HM (ed): *Pathophysiology of Severe Ischemic Myocardial Injury*. Boston, Kluwer Academic Publishers, 1990, pp 269–280.
68. McCord JM: Oxygen-derived free-radicals in post-ischemic tissue injury. *N Engl J Med* 1985; 312:159–163.
69. Przyklenk K, Kloner RA: "Reperfusion injury" by oxygen-derived free radicals: Effect of superoxide dismutase plus catalase, given at the time of reperfusion, on myocardial infarct size, contractile function, coronary microvaculature, and regional myocardial blood flow. *Circ Res* 1989; 64:86–96.
70. Zweier JL, Kuppusamy P, Lutty GA: Measurement of endothelial cell free radical generation: Evidence for a central mechanism of free radical injury in postischemic tissue. *Proc Natl Acad Sci U S A* 1988; 85:4046–4050.
71. Uraizee A, Reimer KA, Murry CE, et al: Failure of superoxide dismutase to limit size of myocardial infarction after 40 minutes of ischemia and 4 days of reperfusion in dogs. *Circulation* 1987; 75:1237–1248.
72. Gallagher KP, Buda AJ, Pace D, et al: Failure of superoxide dismutase and

catalase to alter size of infarction in conscious dogs after 4 hours of occlusion followed by reperfusion. *Circulation* 1986; 73:1065–1076.

73. Richard VJH, Murry CE, Jennings RB, et al: Therapy to reduce free radicals during early reperfusion does not limit the size of myocardial infarcts caused by 90 minutes of ischemia in dogs. *Circulation* 1988; 78:473–480.

74. Jolly SR, Kane WJ, Bailie WB, et al: Canine myocardial reperfusion injury: Its reduction by the combined administration of superoxide dismutase and catalase. *Circ Res 1984; 54:227–285.*

75. Badylak SF, Simmons A, Rursk J, et al: Protection from reperfusion injury in the isolated rat heart by post-ischemic defroxamine and oxypurinol administration. *Cardiovasc Res* 1987; 21:500–506.

76. Jolly SR, Kane WJ, Hook BG, et al: Reduction of myocardial infarct size by neutrophil depletion: Effect of duration of occlusion. *Am Heart J* 1986; 112:682–690.

77. Dworkin GH, Abd-Elfattah AS, Yeh T Jr, et al: Effect of recombinant human superoxide dismutase (rHSOD) on left ventricular contractility after global myocardial ischemia. *Circulation* 1990; 82(suppl V):359–366.

78. Shlafer M, Kane PF, Kirsh MM: Superoxide dismutase plus catalase enhances the efficacy of hypothermic cardioplegia to protect the globally ischemic, reperfused heart. *J Thorac Cardiovasc Surg* 1982; 83:830–839.

79. Miura T, Ogawa S, Ociwa H, et al: Human superoxide dismutase failed to limit the size of myocardial infarct after 20-, 30-, or 60-minute ischemia and 72-hour reperfusion in the rabbit. *Jpn Circ J* 1989; 53:786–794.

80. Tasmura Y, Chi LG, Driscoll EM Jr, et al: Superoxide dismutase conjugated to polyethylene glycol provides sustained protection against myocardial ischemia/reperfusion injury in canine heart. *Circ Res* 1988; 63:944–959.

81. Chi L, Tamura Y, Hoff PT, et al: Effect of superoxide dismutase on myocardial infarct size in the canine heart after 6 hours of regional ischemia and reperfusion: A demonstration of myocardial salvage. *Circ Res* 1989; 64:665–675.

82. Hanan S, Tuchy G, Abd-Elfattah AS: Efficacy of polyethylene glycol-superoxide dismutase on myocardial functional and metabolic recovery following normothermic ischemia and cardioplegic arrest. *J Thorac Cardiovasc Surg*, in press.

83. Lehman J, Dyke C, Abd-Elfattah AS, et al: Preadministration of polyethylene glycol-conjugated superoxide dismutase (PEG-SOD) attenuates reperfusion injury when administered 24 hours before ischemia. *J Thorac Cardiovasc Surg*, in press.

84. Lolley DM, Hewitt RL, Drapanas T: Retroperfusion of the heart with a solution of glucose, insulin potassium during anoxic arrest. *J Thorac Cardiovasc Surg* 1974; 67:364.

85. Clark RE: Verapamil, cardioplegia, and coronary artery bypass grafting. *Ann Thorac Surg* 1986; 41:585.

86. Hammerman H, Kloner RA, Briggs LL, et al: Enhancement of salvage of reperfusion myocardium by early beta-adrenergic blockage (timolol). *J Am Coll Cardiol* 1984; 3:1438–1443.

87. Lesnefsky EJ, VanBenthuysen KM, McMurtry IF, et al: Lidocaine reduces canine infarct size and decreases release of a lipid peroxidation product. *J Cardiovasc Pharmacol* 1989; 13:895–901.

88. Borgers M: Loss of sarcolemmal integrity in ischemic myocardium, in Piper HM (ed): *Pathophysiology of Severe Ischemic Myocardial Injury.* Dordrecht, Kluwer Academic Publishers, 1990, pp 69–89.

89. Swanson DK, Pasaoglu I, Berkoff HA, et al: Improved heart reservation with UW preservation solution. *J Heart Transplant* 1988; 7:456–467.
90. Brodeur RD, Storey CJ, Byron AD, et al: Effects of adenosine on functional recovery during reperfusion of the ischemic rabbit myocardium (abstract). *Circulation* 1990; 82(suppl III):III-289.
91. Zimmer H-G, Ibel H, Steinkopff G, et al: Long-term effect of ribose on adenine nucleotide metabolism in isoproterenol-stimulated hearts. *Adv Exp Med Biol* 1980; 122B:45.
92. Rosenkranz ER, Vinten-Johansen J, Buckberg GD, et al: Benefits of normothermic induction of blood cardioplegia in energy-depleted hearts with maintenance of arrest by multidose cold blood cardioplegic infusion. *J Thorac Cardiovasc Surg* 1982; 84:667–677.
93. Rau EE, Shine KI, Gervais A, et al: Enhanced myocardial recovery of anoxic and ischemic myocardium by amino acid perfusion. *Am J Physiol* 1979; 236:H873–H879.
94. Akizuki S, Yoshida S, Chambers DF, et al: Infarct size limitation by the xanthine oxidase inhibitor, allopurinol in closed chest dogs with small infarcts. *Cardiovasc Res* 1985; 19:686–692.
95. Arnold WL, DeWall RA, Kezki P, et al: The effect of allopurinol on the degree of early myocardial ischemia. *Am Heart J* 1980; 99:614–624.
96. Bodenhamer RM, Johnson RG, Randolph JE, et al: The effect of adding mannitol or albumin to a crystalloid cardioplegic solution: A prospective randomized clinical study. *Ann Thorac Surg* 1985; 40:375.
97. Badylak SF, Simmons A, Turek J, et al: Protection from reperfusion injury in the isolated rat heart by post ischemic deferoxamine oxypurinol administration. *Cardiovasc Res* 1987; 21:500–506.
98. Gunn MD, Sen A, Chang A, et al: Mechanisms of accumulation of arachidonic acid in cultured myocardial cells during ATP depletion. *Am J Physiol* 1985; 249:1188–1194.
99. Flynn J, Becker WK, Vercellotti GM, et al: Ibuprofen inhibits granulocyte responses to inflammatory mediators: A proposed mechanism for reduction of experimental myocardial infarct size. *Inflammation* 1984; 8:33–44.
100. Simpson PJ, Tood RF III, Fantone JC, et al: Reduction of experimental canine myocardial reperfusion injury by a monoclonal antibody (anti-Mo1, anti-CD116) that inhibits leukocyte adhesion. *J Clin Invest* 1988; 81:624–629.
101. Yeh T, Hanan SA, Johnson DE, et al: Superior myocardial preservation with modified UW solution after prolonged ischemia in the rat heart. *Ann Thorac Surg* 1990; 49:1–8.
102. Ledingham SJM, Katayama O, Lachno DR, et al: Prolonged cardiac preservation: Evaluation of the University of Wisconsin preservation solution by comparison with St. Thomas Hospital cardioplegic solution in the rats. *Circulation* 1990; 82(suppl IV):IV-351–358.
103. Swain JL, Hines JJ, Sabina RL, et al: Accelerated repletion of ATP and GTP pool in postischemic canine myocardium using a precursor of purine de novo synthesis. *Circ Res* 1982; 51:102–105.
104. Sabina RL, Kernstine KH, Boyd RL, et al: Metabolism of 5-amino-4-imidazolecarboxamide riboside cardiac and skeletal muscle. *J Biol Chem* 1982; 257:10178–10183.
105. Flameng W, Daenen W, Borgers M, et al: Cardioprotective effects of lidoflazine during 1h of normothermic global ischemia. *Circulation* 1981; 64:796–807.
106. Flameng W, Xhonneux R, Van Belle H, et al: Cardioprotective effects of mi-

oflazine during 1h of normothermic global ischemia in the canine heart. *Cardiovasc Res* 1984; 18:528–537.

107. Abd-Elfattah AS, Wechsler AS: Cardioprotective actions of circulating and non-circulating endogenous adenosine generated during myocardial ischemia (abstract). *J Mol Cell Cardiol,*1991; 23(suppl 3):S76.

108. Rouslin W, Erickson JL, Solaro RJ: Effects of oligomycin and acidosis on rates of ATP depletion in ischemic heart muscle. *Am J Physiol* 1986; 250:H503–H508.

109. Ferrari R, Lissa F, Raddino R, et al: The effect of ruthenium red on mitochondrial function during post-ischemic reperfusion. *J Mol Cell Cardiol* 1982; 14:737–740.

110. Cunningham JN, Adams PX, Knopp EA, et al: Preservation of ATP ultrastructural and ventricular function after aortic cross-clamping and reperfusion. *J Thorac Cardiovasc Surg* 1979; 78:72–78.

111. Bretschneider H, Hunber G, Knoll D: Myocardial resistance and tolerance to ischemia: Physiological and biochemical bases. *J Thorac Cardiovasc Surg* 1975; 16:241–260.

112. Chiu RCJ, Blendall PE, Scott HJ, et al: The importance of monitoring intramyocardial temperature during hypothermic myocardial protection. *Ann Thorac Surg* 1979; 28:317–272.

113. Melrose DA, Dreyer B, Bentall HH, et al: Elective cardiac arrest. *Lancet* 1955; 2:21–22.

114. Helmworth JA, Kaplan S, Clark L Jr, et al: Myocardial injury associated with systole induced with potassium citrate. *Ann Surg* 1959; 149:200.

115. Bjork V, Fors B: Induced cardiac arrest. *J Thorac Cardiovasc Surg* 1961; 42:387.

116. Rau EE, Shine KI, Gervais A, et al: Enhanced myocardial recovery of anoxic and ischemic myocardium by amino acid perfusion. *Am J Physiol* 1979; 236:H873.

117. Lazar HL, Buckberg GD, Manganaro AJ, et al: Reversal of ischemic damage with amino acid substrate enhancement. *J Thorac Cardiovasc Surg* 1980; 88:700–709.

118. Rosenkranz ER, Okamoto F, Buckberg GD, et al: Safety of prolonged aortic clamping with cardioplegia. III. Aspartate enhancement of glutamate-blood cardioplegia in energy-depleted hearts after ischemic and reperfusion injury. *J Thorac Cardiovasc Surg* 1986; 91:428–435.

119. Hass GS, DeBoer LWV, O'Keefe DD, et al: Reduction of post-ischemic myocardial dysfunction by substrate repletion during reperfusion. *Circulation* 1984; 70(suppl I):65.

120. Rosenkranz ER, Buckberg GD, Laks H, et al: Warm induction of cardioplegia with glutamate-enhancer blood in coronary patients with cardiogenic shock who are dependent on inotropic drugs and intra-aortic bypass support. *J Thorac Cardiovasc Surg* 1983; 86:507–518.

121. Abd-Elfattah AS, Salter DR, Murphy CE, et al: Metabolic differences between retrograde and antegrade cardioplegia following reversible normothermic global ischemic injury. *Surg Forum* 1986; 37:267–270.

122. Gundry SR, Kirsh MM: Comparison of retrograde cardioplegia versus antegrade cardioplegia in the presence of coronary artery obstruction *Ann Thorac Surg* 1984; 38:114–127.

123. Silverman NA, Schmitt G, Levitsky S, et al: Effect of coronary artery occlusion on myocardial protection by retroperfusion of cardioplegic solution. *J Surg Res* 1985; 39:164.

124. Goldstein JP, Salter DR, Murphy CE, et al: The efficacy of blood versus crystalloid coronary sinus cardioplegia during global myocardial ischemia. *Circulation* 1986; 74(suppl III):III-99.
125. Salter DR, Goldstein JP, Abd-Elfattah AS, et al: Efficacy of continuous retrograde coronary sinus cardioplegia without topical hypothermia in the normal and hypertrophic canine ventricle. *Surg Forum* 1985; 36:192.
126. Shumway NE: Forward versus retrograde coronary perfusion for direct vision surgery of acquired aortic valvular disease. *J Thorac Cardiovasc Surg* 1959; 38:75.
127. Menasche P, Kural S, Fauchet M, et al: Retrograde coronary sinus perfusion: A safe alternative for ensuring cardioplegic delivery in aortic valve surgery. *Ann Thorac Surg* 1982; 34:647.
128. Rebeyka IM, Hanan SA, Borges MR, et al: Rapid cooling contracture of the myocardium: Adverse effect of rearrest cardiac cooling. *Surg Forum* 1989; 40:243–245.
129. Lofland GK, Abd-Elfattah AS, Wyse R, et al: Myocardial adenine nucleotide pool metabolism in human infants and children during hypothermic cardioplegic arrest and normothermic ischemia. *Ann Surg* 1989; 47:663–668.
130. Baker JE, Boerboom LE, Olinger GN: Age-related changes in the ability of hypothermia and cardioplegia to protect ischemic rabbit myocardium. *J Thorac Cardiovasc Surg* 1987; 93:163–172.
131. Kepsford RD, Hearse DJ: Protection of the immature heart: Temperature-dependent beneficial or detrimental effects of multidase crystalloid cardioplegia in the neonatal rabbit heart. *J Thorac Cardiovasc Surg* 1990; 99:269–279.
132. Abd-Elfattah AS, Godwin CK, McRae RL, et al: Biochemical bases for tolerance of newborn hearts at ischemic injury: Developmental differences in adenine nucleotide degradation in ischemic immature and adult myocardium: A possible role of sarcolemmal 5'-nucleotidase. *Pediatr Res* 1985; 9:122A.
133. Abd-Elfattah AS, Murphy CE, Salter DR, et al: Age- and species-related differences in adenine nucleotide degradation during myocardial global ischemia. *Fed Proc* 1986; 45:1039.
134. Abd-Elfattah AS, Murphy CE, Salter DR, et al: Maturational role of myocardial 5'-nucleotidase and AMP-deaminase isoenzymes in the increased tolerance of immature hearts to ischemic injury. *Circulation* 1986; 74(suppl II):II-492.
135. Jessen ME, Abd-Elfattah AS, Lekven J, et al: Sensitivity of neonatal hearts to ischemia: Confusion from failure to control the bathing media during ischemia. *Surg Forum* 1987; 38:226–227.
136. Abd-Elfattah AS, Wechsler AS: Superiority of HPLC to assay for enzymes regulating adenine nucleotidase pool intermediates metabolism: 5'-Nucleotidase, adenylate deaminase, adenosine deaminase and adenylosuccinate layase: A simple and rapid determination of adenosine. *J Liquid Chromatography* 1987; 10:2653–2694.
137. Morris JJ III, Hamm DD, Pellom GL, et al: Differential ventricular ischemic injury: An experimental model of right ventricular failure with a variable degree of left ventricular dysfunction. *J Thorac Cardiovasc Surg* 1988; 96:590–599.
138. Teoh KH, Christakis GT, Weisel RD, et al: Accelerated myocardial metabolic recovery with terminal warm blood cardioplegia. *J Thorac Cardiovasc Surg* 1986; 91:888.
139. Roberts AJ, Woodhall DD, Knauf DG, et al: Coronary artery bypass graft surgery: Clinical comparison of cold blood potassium cardioplegia, with car-

dioplegic reduction and secondary cardioplegia. *Ann Thorac Surg* 1985; 40:483.

140. Porterfield JK, Kusuoka H, Weisman HF, et al: Ryanodine prevents the changes in myocardial function and morphology induced by reperfusion after brief periods of ischemia (abstract). *Circ Res* 1987; 35:315A.

141. Geisbucheler T, Altschuld RA, Trewyn RW, et al: Adenine nucleotides metabolism compartmentalization in isolated rat heart. *Circ Res* 1984; 54:536–546.

142. Dow JW: Metabolism of purines by adult cardiomyocytes, in Piper HM, Isenberg G (eds): *Isolated Adult Cardiomyocytes.* New York, Raven Press, 1986, pp 216–237.

143. Becker BF, Gerlach E: Uric acid, the major adenine nucleotide catabolite released from isolated perfused guinea pig hearts, is formed in the coronary endothelium (abstract). *J Mol Cell Cardiol* 1986; 18(suppl):157.

144. Vicker S, Hildreth J, Kajada F, et al: Localization of the free radical-generating enzyme xanthine oxidase in the microvascular endothelium of the canine and human heart (abstract). *Assoc Academic Surgery* 1990; :31.

145. Hori M, Kitakaje T: AICA-riboside (5-amino-4-imidazole carbosamide riboside 100) a novel adenosine poleutiater attenuates myocardial stunning (abstract). *Circulation* 1990; 82(suppl III):III-466.

146. Molina-Viamonte V, Rosen MR: AIC-riboside suppresses arrhythmias induced by coronary artery occlusion and reperfusion (abstract). *Circulation* 1990; 82(suppl III):III-645.

147. Abd-Elfattah AS, Sheffield C, Forsberg DA, et al: Myocardial protection with brono-adenosine monophosphate (Br-AMP) during global ischemia and reperfusion. A novel inhibition of 5'-nucleotidase in cardiomyocytes. *Circulation* 1986; 74(suppl II):II-357.

148. Frick GP, Lowenstein JM: Studies of 5'-nucleotidase of the heart. *J Biol Chem* 1976; 250:6372.

149. Okamura T, Nakagawa A, Susuki A: Myocardial protection with bromo-adenosine monophosphate (Br-AMP) as an adjunct to cardioplegic solution (abstract). *J Mol Cell Cardiol* 1989; 21(suppl):S.121.

150. Newby AC, Worku Y, Holmquist CA: Adenosine formation, evidence for a direct biochemical link with energy metabolism. *Adv Myocardial* 1984; 6:273–284.

151. Imai S, Nakazawa H, Imai H, et al: 5'-Nucleotidase inhibitors and myocardial reactive hyperemia and adenosine content, in Gerlach E, Becker BF (eds): *Topics and Perspectives in Adenosine Research.* New York, Springer-Verlag, 1987, pp 155–169.

152. Newby AC, Worku Y, Meghji P: Critical elevation of the role of ecto- and cytosolic 5'-nucleotidase in adenosine formation, in Gerlach E, Becker BF (eds); *Topics and Perspectives in Adenosine Research.* Springer-Verlag, 1987, pp 155–169.

153. Dendorfer A, Lauk S, Schaff A, et al: New insight into the mechanism of myocardial adenosine formation, in Gerlach E, Becker BF (eds): *Topics and Perspectives in Adenosine Research.* New York, Springer-Verlag, 1987, pp 170–189.

154. Ward JB, Wang MC, Einzig S, et al: Prevention of ATP catabolism during myocardial ischemia: A preliminary report. *J Surg Res* 1983; 34:292.

155. Henry PD, Sobel BE, Braunwald E: Protection of hypoxic guinea pig hearts with glucose and insulin. *Am J Physiol* 1974; 226:309.

156. Hewitt RL, Lolley DM, Androuny GA, et al: Protective effect of glycogen and glucose on the anoxic arrested heart. *Surgery* 1974; 75:1.
157. Hearse DJ, Steward A, Braimbridge MV: Myocardial protection during ischemic arrest, possible deleterious effects of glucose and mannitol in coronary infusates. *J Thorac Cardiovasc Surg* 1978; 76:16.
158. Wechsler AS, Abd-Elfattah AS, Murphy CE, et al: Myocardial protection. *J Cardiovasc Surg* 1986; 1:271–306.
159. McDonagh PF, Laks H, Chaudry IH, et al: Improved myocardial recovery for ischemia: Treatment with low dose adenosine triphosphate-magnesium chloride. *Arch Surg* 1984; 119:1379–1384.
160. Kopf GS, Chaudry IH, Condos SG, et al: Improved myocardial performance after prolonged ischemia with ATP-MgCl$_2$ cardioplegia. *Surg Forum* 1986; 37:234–236.
161. Robinson LA, Braimbridge MV, Hearse DJ, et al: Creatine phosphate: An additive myocardial protective and antiarrhythmic agent in cardioplegia. *J Thorac Cardiovasc Surg* 1984; 87:190–200.
162. Mankad PS, Cheslir AH, Yacoub MH: Role of potassium concentration in cardioplegic solution in mediating endothelial damage. *Ann Thorac Surg* 1991; 51:89–93.
163. Ely SW, Mentzer RM, Lasley RD, et al: Functional and metabolic evidence of enhanced myocardial tolerance to ischemia and reperfusion. *J Thorac Cardiovasc Surg* 1985; 90:549–556.
164. Olafsson B, Forman MB, Puett DW, et al: Reduction of reperfusion injury in the canine preparation by intracoronary adenosine: Importance of the endothelium and the no-reflow phenomenon. *Circulation* 1987; 76:1135–1145.
165. Babbitt OG, Virmani R, Forman M: Intracoronary adenosine administered after reperfusion limits vascular injury after prolonged ischemia in the canine model. *Circulation* 1989; 80:1388–1399.
166. Abd-Elfattah AS, Maddox R, Hanan S, et al: [³H] adenosine uptake in ischemically injured myocardium during reperfusion: Role of outward flux via nucleoside transport (abstract). *J Mol Cell Cardiol* 1989; 21(suppl II):S143.
167. Ramos-Salazer A, Baines AD: Role of 5′-nucleotidase in adenosine-mediated renal vasoconstriction during hypoxia. *J Pharmacol Exp Ther* 1986; 230:494–499.
168. Ceccarelli M, Ciompi ML, Pasero G: Acute renal failure during adenine therapy in the lesch-nyhan syndrome, in Sperling P, De Vries AS, Wyngaarden JB (eds): *Purine Metabolism in Man.* New York, Raven Press, 1974, pp 671–679.
169. Smiseth OA: Inosine infusion in dogs with acute ischemic left ventricular function: Favorable effects on myocardial performance and metabolism. *Cardiovasc Res* 1983; 17:192.
170. Silverman NA, Kohler J, Finberg H, et al: Beneficial metabolic effect of nucleoside augmentation on reperfusion injury following cardioplegic arrest. *Chest* 1983; 83:787.
171. Robinson LA, Haywood DL: Nucleoside-enriched cardioplegia: Metabolic protection during ischemia (abstract). *J Mol Cell Cardiol* 1989; 21(suppl II):S121.
172. Zimmer HG, Ibel H, Steinkopff G, et al: Reduction of isoproterenol-induced alteration in cardiac adenine nucleotide and morphology by ribose. *Science* 1980; 207:319.
173. Zimmer HG: Acceleration of adenine nucleotide biosynthesis after ischemic

insult, in de Jong JW (eds): *Myocardial Energy Metabolism*. Dordrecht, The Netherlands, Martinus Niihoff Publisher, 1988, pp 105–114.

174. Zimmer HG, Gerlach E: Studies on the regulation of the biosynthesis of myocardial adenine nucleotides. *Adv Exp Med Biol* 1977; 70A:40.

175. Zimmer GH, Gerlach E: Effect of beta adrenergic stimulation on myocardial adenine nucleotide metabolism. *Circ Res* 1974; 35:536.

176. Pasque MK, Spray TL, Pellom GL, et al: Ribose-enhanced myocardial recovery following ischemia in isolated working rat heart. *J Thorac Cardiovasc Surg* 1982; 83:390.

177. Sterling K: Direct thyroid hormone activation of mitochondria: The role of adenine nucleotide translocase. *Endocrinology* 1986; 119:292–295.

178. Schrader WP, West C: Localization of adenosine deaminase and adenosine deaminase complex protein in rabbit heart: Implications for adenosine metabolism. *Circ Res* 1990; 66:754–762.

179. Huzer T, De Jong JW, Nelson JA, et al: Urate production by human heart. *J Mol Cell Cardiol* 1989; 21:691–695.

180. Becker BF, Gerlach E: Uric acid, the major adenine nucleotide catabolite released from isolated perfused guinea pig is formed in the coronary endothelium (abstract). *J Mol Cell Cardiol* 1986; 18(suppl I):157.

181. Werns W, Shea MJ, Mitso S, et al: Reduction of the size infarction by allopurinol in the ischemic reperfused canine heart. *Circulation* 1986; 3:518–524.

182. Puitt DW, Forman MB, Cates CU, et al: Oxypurinol limits myocardial stunning but not infarct size after reperfusion. *Circulation* 1987; 76:678–686.

183. Reimer KA, Jennings RB: Failure of xanthine oxidase inhibitor allopurinol to limit infarct size after ischemia and reperfusion in dogs. *Circulation* 1985; 71:1069–1075.

Myocardial Protection in Children

Darryl G. Stein, M.D.

Research Fellow, Division of Cardiothoracic Surgery, University of California, Los Angeles Medical Center, Los Angeles, California

Hillel Laks, M.D.

Professor of Surgery and Chief, Division of Cardiothoracic Surgery, University of California, Los Angeles Medical Center, Los Angeles, California

Davis C. Drinkwater Jr., M.D.

Associate Professor of Surgery, Division of Cardiothoracic Surgery, University of California, Los Angeles Medical Center, Los Angeles, California

Protecting the myocardium at the time of surgery is of paramount importance. When protection is inadequate, poor function occurs postoperatively with resultant abnormal hemodynamics, increased need for inotropic support, and increased risk of perioperative morbidity and mortality. There are special considerations in the pediatric patient. The immature heart has structural, metabolic, and functional differences compared to the adult heart. In addition, the patient with congenital heart disease may have to undergo cardiac surgery after stresses that are different from those seen in the adult and include hypoxemia, pressure overload, and volume overload. The interaction of these stresses with different methods of myocardial protection is not completely understood. Additionally, the conduct of bypass can affect postoperative cardiac function significantly. These considerations often necessitate changes from the methods employed in adult myocardial protection and make protection of the child's heart challenging. An understanding of the pediatric heart's unique properties is essential when choosing a method of myocardial protection for the developing heart.

Structural, Metabolic, and Functional Characteristics of the Developing Heart

Structural Characteristics

Numerous morphologic differences exist between the immature myocyte and the mature cell, the most striking being cell size. In the rat ventricle, cell size increases 90% between the 1st and 5th days of life, 30% to 40%

between the 5th and 11th days, and 500% by maturity.[1, 2] Similar, although slower, cell growth is likely to occur in human hearts. Another characteristic of neonatal myocardium is the absence or paucity of T tubules. T tubules first appear in the rat ventricle at 21 days, in the cat at 16 days, and in the opossum at 43 days.[3-5] The appearance of T tubules, which allow interstitial fluid and thus cardioplegia to be in contact with a greater portion of the myocyte, limits the fall of the surface-to-volume ratio that would be expected otherwise as the cell hypertrophies. These myocyte characteristics may alter myocyte cooling and cardioplegia equilibration, affecting preservation.

The distribution and arrangement of intracellular structures in the neonatal cardiac myocyte also differ from the mature myocyte. Myofibrils are oriented randomly with incomplete sarcomeres[6, 7] and make up a smaller volume density, as a percentage of cell volume, than in the mature myocyte.[8] Mitochondria are dispersed indiscriminately among these myofibrils, are fewer in number, and have less well developed cristae.[6, 9, 10] The sarcoplasmic reticulum, while apparently fully developed at birth,[11] grows in volume relative to the growth of the myocyte during the early neonatal period.[12] Subsequent maturation of these organelles coincides with the metabolic and functional maturity of the heart,[13] and probably corresponds with a change in the heart's tolerance to an ischemic insult.

Metabolic Characteristics

The myocyte's early embryonic life is marked by a lack of enzymes to perform oxidative phosphorylation and dependence upon glycolysis for energy production.[14-16] Glucose, however, provides less than half the energy required to sustain the adult heart.[17] A transition from glucose-dependent to fatty acid–dependent energy production begins in utero as the ability for gas exchange is achieved. This transition continues after birth and is not complete until the myocyte reaches the mature form. The maturation parallels the increases in number and complexity of the mitochondria seen ultrastructurally.[16, 18]

As might be expected from the immature heart's metabolic state, glucose is stored readily as glycogen in the immature heart.[19, 20] The glycogen content of the adult heart, however, is considerably less.[21] These glycogen stores are an advantage for the immature myocyte in that they serve as a ready energy source for the stressed heart.[22] The advantage this conveys to the immature heart has been demonstrated in several investigations, which showed improved recovery of contractility and greater compliance of the immature ventricle as compared to the adult ventricle after an ischemic event.[23-25] Additionally, a direct correlation between survival time during anoxia and myocardial glycogen stores has been observed.[26, 27] The potential advantage the immature myocardium may have to recover from a hypoxic/ischemic insult, however, may not be realized clinically, since most pediatric patients undergoing open heart surgery have abnormal physiologic states that have stressed the heart prior to surgery.

Altered calcium homeostasis in the immature myocardium is another characteristic of the developing heart that affects preservation. Calcium contributes to myocardial cell structure, enzymatic processes, and contraction. Each is altered in the developing myocyte and must be considered when attempting to protect the heart.

The integrity of the glycocalyx, the outermost layer of the cell membrane, is dependent upon calcium bridging.[28] At calcium levels below $25 \mu M$, integrity of the membrane is lost, causing massive injury to the cell.[29] The sarcolemma also binds calcium, which appears to be the primary source for the exchangeable calcium pool.[30, 31] This exchangeable pool plays a role in excitation-contraction coupling and quantitative force development.[32, 33] It may be especially important in the infant heart, since excitation-contraction coupling appears to be more dependent on extracellular calcium in the immature heart than in the adult heart.[32] In addition, calcium serves as a coenzyme for many cellular reactions and regulates crossbridging of myosin to actin.[31] As would be expected, maintaining optimum calcium levels at the time of arrest and reperfusion contributes to improved functional recovery in the newborn heart.[34-36]

Functional Characteristics

Fetal myocardial functional characteristics are altered from those of the adult. Isolated heart muscle preparations reveal a reduced ability to generate active tension by fetal heart muscle.[37] Diminished myocardial shortening velocity and increased myocardial resting tension also are observed. However, these differences from adult myocardium are negated when the observations are normalized for reduced fetal myocyte size and myofibril volume density. The intrinsic fetal sarcomere strength and contraction velocity actually is equivalent to that of the adult sarcomere. The importance of fetal and adult myocyte structural differences and their relation to function, therefore, is clearly evident.

Studies in the intact ventricle reveal similar differences between the newborn and adult heart. The newborn right ventricle is significantly less compliant than the adult right ventricle, although it is more compliant than the left ventricle at all developmental stages.[37] This reduced compliance leads to diminished preload reserve where, upon volume loading, left ventricular stroke volume, stroke work, and mean fiber shortening are reduced.[38] Additionally, volume loading of one ventricle significantly affects the other ventricle's compliance.[37, 39] This phenomenon may account for the newborn's propensity for right ventricular failure in the presence of malformations primarily affecting the left ventricle. The newborn's heart may be limited further by operating under maximal adrenergic stimulation with limited inotropic reserve.[40] These functional disadvantages limit the newborn heart's ability to compensate for certain stress states, emphasizing the necessity for optimal intraoperative myocardial protection to ensure adequate function after surgery.

Preoperative Stress States Associated With Congenital Heart Disease

The congenitally malformed heart is often subject to abnormal preoperative stress states that may significantly affect the heart's recovery after cardiopulmonary bypass. Several clinical studies have shown suboptimal myocardial protection in pediatric patients undergoing corrective procedures.[41, 42] In contrast, many laboratory investigations show improved tolerance to ischemia/hypoxia by immature hearts when compared to adult hearts.[43–45] This discrepancy may be related to the state of the myocardium at the time of surgery. Most laboratory investigations are performed on normal, unstressed hearts, giving them a potential advantage over the congenitally malformed heart. The stress states associated with congenital heart disease include hypoxemia, ischemia, pressure overload, and/or volume overload. Any one can potentially affect preservation of the pediatric heart.

Hypoxemia

Acute Hypoxemia.—Acute hypoxemia occurs as the result of a variety of congenital heart defects, including pulmonary atresia, tricuspid atresia, transposition of the great arteries, and tetralogy of Fallot. The degree of hypoxemia is dependent upon the amount of pulmonary blood flow and the degree of mixing. As hypoxia increases, contractility and myocardial high-energy phosphate levels are reduced.[46, 47] Acidosis may follow, causing further deterioration in function.[48, 49] Resultant increases in anaerobic metabolism reduce glycogen levels, rendering the heart less tolerant to subsequent ischemia.[50] When palliation or corrective procedures are performed, reoxygenation injury may result, further compromising myocardial recovery.[51, 52]

Chronic Hypoxemia.—Chronic hypoxemia may be present in patients with cyanotic congenital heart disease who have mixing of their pulmonary and systemic circulations. Studies in resting cyanotic patients showed no differences in myocardial glucose and free fatty acid uptake or oxygen consumption when compared to acyanotic patients.[50] Myocardial glycogen and triglyceride levels, however, were lower in cyanotic patients,[53] possibly affecting their tolerance to ischemia.[54] Indeed, experimental studies have shown decreased tolerance to protected ischemia in models of chronic hypoxia.

In a chronic canine model of cyanosis, Silverman and colleagues showed that after 3 months, the cyanotic animals' ejection fractions were significantly reduced compared to those of controls.[55] Adenosine triphosphate and creatine phosphate (CP) levels were similar in all groups prior to a period of cardiopulmonary bypass and cardioplegic arrest. At end-ischemia, however, both levels were reduced significantly in the cyanotic animals, with adenosine triphosphate levels remaining low upon reperfusion. Fujiwara confirmed chronic hypoxia's deleterious effects in a neonatal lamb model.[56] Following 2 hours of hypothermic cardioplegic arrest, functional assessments were made using an isolated heart model. Chronically cyanotic hearts showed reduced functional recovery.

The deleterious effect of hypoxemia on myocardial preservation is evident in both the acute and chronic states. In either situation, the heart's altered response to ischemic arrest must be considered when planning surgery.

Ischemia

Altered coronary perfusion in the pediatric patient may be present from an anomalous coronary connection or as the result of reduced systemic diastolic pressure in patients with aorto-pulmonary collaterals. Achieving adequate myocardial protection in these patients may be difficult. The patient with an anomalous left coronary artery from the pulmonary artery is dependent upon right coronary artery collateral flow to maintain adequate myocardial perfusion in the left coronary artery distribution.[57] Therefore, myocardium in the left distribution may be perfused inadequately, with resultant decreased tolerance to ischemia. Patients with extracardiac mixing (truncus arteriosus and hemitruncus arteriosus) and excessive pulmonary blood flow may have difficulty maintaining coronary perfusion after pulmonary vascular resistance falls in the neonatal period. With a fall in pulmonary vascular resistance, systemic diastolic runoff is increased through the pulmonary bed, lowering systemic diastolic pressure and reducing coronary perfusion. The administration of oxygen during the induction of anesthesia can increase pulmonary blood flow further, reducing aortic diastolic pressure, and may cause electrocardiographic signs of ischemia.[58] Care must be taken in these patients to ensure adequate coronary perfusion prior to cardiopulmonary bypass.

Pressure Overload

Obstructive lesions involving outflow (aortic stenosis, coarctation of the aorta, pulmonary stenosis, and tetralogy of Fallot) from the ventricles are common in patients with congenital heart disease. The ability of the immature myocardium to overcome the increased afterload imposed by the obstruction, however, is hindered by the neonatal heart's limited ability to augment the inotropic state over baseline.[59] The lack of well-organized sarcomeres and limited number of myofibrils contribute to the increased reserve. An attempt to compensate through ventricular hypertrophy ensues, with resultant loss in ventricular compliance.[60, 61] Lower high-energy phosphate levels and inefficient oxygen utilization accompanies the hypertrophy.[62] Increased susceptibility to ischemia of such hypertrophied myocardium also has been shown.[63, 64]

Volume Overload

Volume loading of the heart may arise from large left-to-right shunts, valvular insufficiency, or arteriovenous fistulae. Compensation by the Frank-

Starling mechanism may be limited, since the newborn heart functions at a high diastolic volume and, as such, has a limited diastolic reserve.[65, 66] Studies in neonatal lamb hearts show that volume loading of one ventricle profoundly affects the distensibility of the other ventricle, potentially causing biventricular failure.[39] Further compromise in function can occur by ventricular dilation with associated increased wall stress and myocardial oxygen demand. In fact, oxygen consumption has been noted to be increased in infants with cardiac failure secondary to large left-to-right shunts.[67] In patients with truncus arteriosus, the large volume load results in an elevated end-diastolic pressure. This may reduce the coronary perfusion pressure, increasing the risk of ischemia by the mechanism described above. Increased oxygen demands in the patient with volume overload and the other stresses that are often associated may affect preservation adversely.

Methods of Pediatric Myocardial Protection

Numerous strategies have been employed to protect the pediatric heart. Continuous coronary perfusion was an early technique that fell into disfavor due to difficult operating conditions, complications associated with coronary cannulation,[68-70] and potential injury to the fibrillating heart.[71, 72] Intermittent aortic clamping is another technique that was advocated as recently as 1984.[41] The potential for this procedure to injure the myocardium, however, was shown in numerous experimental[73-77] and clinical investigations.[78-81] Current methods almost universally employ cardioplegia.

However, cardioplegia is only one part of a myocardial protective strategy. Attention to the conditions of induction, maintenance, and reperfusion, along with the conduct of bypass are necessary for optimal myocardial recovery. The developing heart's unique properties and often-associated preoperative stress states must be considered when developing a protective strategy. Conditions that favor the pediatric heart in each area of protection will result in superior myocardial protection.

Cardioplegia Formulation

Formulations for cardioplegic solutions are numerous, with most centers utilizing solutions developed locally. The composition of these solutions is based largely on developmental work performed in adult animal models. Not unexpectedly, the application of these solutions to the neonatal animal model has led to mixed results.[82-84] Clinical application has improved outcome, but sometimes achieves less than optimal results.[85, 86]

Recently, several experimental studies have been performed to determine preferred cardioplegic formulations for protection of the immature heart. Kempsford and Hearse compared the efficacy of four adult cardioplegic solutions in an isolated neonatal rabbit heart model.[35] After 50 minutes of normothermic ischemia, hearts arrested with St. Thomas' and

Tyers' solutions recovered significantly better than did hearts preserved with Bretschneider's or Roe's solution. This study emphasizes the altered response of neonatal myocardium to cardioplegic solutions; cardioplegic solutions that work well in adult hearts may not be as effective in immature hearts.

Calcium Concentration.—The calcium concentration may be critical to the observed differences in pediatric and adult myocardium. In the Kempsford and Hearse study, the acalcemic cardioplegic solutions (Bretschneider's and Roe's) fared far worse than did the calcium containing solutions (St. Thomas' and Tyers'). Konishi and Apstein further demonstrated the importance of calcium in pediatric cardioplegia.[87] They examined the preservation of neonatal rabbit hearts arrested with either acalcemic cardioplegia, St. Thomas' Hospital No. 2 (calcium 1.2mM), or Hopital Lariboisiere's cardioplegia (calcium 0.25mM). Improved preservation was observed with the solutions containing calcium.

Zweng and associates specifically studied the effects of different calcium concentrations in St. Thomas' cardioplegia on the preservation of neonatal rabbit hearts.[36] Following 60 minutes of normothermic ischemia, hearts arrested with acalcemic cardioplegia recovered only 10% of baseline dP/dT. Hearts arrested with an optimal calcium concentration of 1.2mM recovered 76% of baseline dP/dt. As demonstrated in this study, the importance of each cardioplegia component can be determined only by similar dose-response investigations.

Blood vs. Crystalloid Cardioplegia.—The original cardioplegia as introduced by Melrose was a sanguineous solution. This blood potassium cardioplegia, however, soon fell into disfavor due to myocyte injury caused by one component of the solution, citrate.[88] Crystalloid cardioplegias were introduced as an alternative and gained acceptance. The benefits of blood cardioplegia, however, were reexamined later and advocated at our institution.[81] The potential advantages of blood cardioplegia include continued oxygen delivery to the myocardium at the time of arrest, improved buffering capacity, improved oncotic properties, and readily controlled reperfusion of the ischemic heart.

Several studies have demonstrated these advantages by showing the superiority of blood cardioplegia over crystalloid cardioplegia. Among the findings are improved preservation of function, retention of high-energy phosphate levels, and reduced ultrastructural injury.[34, 81, 89–93] A recent study by Illes and associates attempted to identify the critical component of blood cardioplegia.[94] Blood cardioplegia was delivered at hematocrits of 17%, 8.2%, and 0%, each with equal amounts of plasma. Following 2 hours of hypothermic arrest, contractile function was equivalent in all groups. Despite similar oxygen availability between the 8.2% and 0% hematocrit groups (achieved by raising the Po_2 in the 0% group), the 0% group had significantly increased basal metabolic oxygen consumption. The authors concluded that the red cell was important not only for its oxygen carrying capacity, but also for its buffering capacity and other as yet unidentified properties.

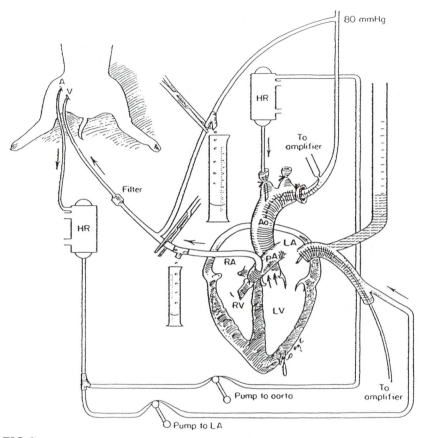

FIG 1.
Perfusion circuit. *A* = femoral artery of the adult support pig; *Ao* = aorta; *HR* = heated reservoir; *LA* = left atrium; *LV* = left ventricle; *PA* = pulmonary artery; *RA* = right atrium; *RV* = right ventricle; *V* = femoral vein of the adult support pig.

The benefits of blood cardioplegia in the developing heart have been studied less extensively. To determine the efficacy of blood cardioplegia in the pediatric heart, we utilized an isolated, blood-perfused neonatal piglet heart model (Fig 1).[34] Topical hypothermia, crystalloid cardioplegia, and blood cardioplegia were examined. After 2 hours of hypothermic or multi-dose cardioplegic arrest, the hearts were reperfused on the isolated circuit. Functional evaluation was performed 30 and 60 minutes after reperfusion. The hearts protected with cold blood cardioplegia recovered complete preischemic function; the other groups recovered less completely. The calcium concentration also was shown to affect preservation significantly, emphasizing the importance of each cardioplegic component.

Several randomized clinical trials have proven the superiority of blood cardioplegia in adults.[95–98] No similar trials, however, have been conducted in children. Nevertheless, we demonstrated significant benefits in the laboratory setting and therefore we have adopted blood cardioplegia as our preferred method for myocardial protection.

Cardioplegia Induction

As discussed earlier, the pediatric heart is often stressed and metabolically depleted prior to surgery, reducing its tolerance to ischemia. Improving the heart's metabolic state during cardioplegic induction should enhance postischemic recovery. Rosenkranz and colleagues studied the benefits of warm amino acid–enriched blood cardioplegia induction on previously ischemic, energy-depleted adult canine hearts.[99, 100] They found that a 5-minute infusion of warm blood cardioplegia enhances high-energy phosphate repletion and improves oxygen utilization during induction. Enrichment with aspartate and glutamate raises oxygen consumption further, indicating increased aerobic metabolism and "active resuscitation" of the heart. Following induction, cold cardioplegia was administered and subsequently reinfused every 20 minutes. Hearts induced with aspartate/glutamate–enriched warm blood cardioplegia recovered fully, while those induced with cold blood cardioplegia recovered less than one half of their baseline function. The application of this technique to the metabolically depleted pediatric heart may enhance postischemic recovery.

Additional considerations at induction include cardioplegic infusion pressure and myocardial distention. Elevated cardioplegic infusion pressure can affect functional recovery adversely in adult animal models.[101, 102] We suspected that the developing heart would be affected similarly and, therefore, examined the effect of elevated cardioplegia infusion pressure on the neonatal heart.[103] Using the previously described neonatal piglet model, baseline function curves were obtained prior to cardioplegia infusion at 120, 150, 180, and 210 mm Hg. Arrest was maintained for 1 hour with intermittent infusions every 20 minutes. Following reperfusion, hearts infused at pressures of 120 and 150 mm Hg returned to near-baseline function, while those perfused at 180 and 210 mm Hg showed markedly depressed recovery of function. In a related study, we examined the neonatal heart's susceptibility to ventricular distention during cardioplegic arrest.[104] After cardioplegic arrest, the left ventricle was distended to a presure of 30, 60, 90, or 120 mm Hg for 5 minutes. Hearts distended to 120 mmHg recovered only 43% of preischemic function. Ultrastructural examination revealed myofibrillar lysis, dissociation of intercellular junctions, and interstitial edema. We concluded that improved myocardial function could be expected by meticulous attention to cardioplegic infusion pressure and adequate ventricular venting.

Cardioplegic Maintenance

All hearts receive noncoronary collateral blood flow. The amount is variable, but may be increased in children with cyanotic congenital heart disease through bronchial-to-coronary collaterals.[105] Canine studies have shown that up to 20% of normal left ventricular coronary blood flow is maintained in hypertrophied hearts after aortic cross-clamping.[106] This flow, which washes out cardioplegia, necessitates repeated cardioplegia infusions to maintain electromechanical arrest. Repeated dosing is necessary even when electromechanical acitivity does not return, because low-level electrical activity can precede visible mechanical activity, leading to impaired ventricular recovery, when administration is delayed.[107] We adopted a policy of reinfusing cardioplegia at a maximum interval of 20 minutes.

Cardioplegic Reperfusion

Reperfusion injury is a well-recognized phenomenon following an ischemic period. The injury alters myocardial structure, metabolism, and function. The mechanism of this injury is not well elucidated, but undoubtedly involves a complex interaction between leukocytes, endothelial cells, complement, and other elements.[108, 109] Preventing or reducing this injury will improve postischemic myocardial recovery. Follette and associates attempted to reduce such injury by modifying the reperfusate.[110] They hypothesized that modification of the reperfusate could allow reparative cellular processes to take place prior to permanent reperfusion injury. Using a canine model, hearts underwent 1 hour of hypothermic arrest before reperfusion with warm hypocalcemic, hypercalemic, alkalotic, and hyperosmolar blood reperfusate. Without temporary reperfusate modification, left ventricular function fell to 60% of baseline and compliance fell 50%. Hearts receiving the modified reperfusate recovered 104% of baseline function, with a 20% decline in compliance.

Mounting evidence has confirmed the leukocyte's extensive role in reperfusion injury. Leukocytes appear to mediate reperfusion injury through the no-reflow phenomenon, release of oxygen free radicals, and release of lysosomal enzymes by degranulation.[111-113] We recently examined the benefits of leukocyte-depleted reperfusion alone and in conjunction with warm aspartate/glutamate−enriched cardioplegic reperfusion.[114] After arrest and static storage with University of Wisconsin solution for 24 hours at 4° C, neonatal porcine hearts were reperfused on the previously described isolated heart circuit. Whole blood reperfused hearts recovered 70% of control function after 50 minutes. Hearts reperfused with leukocyte-depleted blood for 10 minutes regained 83% of control function, while hearts that received leukocyte-depleted aspartate/glutamate−enriched warm blood cardioplegic reperfusate recovered 100% of function. We feel that reperfusion injury is a major cause of myocardial dysfunction postoperatively; therefore, we modify the reperfusate in all of our pediatric cases.

Conduct of Cardiopulmonary Bypass

While the formulation of the cardioplegic solution and the conditions of induction, maintenance, and reperfusion can affect myocardial preservation dramatically, the conduct of bypass can be equally important. Yamaguchi reported improved myocardial function and decreased mortality for patients undergoing repair of tetralogy of Fallot when cardioplegia with deep systemic hypothermia was used in place of cardioplegia with moderate hypothermia.[115] Ganzel confirmed the benefits of deep systemic hypothermia in a neonatal piglet model.[116] He emphasized the importance of the increased surface-to-mass ratio of the neonatal heart, which allows more rapid warming of the heart between cardioplegia doses and subsequent inferior protection. Increased noncoronary collateral blood flow in the cyanotic patient also may play a role, where, during deep hypothermia, less rewarming of the heart occurs between cardioplegic doses. Caution must be taken, however, when cooling the heart rapidly, as this may induce myocardial contracture with resultant irreversible injury.[117, 118] As recently reported by Williams and associates, this contracture can be prevented by the induction of cardioplegic arrest with a warm induction cardioplegia prior to cooling.[119]

The University of California, Los Angeles Experience

The composition of our cardioplegia and our techniques of administration were developed from both our laboratory and clinical experience. They take into consideration the metabolic and physiologic differences between the adult and pediatric heart in an attempt to provide optimal protection for the latter. We find these techniques to be simple and efficient to implement in the operating room.

Cardioplegic Solutions

Three cardioplegic solutions are employed: a high-potassium arresting solution, a low-potassium maintenance solution, and a warm, modified, induction/reperfusion solution (Table 1). All solutions are mixed with blood in a 4:1 blood-to-cardioplegia ratio. Final concentrations of delivered cardioplegia are shown in Table 2. Laboratory values are obtained to confirm the final concentrations. In neonates and in hearts that have sustained preoperative stress or ischemia, warm cardioplegic induction is used and followed by cold blood cardioplegia.

Administration Technique

In patients weighing 6 kg or less, cardioplegia is delivered through a pressure-transduced hand-held syringe. The initial cadioplegia infusion is at 80 mm Hg, with warm, high-potassium cardioplegia until the heart arrests (10 mL/kg). The infusion is subsequently changed to cold, high-potassium cardioplegia and the infusion slowed to maintain a pressure between 60 and 70 mm Hg until a total of 30 mL/kg is delivered. If circulatory arrest is used, additional cardioplegic infusions are not administered until the end of the arrest period. In other patients, low-potassium cardioplegia (15 mL/kg) maintenance doses are given every 20 minutes at 60 to 70 mm Hg. Be-

TABLE 1.
Cardioplegic Solutions

Type of Solution	Amount Administered
High-potassium arresting solution	
5% Dextrose 0.2 sodium chloride	500 mL
Tromethamine solution 1/3M	200 mL
Citrate phosphate dextrose solution	50 mL
Potassium chloride (2 mEq/cc)	30 mL
Low-potassium maintenance and warm reperfusate solution	
5% Dextrose 0.2 sodium chloride	500 mL
Tromethamine solution 1/3M	200 mL
Citrate phosphate dextrose solution	50 mL
Potassium chloride (2 mEq/cc)	15 mL
Modified warm blood induction/reperfusion solution	
5% Dextrose 0.2 sodium chloride	485 mL
Tromethamine solution 1/3M	200 mL
Citrate phosphate dextrose solution	50 mL
Potassium chloride (2 mEq/cc)	15 mL
Aspartate/glutamate 0.46M	250 mL

tween infusions, systemic perfusion pressure is kept at 35 to 50 mm Hg to reduce noncoronary collateral flow, thereby lowering cardioplegic washout. Should cardiac activity resume prior to scheduled cardioplegia doses, an additional infusion is given to induce arrest, the perfusate is cooled further, and the systemic flow is reduced to slow cardioplegic washout by noncoronary collateral flow. Cold saline is used to provide topical hypothermia between cardioplegia doses. Ice is avoided to prevent phrenic nerve injury.

At the end of the intracardiac portion of the operation, warm ($\geq 32°$ C) glutamate/aspartate–enriched cardioplegia is given. A total of 15 mL/kg is administered at a pressure of 50 mm Hg. Lidocaine (2 mg/kg) is administered systemically prior to cross-clamp release.

In children weighing over 6 kg, the technique is altered somewhat. Cardioplegia is delivered into the aortic root by pressure-monitored pumping rather than hand-held infusion. Warm induction is limited to those hearts under preoperative stress or ischemia and is given for 2 minutes followed by 3 minutes of cold, high-potassium cardioplegia. Additional changes include administration of initial cardioplegia dose at 80 mm Hg for 3 minutes, timed maintenance infusion of 1 to 2 minutes rather than volume-dependent infusions, and timed warm aspartate/glutamate–enriched blood reperfusion for 3 minutes. As an adjunct to maintenance cardioplegia doses, retrograde coronary

TABLE 2.
Final Composition of Cardioplegic Solutions When Mixed
With Blood

Type of Solution and Composition	Amount of Each Component
High-potassium solution	
pH	7.5–7.6
Ca++	0.8mM/L
K+	20–24 mEq/L
Osmolarity	380–400 mOsm
Hematocrit	80% of pump hematocrit
Low-potassium solution (non–glutamate/	
aspartate)	
pH	7.5–7.6
Ca++	0.8mM/L
K+	8–10 mEq/L
Osmolarity	340–360 mOsm
Hematocrit	80% of pump hematocrit
Modified warm blood induction/	
reperfusion solution	
pH	7.5–7.6
Ca++	0.8mM/L (neonate); 0.5mML (Older child)
K+	8–10 mEq/L
Aspartate	13mM
Glutamate	13mM
Osmolarity	380–400 mOsm
Hematocrit	80% of pump hematocrit

sinus cardioplegia may be given when the repair is complex, lengthy, and the heart has been preoperatively stressed. When used, retrograde infusions are alternated every 10 minutes with aortic root infusions.

Cardiopulmonary Bypass Technique

Cardiopulmonary bypass may be conducted with deep (18° C) or moderate (24 to 26° C) systemic hypothermia as dictated by the planned repair. For most operations, we prefer bypass with deep hypothermia and low flow to prevent neurologic complications associated with extended circulatory arrest. Moderate hypothermia is used for less complicated repairs. In either case, cardioplegic arrest is induced before cooling below 26° C to prevent hypothermic contracture. Low flow is used between cardioplegia doses and full flow is reinstituted while cardioplegia is being administered to prevent systemic acidosis. The technique may be altered depending on the repair. For example, in the arterial switch procedure, we use deep hypothermic perfusion at low flow with a brief (5-minute) period of circulatory arrest to close the atrial septal or ventricular septal defect. As the repair approaches completion, the patient is rewarmed and a dose of warm cardioplegia is given before cross-clamp release. Pump flow is slowed to reduce systemic perfusion pressure to 40 mm Hg or less prior to and for 2 minutes after cross-clamp release. The heart is kept well vented until it has recovered in order to avoid distention.

Results

Ideally, a prospective, randomized trial is required to compare different methods of myocardial protection. Unfortunately, such a study is not available at this time. A retrospective review, however, is helpful in giving an indication of the efficacy of the myocardial protection. Between January 1989 and December 1990, 293 pediatric open heart procedures were performed at the University of California, Los Angeles. The early (<30 day or hospital) mortality was 3.8% (11 out of 293 patients). The early mortality for the arterial switch procedure in neonates was 5% (1 out of 20 patients). The Fontan procedure, in which systemic ventricular function is critical to survival, was performed in 35 patients, with 2 (6%) early deaths. Truncus arteriosus was repaired in 11 infants, with 1 early death (9%) in a patient with an interrupted aortic arch.

Although improved results of pediatric cardiac surgical procedures are dependent on successful surgical repair,[120] myocardial protection plays a critical role. We feel that the techniques outlined contribute significantly to improved patient outcome.

Conclusions

Optimal pediatric myocardial protection requires an understanding of both the unique properties of the developing myocardium and the unique pathophysiology of congenital heart disease. Pediatric myocardium is structurally, metabolically, and functionally different from adult myocardium. In addition, the heart is often under stress from one or more of the following states: hypoxemia, ischemia, pressure overload, or volume overload. In addition, the heart may have been affected chronically by hypertrophy and cyanosis. Continued investigations to determine the immature heart's response to acute and chronic stress and to determine optimal methods to protect these hearts will lead to improved postoperative cardiac function and, ultimately, to improved patient survival.

References

1. Anversa P, Olivetti G, Loud A: Morphometric study of early postnatal development in the left and right ventricular myocardium of the rat. I. Hypertro-

phy, hyperplasia, and binucleation of myocytes. *Circ Res* 1980; 46:495–502.

2. Korecky B, Rakusan K: Normal and hypertrophic growth of the rat heart: Changes in cell dimensions and number. *Am J Physiol* 1978; 234:H123–128.

3. Page E, Early J, Power B: Normal growth of ultrastructures in rat left ventricular myocardial cells. *Circ Res* 1974; (suppl II):34–35.

4. Gotoh T: Quantitative studies on the ultrastructural differentiation and growth of mammalian cardiac muscle cells. The atria and ventricles of the cat. *Acta Anat (Basel)* 1983; 115:168–177.

5. Hirakow R, Krause W: Postnatal differentiation of ventricular myocardial cells of the opossum and T-tubule formation. *Cell Tissue Res* 1980; 210:95–100.

6. Legato M: Ultrastructural changes during normal growth in the dog and rat ventricular myofiber, in Lieberman M, Sano T (eds): *Developmental and Physiological Correlates of Cardiac Muscle*. New York, Raven Press, 1975, pp 249–273.

7. Legato M: Cellular mechanisms of normal growth in the mammalian heart. I. Qualitative and quantitative features of ventricular architecture in the dog from birth to five months of age. *Circ Res* 1979; 44:250–262.

8. Park I, Michael LH, Driscoll DJ: Comparative response to the developing canine myocardium to inotropic agents. *Am J Physiol* 1982; 242:H13–H18.

9. Legato M: Cellular mechanisms of normal growth in the mammalian heart. II. A quantitative and qualitative comparison between the right and left ventricular myocytes in the dog from birth to five months of age. *Circ Res* 1979; 44:263–279.

10. Smith H, Page E: Ultrastructural changes in rabbit heart mitochondria during the perinatal period. Neonatal transition to aerobic metabolism. *Dev Biol* 1977; 57:109–117.

11. Forbes M, Sperelakis N: The presence of transverse and axial tubules in the ventricular myocardium of embryonic and neonatal guinea pigs. *Cell Tissue Res* 1976; 166:83–90.

12. Colgan J, Lazarus M, Sachs H: Post-natal development of the normal and cardiomyopathic syrian hamster heart: A quantitative electron microscopic study. *J Mol Cell Cardiol* 1978; 10:43–54.

13. Hopkins S, McCutcheon E, Wekstein D: Postnatal changes in rat ventricular function. *Circ Res* 1973; 32:685–691.

14. Girard JR: Metabolic fuels of the fetus. *Isr J Med Sci* 1975; 11:591–600.

15. Battaglia FC, Meschia G: Principle substrates of fetal metabolism. *Physiol Rev* 1978; 58:499–527.

16. Barrie SE, Harris P: Myocardial enzyme activities in guinea pigs during development. *Am J Physiol* 1977; 233:H707–H710.

17. Jones CT (ed): *The Biochemical Development of the Fetus and Neonate*. New York, Elsevier Biomedical Press, 1982.

18. Smith HE, Page E: Ultrastructural changes in rabbit heart mitochondria during the perinatal period. *Dev Biol* 1977; 57:109–117.

19. Clark CM Jr: Characterization of glucose metabolism in the isolated rat heart during fetal and early neonatal development. *Diabetes* 1973; 22:41–49.

20. Clark CM Jr: Carbohydrate metabolism in the isolated fetal rat heart. *Am J Physiol* 1971; 220:583–588.

21. Shelley H: Glycogen reserves and their changes at birth and in anoxia. *Br Med Bull* 1961; 17:137–143.

22. Hoerter J: Changes in the sensitivity to hypoxia and glucose deprivation in

the isolated perfused rabbit heart during perinatal development. *Pflugers Arch* 1976; 363:1–6.

23. Gennser G: Influence of hypoxia and glucose on contractility of papillary muscles from adult and neonatal rabbits. *Biol Neonate* 1972; 21:90.

24. Yee ES, Ebert PA: Effect of ischemia on ventricular function, compliance, and edema in immature and adult canine hearts. *Surg Forum* 1979; 30:250.

25. Bove EL, Stammers AH: Recovery of left ventricular function after hypothermic global ischemia: Age-related differences in the isolated working rabbit heart. *J Thorac Cardiovasc Surg* 1986; 91:115–122.

26. Opie LH: The glucose hypothesis: Relation to acute myocardial ischemia. *J Mol Cell Cardiol* 1970; 1:107.

27. Gelli MG, Enhorning G, Hultman E, et al: Glucose infusion in pregnant rabbit and its effect on glycogen content and activity of fetal heart under anoxia. *Acta Paediatr Scand* 1968; 57:209.

28. Langer GA, Frank JS, Nudd LM, et al: Sialic acid: Effect of removal on calcium exchangeability of cultured heart cells. *Science* 1976; 193:1013–1015.

29. Crevey BJ, Langer GA, Frank JS: Role of calcium in maintenance of rabbit myocardial cell membrane structural and functional integrity. *J Mol Cell Cardiol* 1978; 10:1081–1100.

30. Langer GA, Frank JS, Philipson KD: Ultrastructure and calcium exchange of the sarcolemma, sarcoplasmic reticulum, and mitochondria of the myocardium. *Pharmacol Ther* 1982; 16:331–376.

31. Langer GA: Calcium and the myocardium: Physiologic and pathologic processes, in Karp RB, Kouchoukos NT, Laks H, et al (eds): *Advances in Cardiac Surgery,* vol 1. Chicago, Year Book Medical Publishers, Inc, 1990, pp 55–75.

32. Nakanishi T, Seguchi M, Takao A: Development of the myocardial contractile system. *Experientia* 1988; 44:936–944.

33. Bers DM, Langer GA: Uncoupling cation effects on cardiac contractility and sarcolemma Ca^{+2} binding. *Am J Physiol* 1979; 237:H332–H341.

34. Corno AF, Bethencourt DM, Laks H, et al: Myocardial protection in the neonatal heart: A comparison of topical hypothermia and crystalloid and blood cardioplegic solutions. *J Thorac Cardiovasc Surg* 1987; 93:163–172.

35. Kempsford RD, Hearse DJ: Protection of the immature myocardium during global ischemia: A comparison of four clinical cardioplegic solutions in the rabbit heart. *J Thorac Cardiovasc Surg* 1989; 97:856–863.

36. Zweng TN, Iannettoni MD, Bove EL, et al: The concentration of calcium in neonatal cardioplegia. *Ann Thorac Surg* 1990; 50:262–267.

37. Friedman WF: The intrinsic physiologic properties of the developing heart. *Prog Cardiovasc Dis* 1972; 15:87–111.

38. Romero TE, Friedman WF: Limited left ventricular response to volume overload in the neonatal period: A comparative study with the adult animal. *Pediatr Res* 1979; 13:910–915.

39. Romero T, Covell J, Friedman WFA: Comparison of pressure-volume relations of the fetal, newborn, and adult heart. *Am J Physiol* 1972; 222:1285.

40. Teitel D, Chin T, Heyman MA: Developmental changes in myocardial contractility (abstract). J Am Coll Cardiol 1983; 1:1183.

41. Bull C, Cooper J, Stark J: Cardioplegic protection of the child's heart. *J Thorac Cardiovasc Surg* 1984; 88:287–293.

42. Nido P, Mickle D, Wilson G, et al: Inadequate myocardial protection with cold cardioplegic arrest during repair of tetralogy of Fallot. *J Thorac Cardiovasc Surg* 1988; 95:223–229.

43. Yano Y, Braimbridge M, Hearse D: Protection of the pediatric myocardium. Differential susceptibility to ischemic injury of the neonatal rat heart. *J Thorac Cardiovasc Surg* 1987; 94:887–896.

44. Grice W, Konishi T, Apstein C: Resistance of neonatal myocardium to injury during normothermic and hypothermic ischemic arrest and reperfusion. *Circulation* 1987; 76(suppl V):V150–V155.

45. Baker J, Boerboom L, Olinger G: Age-related changes in the ability of hypothermia and cardioplegia to protect ischemic rabbit myocardium. *J Thorac Cardiovasc Surg* 1988; 96:717–724.

46. Jarmakani J, Nakazawa M, Nagatomo T, et al: Effect of hypoxia on mechanical function in the neonatal mammalian heart. *Am J Physiol* 1978; 235:H469–474.

47. Jarmakani J, Nakazawa M, Nagatomo T, et al: Effect of hypoxia on myocardial high-energy phosphates in the neonatal mammalian heart. *Am J Physiol* 1978; 235:H475–481.

48. Lee J, Halloran K, Taylor J, et al: Coronary flow and myocardial metabolism in newborn lambs: Effect of hypoxia and acidemia. *Am J Physiol* 1973; 224:1381.

49. Downing S, Talner N, Gardner T: Influences of arterial oxygen tensin and pH on cardiac function in the newborn lamb. *Am J Physiol* 1966; 211:1203.

50. Scheuer J, Shaver J, Kroetz F, et al: Myocardial metabolism in cyanotic congenital heart disease studied by arteriovenous differences of lactase, phosphate, and potassium at rest and during atrial pacing. *Circulation* 1976; 55:647.

51. Guarnieri C, Flamigni F, Caldarera C: Role of oxygen in the cellular damage induced by re-oxygenation of hypoxic heart. *J Mol Cell Biol* 1980; 12:797.

52. Hearse D, Humphrey S, Bullock G: The oxygen paradox and the calcium paradox: Two facets of the same problem? *J Mol Cell Biol* 1978; 10:641.

53. Scheuer J: Studies in the human heart exposed to chronic hypoxemia. *Cardiology* 1972; 56:215.

54. Dawes G, Mott J, Shelley H: The importance of cardiac glycogen for the maintenance of life in fetal lambs and newborn animals during anoxia. *J Physiol (Lond)* 1959; 146:516–538.

55. Silverman NA, Kohler J, Levitsky S, et al: Chronic hypoxemia depresses global ventricular function and predisposes to the depletion of high-energy phosphates during cardioplegic arrest: Implications for surgical repair of cyanotic congenital heart defects. *Ann Thorac Surg* 1984; 347:304–308.

56. Fujiwara T, Kurtts T, Anderson W, et al: Myocardial protection in cyanotic neonatal lambs. *J Thorac Cardiovasc Surg* 1988; 96:700–710.

57. Tulner N, Hellenbrand W, Kleinman C, et al: The functional and structural diagnosis of congenital heart disease, in Glenn WWL (ed): *Thoracic and Cardiovascular Surgery*, ed 4. Norwalk, Conn, Appleton-Century-Crofts, 1983, pp 597–625.

58. Wong RS, Baum VC, Sangwan S: Truncus arteriosus: Recognition and therapy of intraoperative cardiac ischemia. *Anesthesiology* 1991; 74:378–380.

59. Teitel D, Sidi D, Chin T, et al: Developmental changes in myocardial contractile reserve in the lamb. *Pediatr Res* 1985; 19:948–955.

60. Grossman W, Barry W: Diastolic pressure-volume relations in the diseased heart. *Fed Proc* 1980; 39:148–155.

61. Gaasch W, Levine H, Quinones M, et al: Left ventricular compliance: Mechanisms and clinical implications. *Am J Cardiol* 1976; 38:645–653.

62. Peyton RB, Hones RN, Attarian D, et al: Depressed high-energy phosphate

content in hypertrophied ventricles of animals and man. *Ann Surg* 1982; 196:278.

63. Sink J, Pellon G, Currie W, et al: Response of hypertrophied myocardium to ischemia. *J Thorac Cardiovasc Surg* 1981; 81:865.
64. Buckberg G: Left ventricular subendocardial necrosis. *Ann Thorac Surg* 1977; 24:379–393.
65. Klopfenstein H, Rudolph A: Postnatal changes in the circulation and responses to volume loading in sheep. *Circ Res* 1978; 42:839–845.
66. Downing S, Talner N, Gardner T: Ventricular function in the newborn lamb. *Am J Physiol* 1965; 208:931–937.
67. Lees M, Bristow J, Griswold H, et al: Relative hypermetabolism in infants with congenital heart disease and undernutrition. *Pediatrics* 1965; 36:183–191.
68. Hahn C, Simonet F: Resistance and tolerance of the myocardium to ischemia. *J Cardiovasc Surg (Torino)* 1975; 16:265–267.
69. Morales A, Fine G, Taber R: Cardiac surgery and myocardial necrosis. *Arch Pathol* 1967; 83:71–79.
70. Taber R, Morales A, Fine G: Myocardial necrosis and the postoperative low-cardiac-output syndrome. *Ann Thorac Surg* 1967; 4:12–28.
71. Hottenrott C, Maloney J, Buckberg G: Studies of the effects of ventricular fibrillation on the adequacy of regional myocardial flow: I. Electrical vs. spontaneous fibrillation. *J Thorac Cardiovasc Surg* 1974; 68:615–625.
72. Hottenrott C, Buckberg G: Studies on the effects of ventricular fibrillation on the adequacy of regional myocardial flow: II. Effects of ventricular distention. *J Thorac Cardiovasc Surg* 1974; 68:626–633.
73. Katz AM: Effects of interrupted coronary flow upon myocardial metabolism and contractility. *Prog Cardiovasc Dis* 1968; 10:450.
74. Brown A, Braimbridge M, Darracott S, et al: An experimental evaluation of continuous normothermic, intermittent hypothermic, and intermittent normothermic coronary perfusion. *Thorax* 1974; 29:38–50.
75. Engelman R, Adler S, Gouge T, et al: The effect of normothermic anoxic arrest and ventricular fibrillation on the coronary blood flow distribution of the pig. *J Thorac Cardiovasc Surg* 1975; 69:858–869.
76. Hearse D, Stewart D, Chain E: Recovery from cardiac bypass and elective cardiac arrest: The metabolic consequences of various cardioplegic procedures in the isolated rat heart. *Circ Res* 1974; 35:448–457.
77. Levitsky S, Wright R, Rao K, et al: Does intermittent coronary perfusion offer greater myocardial protection than continuous aortic cross-clamping? *Surgery* 1977; 82:51–59.
78. Bercot M, Deloche A, Piwnica A, et al: Selective cardiac hypothermia versus coronary perfusion: A study of ischemic complications in two series of 100 consecutive valvular patients. *J Cardiovasc Surg (Torino)* 1975; 16:232–240.
79. Braimbridge M, Darracott S, Clement A, et al: Myocardial deterioration during aortic valve replacement assessed by cellular biological tests. *J Thorac Cardiovasc Surg* 1973; 66:241–246.
80. Cankovic-Darracott S, Braimbridge M, Williams B, et al: Myocardial preservation during aortic valve surgery: Assessment of five techniques by cellular chemical and biophysical methods. *J Thorac Cardiovasc Surg* 1977; 73:699–706.
81. Follette D, Mulder D, Maloney J, et al: Advantages of blood cardioplegia over

continuous coronary perfusion or intermittent ischemia: Experimental and clinical study. *J Thorac Cardiovasc Surg* 1978; 76:604–619.

82. Baker J, Boerboom L, Olinger G: Age-related changes in the ability of hypothermia and cardioplegia to protect ischemic rabbit myocardium. *J Thorac Cardiovasc Surg* 1988; 96:717–724.

83. Watanabe H, Yokosawa T, Eguchi S, et al: Functional and metabolic protection of the neonatal, myocardium and ischemia. *J Thorac Cardiovasc Surg* 1989; 97:50–58.

84. Baker J, Boerboom L, Olinger G: Cardioplegia-induced damage to ischemic immature myocardium is independent of oxygen availability. *Ann Thorac Surg* 1990; 50:934–939.

85. del Nido PJ, Mickle DA, Wilson GJ, et al: Inadequate myocardial protection with cold cardioplegic arrest during repair of tetralogy of Fallot. *J Thorac Cardiovasc Surg* 1988; 95:223–229.

86. Sawa Y, Matsuda H, Shimazaki Y, et al: Ultrastructural assessment of the infant myocardium receiving crystalloid cardioplegia. *Circulation* 1987; 76 (suppl V):141.

87. Konishi T, Apstein C: Comparison of three cardioplegic solutions during hypothermic ischemic arrest in neonatal blood-perfused rabbit hearts. *J Thorac Cardiovasc Surg* 1989; 98:1132–1137.

88. Helmsworth JA, Kaplan S, Clark LC, et al: Myocardial injury associated with asystole induced with potassium citrate. *Ann Surg* 1959; 149:200–206.

89. Takamoto S, Levine F, LaRaia P, et al: Comparison of single-dose and multiple-dose crystalloid and blood potassium cardioplegia during prolonged hypothermic aortic occlusion. *J Thorac Cardiovasc Surg* 1980; 79:19–28.

90. Chen Y, Lin Y: Comparison of blood cardioplegia to electrolyte cardioplegia on the effectiveness of preservation of right atrial myocardium: Mitochondrial morphometric study. *Ann Thorac Surg* 1985; 39:134–138.

91. Feindel C, Tiat G, Wilson G, et al: Multidose blood versus crystalloid cardioplegia: Comparison by quantitative assessment of irreversible myocardial injury. *J Thorac Cardiovasc Surg* 1984; 87:585–595.

92. Engelman R, Rousou J, Dobbs W, et al: The superiority of blood cardioplegia in myocardial preservation. *Circulation* 1980; 62(suppl I):I-62–6.

93. Catinella F, Cunningham J, Knopp E, et al: Preservation of myocardial ATP: Comparison of blood vs. crystalloid cardioplegia. *Chest* 1983; 4:650–654.

94. Illes R, Silverman N, Krukenkamp I, et al: The efficacy of blood cardioplegia is not due to oxygen delivery. *J Thorac Cardiovasc Surg* 1989; 98:1051–1056.

95. Singh A, Farrugia R, Teplitz C, et al: Electrolyte versus blood cardioplegia: Randomized clinical and myocardial ultrastructural study. *Ann Thorac Surg* 1982; 33:218–227.

96. Iverson L, Young J, Ennix C, et al: Myocardial protection: A comparison of cold blood and cold crystalloid cardioplegia. *J Thorac Cardiovasc Surg* 1984; 87:509–516.

97. Fremes S, Christakis G, Weisel R, et al: A clinical trial of blood and crystalloid cardioplegia. *J Thorac Cardiovasc Surg* 1984; 88:726–741.

98. Beyersdorf F, Krause E, Sarai K, et al: Clinical evaluation of hypothermic ventricular fibrillation, multi-dose blood cardioplegia, and single-dose Bretschneider cardioplegia in coronary surgery. *Thorac Cardiovasc Surg* 1990; 38:20.

99. Rosenkranz ER, Vinten-Johansen J, Buckberg GD, et al: Benefits of normo-

thermic induction of cardioplegia in energy depleted hearts, with maintenance of arrest by multidose cold blood cardioplegic infusion. *J Thorac Cardiovasc Surg* 1982; 84:667–677.

100. Rosenkranz ER, Okamoto F, Buckberg GD, et al: Safety of prolonged aortic
clamping with blood cardioplegia. III. Aspartate enrichment of glutamate
blood cardioplegia in energy depleted hearts after ischemic and reperfusion
injury. *J Thorac Cardiovasc Surg* 1986; 91:428–435.

101. Brown A, Braimbridge M, Niles M, et al: The effect of excessively high perfusion pressures on the histology, histochemistry, birefringence, and function of
the myocardium. *J Thorac Cardiovasc Surg* 1969; 58:655–663.

102. Shaw R, Mosher P, Ross J, et al: Physiologic principles of coronary perfusion.
J Thorac Cardiovasc Surg 1962; 44:608–616.

103. Haas G, Bhuta S, Laks H: The effect of elevated cardioplegia infusion pressures on the neonate's heart. Submitted for publication.

104. Haas G, Laks H, Bhuta S: Ventricular distension and myocardial injury in the
neonatal heart. Submitted for publication.

105. Zureikat H: Collateral vessels between the coronary and bronchial arteries in
patients with cyanotic congenital heart disease. *Am J Cardiol* 1980;
45:599–603.

106. Brazier J, Hottenrott C, Buckberg G: Noncoronary collateral myocardial
blood flow. *Ann Thorac Surg* 1975; 19:426.

107. Ferguson TB, Smith PK, Buhrman WC, et al: Studies on the physiology of
the conduction system during hyperkalemic, hypothermic cardioplegic arrest.
Surg Forum 1983; 34:302–304.

108. Lucchessi BR: Role of leukocytes in ischemic heart disease: Pathophysiologic
role in myocardial ischemia and coronary artery reperfusion, in Mehta JL
(ed): *Thrombosis and Platelets in Myocardial Ischemia*. Philadelphia, FA
Davis, 1987, pp 35–48.

109. Engler RL, Schmid-Schonbein GW, Pavelec RS: Leukocyte capillary plugging in myocardial ischemia and reperfusion in the dog. *Am J Physiol* 1983;
3:98–111.

110. Follette D, Fey K, Buckberg G, et al: Reducing postischemic damage by temporary modification of reperfusate calcium, potassium, pH, and osmolarity. *J
Thorac Cardiovasc Surg* 1981; 82:221–238.

111. Schmid-Schonbein GW: Capillary plugging by granulocytes and the no-reflow phenomenon in the microcirculation. *Fed Proc* 1987; 46:2397–2401.

112. McCord JM: Superoxide radical: A link betwen reperfusion injury and inflammation. *Adv Free Radical Biol Med* 1986; 2:325–345.

113. Weiss SJ: Tissue destruction by neutrophils. *N Engl J Med* 1989;
320:365–376.

114. Stein D, Permut L, Drinkwater D, et al: Complete functional recovery after
24 hour heart preservation with University of Wisconsin solution and modified reperfusion. *Circulation,* in press.

115. Yamaguchi M, Imai M, Ohashi H, et al: Enhanced myocardial protection by
systemic deep hypothermia in children undergoing total correction of tetralogy of Fallot. *Ann Thorac Surg* 1986; 41:639–647.

116. Ganzel B, Katzmark S, Mavroudis C: Myocardial preservation in the neonate:
Beneficial effects of cardioplegia and systemic hypothermia on piglets undergoing cardiopulmonary bypass and myocardial ischemia. *J Thorac Cardiovasc Surg* 1988; 96:414–422.

117. Sakai T, Kurihara S: The rapid cooling contracture of toad cardiac muscles. *Jpn J Physiol* 1974; 24:649–666.
118. Konishi M, Kurihara S, Sakai T: Changes in intracellular calcium ion concentration induced by caffeine and rapid cooling in frog skeletal muscle fibers. *J Physiol (Lond)* 1985; 365:131–146.
119. Williams WG, Rebeyka IM, Tibshirani RJ, et al: Warm induction blood cardioplegia in the infant: A technique to avoid rapid cooling myocardial contracture. *J Thorac Cardiovasc Surg* 1990; 100:896–901.
120. Jonas RA, Krsna M, Sell JE, et al: Myocardial failure is a rare cause of death after pediatric cardiac surgery (abstract). *J Am Coll Cardiol* 1991; 17:110A.

Warm Heart Surgery: Theory and Current Practice

Samuel V. Lichtenstein, M.D., Ph.D.

Assistant Professor, Cardiovascular Surgery, St. Michael's Hospital; Department of Surgery, University of Toronto, Toronto, Ontario, Canada

James G. Abel, M.D., M.Sc.

Senior Resident, Cardiovascular Surgery, St. Michael's Hospital; Department of Surgery, University of Toronto, Toronto, Ontario, Canada

In Toronto in 1950, Dr. William Bigelow ushered in the era of open heart surgery under direct vision when he introduced systemic hypothermia for cerebral and myocardial protection.[1] Following this, advances in cardiac surgery paralleled technical developments that enabled surgeons to assume temporarily the physiologic functions of the heart and lungs. Total cardiopulmonary bypass with an in-line oxygenator permitted operation on the beating, continuously perfused heart.[2] Melrose[3] added elective pharmacologic cardiac arrest shortly thereafter, to provide a quiet operating field. Early results were disappointing, however,[4] and it was clear that the challenge of maintaining cardiac structure and physiologic integrity following arrest was substantial. Indeed, the ideal method of myocardial protection is still elusive, nearly 40 years later.

The importance of cardioplegic preservation in the operating room stems from the clinician's desire to afford the heart maximal protection from ischemic damage. It is accepted that cold arrest of the heart contributes to this goal by minimizing myocardial oxygen consumption (MVO_2) while conserving myocardial energy stores for subsequent cellular upkeep and repair. Debate now centers around the composition of both the cardioplegic solution and the reperfusate: what additives, if any, should be included in these solutions, the route and technique of infusion, and the optimal hypothermic temperature. Despite these controversies, the principles established by Bigelow and Melrose in the 1950s form the basis of the current standard approach to myocardial protection in cardiac surgery—*cold anaerobic arrest*.

Previous work has suggested that blood cardioplegia affords a higher degree of myocardial protection than does crystalloid.[5–9] In addition, hypothermia has a number of serious detrimental effects[10–15] that have not been well appreciated. These facts, and the central concept that the major reduction of myocardial oxygen requirements occurs with cardiac arrest, have led our group to initiate the clinical use of "continuous" warm blood cardioplegia[16] as an alternative method of myocardial protection during open heart surgery. This utilizes the principle of *warm aerobic arrest.*

Cardiac surgery with normothermic coronary perfusion is certainly not a new concept but one that has fallen into disrepute because it was always used in settings where myocardial oxygen demands were high, such as with a fibrillating or beating heart.[17] Prolonged normothermic ischemia greater than 45 minutes without rapid initial chemical arrest led to the occurrence of stone heart.[18] Apparently, normothermic coronary perfusion with blood combined with chemically induced electromechanical standstill has been overlooked as a viable possibility.

The initial, yet ongoing, goal of myocardial protection during cardiac surgery has been to prolong safe operating time by minimizing ischemic damage to the heart. This goal ultimately becomes an attempt to maintain myocardial energy supply at a level greater than its needs during the time of operation. Cardioplegic preservation must optimize the ratio of energy supply to consumption, and the capacity of the heart to utilize oxygen and substrate, whether aerobic or anaerobic. This capacity will be determined by the temperature and composition of the perfusate, and the distribution, adequacy, and duration of the infusion.

This review outlines the historic, experimental, and theoretic precedents for our approach, and describes the technical aspects and initial encouraging clinical results.[19]

Hypothermia and Myocardial Oxygen Consumption

The use of hypothermia during open heart surgery antedates the development of cardiopulmonary bypass and has been employed since the discovery by Bigelow that temperature and whole-body metabolic rate were directly related.[1] He showed that in animals anesthetized with thiopental (Pentothal) and cooled to 20° C by surface immersion, and in whom shivering was controlled by curare, the heart could be excluded safely from the rest of the circulation to permit operation for up to 25 minutes. John Lewis of the University of Minnesota used Bigelow's technique to close a large atrial septal defect in a 5-year-old girl, performing the first intracardiac operation under direct vision with a dry operating field in 1952.[20] Others followed suit, using the same method to close similar atrial defects and relieve pulmonary outflow obstruction.[21] Although the true goal of this technique was cerebral protection, the success of these early cardiac operations, which previously had been limited to 2 minutes of inflow occlusion, led to a surge of interest in the use of hypothermia for cardiac surgery that has persisted to the present day. Strategies to improve myocardial cooling, such as topical hypothermia,[22, 23] cooling jackets, high-volume crystalloid cardioplegia,[24] retrograde delivery of hypothermic cardioplegia via the coronary sinus,[25] and continuous administration of cold cardioplegia,[9] have been adopted to improve the extent and distribution of cooling. A large body of evidence demonstrating that hypothermia diminishes MVO_2, thereby increasing the tolerance to ischemia, has established hypothermia as the single most important component of myocardial protection.[26, 27] This concept is so ingrained in the practice of cardiac surgery that two major pathophysiologic effects of hypothermia have not been appreciated or have been ignored.

The first is that hypothermia induces a number of changes that may result in significant cellular damage. The second relates to the observation that the oxygen consumption of an arrested normothermic heart is not very different from that of an arrested hypothermic heart. We will discuss each of these in some detail.

Hypothermia has been shown to inactivate both the sodium-potassium adenosine triphosphatase (ATPase) and calcium ATPase enzyme systems of the sarcoplasmic reticulum.[28] The impairment in cell volume control through ionic changes results in cell swelling and mitochondrial rupture.[12, 13, 28] Hypothermia induces cell membrane phase transition[14] by decreasing the fluidity of the membrane lipid layer and the functional capacity of membrane-bound enzymes, impairing membrane electrical and transport function.[29, 30] Injury results as temperatures decrease below 25° C because of ion pump inactivation, unfolding and denaturization of proteins through the disruption of covalent bonds, and loss of tertiary structure. As various ion complexes precipitate out at different temperatures, fluctuating intracellular pH and osmotic shifts are deleterious to cellular integrity.[12, 31] One could conclude, therefore, that other than its apparent ability to decrease MVO_2 and energy requirements somewhat, most other effects of hypothermia are at the very least potentially harmful.

Although these detrimental effects of hypothermia have been well appreciated in the physiologic literature, these concepts have not had an impact on surgical practice. This has been due largely to the surgeon's belief that the oxygen requirements of a hypothermic heart are so markedly lower than those of a normothermic heart that its benefit (making operative intervention possible) outweighs its harm.

It generally is not well recognized that 80% to 90% of myocardial energy consumption is due to the mechanical work of pumping blood.[32, 33] Although it had been appreciated for some time that myocardial fiber shortening and cardiac work, inotropic state, and the frequency of contraction were important determinants of MVO_2 in the working heart, their relative contribution was not easily determined until Melrose reported that electromechanical activity could be abolished with the potassium ion.[3] By perfusing the chemically stilled heart with blood, Bernhard et al.,[34] more recently Buckberg et al.,[35] and others[36, 37] have demonstrated that electromechanical arrest of a working heart at normothermia decreases O_2 consumption by nearly 90% with only a slight further decrease attributable to lowering myocardial temperature to 11° C (Fig 1). In this regard, it should be pointed out that, during hypothermia, a calculated decrease in myocardial O_2 consumption, particularly at constant coronary flow as in the aforementioned experiments, may be due more to a decrease in O_2 delivery to the

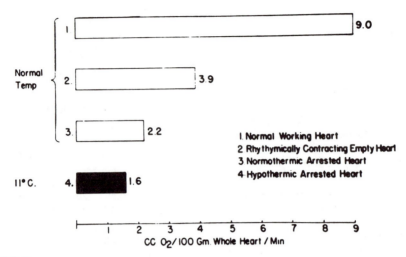

FIG 1.
Oxygen utilization of working, nonworking, and arrested hearts at normothermia, compared to hearts in hypothermic arrest. Note that the single largest decrease in myocardial O_2 consumption is due to electromechanical arrest at normothermia, with only a meager further decrease with profound hypothermia (11° C). (From Bernhard WF, Schwarz HF, Malick NP: *Ann Surg* 1961; 153:43–51. Used by permission.)

tissue caused by an increase in the affinity of hemoglobin for O_2 at low temperatures[38] rather than to a decrease in actual myocardial O_2 needs (see later).

The normal left ventricle, pumping adequate blood to the periphery, consumes approximately 9 to 10 mL of O_2 per 100 g per minute.[33] The energy for electrical activation is negligible and less than 1% of total MVO_2.[39] The basal metabolism required for the maintenance of ionic gradients and organelle structure is approximately 1 mL of O_2 per 100 g per minute and is independent of end-diastolic volume,[40] catecholamine state,[40] ionic calcium,[40] and even, to a large degree, temperature.[34] By far the largest decrease in MVO_2 is provided for by cessation of electromechanical work, and since this can be achieved easily with potassium, the conventional need for hypothermia must be reexamined. Braunwald[32] has shown that in the potassium-arrested heart, lowering temperatures to 20° C could reduce MVO_2 from normothermic arrest by only a further 10%. Below this temperature, debilitating effects of cooling the heart tissue have been noted extensively. Lower temperatures inhibit different biochemical pathways with varying efficiency,[10] and thus can induce an imbalance in homeostasis within the cell. Of particular importance is blocking of the glycolytic pathway at temperatures in the 10° C range,[10] effectively shutting down adenosine triphosphate (ATP) production. Thus, although lower temperatures decrease O_2 demand somewhat, they also decrease or even halt energy production. This permits the cell only those energy stores remaining within it at the time of cooling. Similarly, the hypothermic cell cannot produce ATP efficiently if it subsequently is presented with oxygen after the arrest period,[41] and this further extends the duration of ischemia.[11] Other consequences of hypothermia, already discussed, include cell swelling and mitochondrial rupture due to ionic imbalance,[12, 13] cell membrane phase transition,[14] and eventual lactic acidosis as available oxygen supplies are consumed. Since all induced cellular damage in itself requires energy for repair,[15] it follows that marked cooling ($<15°$ C) in the chemically arrested heart may produce serious consequences that are not outweighed by the small decrease in energy demand.

Although hypothermia decreases basal cellular metabolism slightly, and thereby reduces myocardial O_2 requirements, interpretation of the effects of hypothermia on metabolic rate and MVO_2 has been confounded by its effect on electromechanical coupling. Hypothermia actually increases MVO_2 per beat due to an associated increase in contractility.[35] This is reflected in an increased E_{max} of the pressure-volume relationship with cooling.[42] In other words, if heart rate were kept constant, MVO_2 would increase nearly twofold as temperature approached $20°$ C (Fig 2). Thus, the diminished MVO_2 with cooling actually is due to a decrease in heart rate. If temperature is decreased below $20°$ C, heart rate slows to zero and a state of electromechanical arrest exists. It is the electromechanical arrest and not

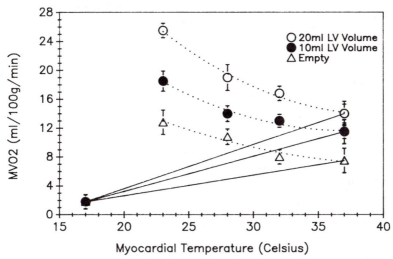

FIG 2.
Myocardial O_2 consumption vs. temperature in swine hearts. The *dotted lines* demonstrate the relationship between myocardial O_2 consumption and temperature at three loading conditions if the heart rate is maintained constant by pacing. Note the increase in myocardial O_2 consumption with hypothermia at a constant heart rate. If the heart rate is allowed to decrease with hypothermia (*solid lines*), electromechanical arrest is achieved below $20°$ C and this is associated with a correspondingly low myocardial O_2 consumption.

hypothermia that is associated with a marked reduction in O_2 requirements (see Fig 2). The marked decrease in O_2 consumption, therefore, is coincident with the decrease in temperature, but is a direct consequence of electromechanical arrest.

Normothermia and Oxygen Delivery

The discussion to this point has dealt with the "demand" side of the energy equation, i.e., how to decrease metabolic O_2 requirements of the heart. Since myocardial oxygen demand in the arrested heart is relatively independent of temperature, it seems logical to look at the "supply" side of the energy equation in an attempt to increase oxygen delivery through the use of oxygenated perfusates. Coetzee[43] has shown that rat hearts perfused with oxygenated crystalloid cardioplegia at 20° C possess greater postperfusion ATP levels and contractility than do similar nonoxygenated preparations. A comparable experiment at perfusion temperatures of 4° C showed no difference in preservation or function, suggesting inhibition of the glycolytic pathway at this temperature. These findings confirm Guyton's[44] experimental and clinical observations of a similar design. Thus, oxygenation of cardioplegic solutions seemingly is beneficial, provided the perfusate temperature is sufficiently high to allow the delivery and utilization of the added O_2.

The extent of tissue oxygenation is dependent upon both the oxygen-carrying capacity of the perfusate and its ability to release O_2. Crystalloid and colloid perfusates utilizing perfluorocarbons to carry O_2 possess a linear oxygen dissociation curve (ODC) and are only moderately able to deliver O_2 to the tissue, being limited by their own oxygen-carrying capacity. It is important to note that MVO_2 normally is determined indirectly from myocardial arteriovenous oxygen extraction. However, if the unloading of oxygen from hemoglobin is limited at low temperatures by the increased affinity of O_2 for hemoglobin,[38, 45] then actual MVO_2 at constant coronary blood flow may be underestimated. There is some experimental evidence for this that indicates high-energy phosphate loss and continued production of lactate and CO_2 by anaerobic glycolysis at low temperatures.[46, 48] Blood at normothermia, however, is better able to unload O_2 at the tissue site, due to both the sigmoidal shape of the hemoglobin-ODC and the influence of local pH and CO_2 changes on oxygen-hemoglobin affinity. Blood also provides excellent buffering ability and an optimal ionic and osmotic environment. Therefore, the use of blood as a protective perfusate with potassium arrest was suggested by Buckberg,[26] and has been studied extensively since. Magovern,[47] in comparing aerated crystalloid vs. blood cardioplegia, found that the ability of perfused canine hearts in vivo to return to the prearrest level of function was proportional to the perfusate temperature. Hearts perfused with blood at 4° C exhibited the poorest function after rewarming compared to aerated crystalloid, with function improving at higher temperatures. This suggests that blood cardioplegia is less effective than crystalloid in preventing ischemic damage if used at very low temperatures.

Consideration of the physical properties of blood allows for explanation of its ineffectiveness at low temperatures. Since cooler temperatures shift hemoglobin's ODC to the left, oxygen dissociation from the hemoglobin molecule, and thus the gradient for oxygen delivery to the tissue, is hindered during hypothermia. Also, the viscosity of blood increases with hypothermia, producing sludging and potential vessel occlusion at lower temperatures. Attempts to reduce sludging of cold blood perfusate through dilution have been only moderately successful,[49] and do not address the problem of hindering hemoglobin-oxygen dissociation.

Recent work dealing with cardioplegic washout with warm blood has shown that the use of normothermic blood upon initial reperfusion elicits a switchover from anaerobic to aerobic metabolism, and an improvement in intracellular high-energy phosphate concentration.[50, 51] These effects were not observed with hypothermic saline reperfusion. In an elegant series of experiments in isolated rat hearts, Hearse et al.[52] demonstrated that electromechanical arrest maintained by normothermic hyperkalemic continuous perfusion was superior to any other form of myocardial protection tested and resulted in recovery of myocardial function to 115% of the pre-arrest control value, with an increase in myocardial energy stores to 170% of control. Rosenkranz[53] and Peyton[54] emphasized the potential benefits of maintaining aerobic metabolism in the arrested heart with warm blood cardioplegia induction and terminal warm blood cardioplegia before removal of the aortic cross-clamp. All of these experiments point to a reinstatement of homeostatic metabolism with warm blood infusion—reversing the combination of decreased delivery and decreased capacity for utilization by the tissues at low temperatures.

Rationale for Warm Heart Surgery

Based on the literature and reasoning cited previously, our group has considered the effects of the use of potassium-containing blood cardioplegia at normothermic temperatures as an adequate perfusate for the prevention of ischemia. Logically, the optimal temperature at which blood cardioplegia should be administered is 37° C, since all exploitable biochemical and biophysical aspects of blood for organ perfusion are employed at this temperature in vivo. At 37° C, oxygen delivery and perfusion of heart tissue is maximal, while the detrimental effects of hypothermia are avoided. Chemical arrest with warm blood perfusion, without contraction, theoretically should allow intracellular aerobic energy production through metabolism of glucose and oxygen to be redirected to cellular repair.

Continuous aerobic perfusion of the arrested heart is the theoretic ideal state that maximizes oxygen supply and minimizes demand. As will be described later, in procedures other than coronary bypass surgery, virtually continuous antegrade or retrograde perfusion of the heart can be achieved. The cardioplegic blood flow rate required to supply the actual requirements of the arrested normothermic heart can be calculated readily. The calculation uses conservative estimates of hemoglobin, oxygen extraction ratio, and dissolved oxygen concentration to overestimate the cardioplegic flow required. Assuming a hemoglobin of 8 g/dL, an oxygen saturation of 100%, and neglecting dissolved O_2, the oxygen content (1.34 mL of O_2 per gram of hemoglobin) is approximately 11 mL of O_2 per 100 mL of cardioplegia. Coronary sinus oxygen saturation in resting human volunteers with coronary artery disease has been measured at 35% to 45%,[55] corresponding to an O_2 extraction of 60%, or about 6 mL of O_2 per 100 mL of cardioplegia in this example. For a heart of 300 g, basal MVO_2 after chemical arrest at normothermia is about 1 mL of O_2 per 100 g per minute; therefore, calculated MVO_2 is 3 mL of O_2 per minute. At a 60% extraction ratio, this demand is met easily, assuming uniform distribution, by a flow of 50 mL/min. A severely hypertrophic heart of 600 g would require a flow of less than 100 mL/min at this extraction ratio to meet basal oxygen requirements.

One might think that the administration of warm blood cardioplegia potentially requires a continuous flow of blood to avoid ischemic damage. The technical constraints of coronary artery surgery may necessitate on occasion either an interruption in global perfusion, or local vessel control, which results in a transient period of normothermic regional or global ischemia and potential reperfusion injury. Intuitively, this would seem particularly detrimental; however, as discussed earlier, there is only a slight decrease in MVO_2 in hearts arrested cold compared to those arrested warm. This implies that, as during intermittent hypothermic cardioplegia, equally safe durations of ischemia (<15 min) are possible with warm electromechanical arrest, as was demonstrated originally by Melrose.[3] Warm blood cardioplegia, therefore, can be administered intermittently if necessary, with safety. The calculated oxygen debt, assuming a constant metabolic rate of 1 mL of O_2 per 100 g per minute, for a 15-minute period of ischemic arrest in a 300-g heart is 45 mL of O_2. A similarly arrested heart at 15° C would have at best an O_2 debt of 20 mL. This oxygen debt very likely can be repaid more easily at normothermia than can a slightly smaller debt at hypothermia. A successful surgical outcome demands a cardioplegic technique that permits a superior technical result (intermittent if necessary) while maximizing myocardial preservation.

It is interesting to speculate that maintaining the integrity of basal metabolism under normothermic conditions may enhance its tolerance to ischemia, as well as its ability to shift from aerobic to anaerobic metabolism and its capacity to deal with reperfusion following short periods of ischemia. Given that continuous perfusion cannot be achieved in all cardiac procedures (i.e., coronary bypass surgery), is a benefit conferred during ischemia at 37° C that offsets the slightly higher oxygen consumption? Is intermittent ischemia and reperfusion in the normothermic arrested heart superior to that in the cold heart? Several indirect pieces of evidence support this contention.

Opie has suggested that the rate of anaerobic metabolism during ischemia ultimately determines cell viability.[56] This effect may be mediated through glycolytic regulation of key membrane enzymes that maintain function.[57] We would postulate that intermittent normothermic ischemia permits the highest rate of anaerobic glycolysis and is the best adaptive state of the myocardium. Schaper has calculated that, in the absence of electromechanical activity, anaerobic energy-producing pathways and cellular energy stores should be able to maintain the viability of tissue for many hours.[58] Alternatively, intermittent warm ischemia and reperfusion may precondition the myocardium, improving the tolerance to ischemia.[59-61] The mechanisms responsible for this tolerance are likely temperature-dependent. The definitive comparisons of warm and cold ischemia that are relevant to the pathophysiology of the arrested heart during cardiac surgery have yet to be carried out.

Technical Aspects

Cardiopulmonary Bypass

Nonpulsatile, heparinized cardiopulmonary bypass is conducted at 37° C, which requires active warming of the systemic perfusate through the membrane oxygenator-heat exchanger. Flow is maintained at predicted rates of 2.2 L/m², and mean systemic pressure is maintained at 50 to 80 mm Hg. Warm perfusion is not associated with requirements for vasoactive or anesthetic agents significantly different from those of hypothermic perfusion. If the predicted hematocrit is less than 0.25, the reservoir is primed with blood and the hematocrit during bypass is kept above 0.20. In operations requiring total circulatory arrest, systemic hypothermia of 18 to 20° C is employed, but the heart is perfused at 37° C through a separate heat exchanger circuit while the systemic circulation is interrupted. The concern of a reduced safety margin for cerebral ischemia at normothermia if a pump or circuit failure requiring a brief period of circulatory arrest occurs is real; however, the incidence of this complication is extremely low (0.1%). In the event of such a mishap, the cardiopulmonary bypass cannulas can be clamped, and internal cardiac massage and lung ventilation instituted until repair is realized. Postoperative shivering, which results in hypercarbia, metabolic and respiratory acidosis, and pulmonary hypertension, is eliminated using normothermic perfusion. Low systemic vascular resistance postoperatively is common, and usually is treated with low-dose norepinephrine infusion.

Cardioplegia Delivery

Cardioplegic composition is shown in Table 1. Oxygenated blood is diluted 4:1 with cardioplegia to give the final approximate compositions shown. The final potassium concentration in the low-potassium solution is more important dependent on the patient's serum potassium. The solution is more hyperglycemic (greater than 50mM) than the solution used in Buckberg's animal experiments (greater than 22mM).[62] Ionized calcium concentration is somewhat higher (0.7mM vs. 0.15 to 2.5mM).

Antegrade cardioplegia to induce arrest is given in the aortic root via a Y

TABLE 1.
Crystalloid Constituents and Final Composition of Blood Cardioplegia*

Crystalloid Constituent		Final Concentration Delivered	
D5W	1,000 mL	Glucose	50mM
Potassium chloride			
High	100 mEq/L		18 + 0.8×(serum potassium)
Low	30 mEq/L		5.6 + 0.8×(serum potassium)
Magnesium sulfate	18 mEq/L	Magnesium	3.0mM
Tromethamine	12 mEq/L	Ionic Ca^{++}	0.7mM
Citrate phosphate dextrose adenine	20 mL	Hematocrit	0.17 to 0.25
Osmolality	425 mOsm/L		
pH	7.95		

*4:1 blood to crystalloid dilution.

cannula (DLP, Grand Rapids, Michigan), which also allows aortic root venting. Initial high-potassium cardioplegia is given at approximately 300 mL/min for 5 minutes. Arrest usually occurs promptly. The infusion then is switched to low-potassium cardioplegia at 75 to 125 mL/min for the duration of the procedure, unless electromechanical activity necessitates a brief return to high-potassium administration.

An alternative technique with which we are gaining increasing experience is continuous retrograde coronary sinus low-potassium warm blood cardioplegia, delivered at 100 to 150 mL/min, following initial antegrade arrest as described above.[63, 64] The retrograde cannula is inserted transatrially while on partial bypass to avoid the hemodynamic fluctuation associated with cardiac manipulation. The catheter is advanced to the inferior border of the left atrial appendage and secured in place with a pursestring suture. Cardioplegia is infused continuously if visualization of the operative field is not compromised and coronary sinus pressure remains below 40 mm Hg.

Coronary Artery Bypass

A single double-stage venous cannula and standard aortic cannulation are used. Following the initial arrest, distal anastomoses of vein grafts are performed to ischemic regions in order of importance, based on the severity of the stenosis and the size of the region at risk as judged by preoperative angiograms. If an arterial conduit such as an internal mammary or gastro-

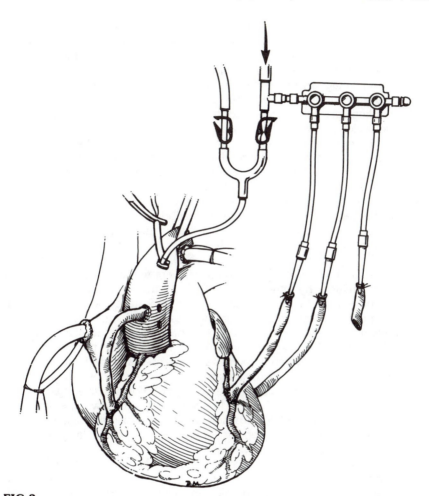

FIG 3.
Technique of coronary artery bypass using antegrade aortic root cardioplegia and vein graft perfusion via a manifold. This allows the independent control of aortic root and regional cardioplegia perfusion following distal anastomoses. Proximal anastomoses are performed with a single aortic cross-clamp and aortic root venting as shown. (From Lichtenstein SV, Fremes SE, Abel JG, et al: *J Card Surg* 1991; 6:1–8. Used by permission.)

epiploic artery is to be used, these anastomoses are performed last. Proximal and distal anastomoses are performed during a single aortic cross-clamp period.[65, 66] Distal anastomoses are performed first and vein grafts are attached to cannulas from a perfusion manifold that comes off the afferent cardioplegia line proximal to the aortic root (Fig 3). This manifold system permits independent control of distal coronary and aortic root perfusion, and is an essential component of the technique. In the arrested heart, continuous aortic root perfusion may cause left ventricular distention in the presence of even mild aortic insufficiency from aortic valve disease, or during displacement of the heart. Independent control of the distal coronary circulation so that it can be dissociated from aortic root perfusion is a distinct advantage of our technique over those in which proximal anastomoses are performed first, or distal followed by proximal followed by aortic root cardioplegia. Independent control of regional perfusion allows one to perfuse regions of the heart distant from the vessel of interest while performing other distal anastomoses. Intermittent regional, rather than global, ischemia is produced, and the total ischemic insult is reduced. We attempt to perfuse with cardioplegia as continuously as possible. This may lead to technical difficulty in visualizing the coronary anastomosis. In this case, aortic root perfusion frequently is stopped while distal vein perfusion continues, or the regional perfusion is varied. Periods of up to 15 minutes of normothermic ischemia with cardioplegia totally turned off have been used without apparent difficulty. Whenever the heart is returned to the pericardial cradle (in between distal anastomoses), aortic root cardioplegia is resumed at about 125 to 175 mL/min with appropriate root pressure, not unlike intermittent hypothermic bolus administration. Proximal anastomoses are performed in the reverse order of importance so that distal vein graft perfusion in the most important vessels is maintained to minimize ischemic time. Following each proximal anastomosis, if aortic insufficiency is not present, cardioplegia may be given in the aortic root to reperfuse those vein grafts in which proximal anastomoses already have been performed. In contrast, all proximal anastomosis can be performed without intermittent perfusion, in which case a short period of selective regional ischemia occurs as each is performed. In either case, zero-flow ischemic time is confined to the period of construction of the last proximal anastomosis. Arterial conduit bypasses are kept occluded to avoid ventricular activity until just prior to cross-clamp removal.

An alternative technique for coronary artery bypass is continuous, normothermic retrograde coronary sinus cardioplegia with low-potassium blood at 100 to 125 mL/min following initial antegrade arrest.[63, 64] In many ways, this is a simpler technique than antegrade root and vein graft perfusion, and may obviate the regional inequalities in perfusion that occur during both distal and proximal anastomoses with the antegrade technique. Care must be taken, however, in identifying the coronary arteries, which contain blue deoxygenated blood at 37° C during retrograde perfusion, while the veins are pink with oxygenated blood. Nevertheless, visualization still may be impaired and intermittent periods of ischemia with either reduced or totally interrupted coronary sinus flow may be required. Although this technique lends itself to continuous perfusion during both distal and proximal anastomosis, irrespective of order, its place in routine coronary bypass procedures using normothermic arrest awaits definition.

Aortic Valve Surgery

In purely stenotic lesions, antegrade aortic arrest is performed in the standard manner. A left ventricular vent is placed through the right superior pulmonary vein following arrest. In mixed lesions or aortic insufficiency, antegrade arrest may be slightly more difficult, but is preferable to the ischemia that occurs when the aortic root is opened with the heart beating. Antegrade diastolic arrest can be achieved almost always, even with moderate to severe aortic insufficiency, without persistent left ventricular distention, by applying manual counterpressure on the left ventricle after cardiac standstill. At this point, antegrade cardioplegia is discontinued, the aortotomy is made, and soft coronary cannulas with self-inflating balloons (Polystan, A/S, Copenhagen, Denmark) connected to a manifold are inserted for continuous perfusion. These are tacked along the anterior and posterior aortic walls in order to remove them from the operative field during valve replacement. Low-potassium cardioplegia is administered continuously at 100 to 150 mL/min. In aortic valve surgery combined with aortocoronary bypass, the vein grafts are constructed first and perfused via the manifold, in addition to the coronary ostia. Alternatively, low-potassium, warm blood cardioplegia can be administered retrogradely via the coronary sinus at 125 mL/min after antegrade arrest. This is particularly useful when the aortic root is small, and root enlargement or replacement with or without coronary reimplantation or concomitant aortocoronary bypass is planned.

Mitral Valve Surgery

Prior to 1989, mitral valve surgery was performed with continuous antegrade aortic root cardioplegia. Mild aortic insufficiency not requiring valve replacement, or the retraction required for adequate exposure (which induced aortic insufficiency) diminished the delivery of cardioplegia. We initially introduced continuous retrograde cardioplegia at our institution to circumvent this problem.[19,63,64] We now perform all mitral valve surgery with continuous retrograde coronary sinus warm blood cardioplegia. The coronary sinus catheter is inserted while on partial bypass via a right atrial pursestring suture after standard aortic and double venous cannulation. The coronary sinus is cannulated directly if a right atriotomy is required. Cardioplegia is administered continuously, keeping the coronary sinus pressure less than 40 mm Hg. This typically permits flow rates of 100 to 150 mL/min. Exposure of the mitral valve for repair or replacement can be maintained without the interruption required for intermittent aortic root cardioplegia. The aortic root cardioplegia cannula may be infused with cardioplegia at the end of the procedure to test the integrity of valve repair. Despite concerns regarding the adequacy of right ventricular delivery of retrograde cardioplegia,[67] excellent clinical results have been obtained without the use of hypothermia, even with suprasystemic pulmonary hypertension and right ventricular hypertrophy.[64]

Preliminary Clinical Results

Based on the theoretic framework discussed, the warm blood cardioplegia and warm systemic perfusion technique was introduced into clinical practice in a nonrandomized manner. The clinical experience has been analyzed prospectively and retrospectively in two clinical groups: patients undergoing coronary artery bypass and patients with long aortic cross-clamp times undergoing complex procedures who received antegrade cardioplegia or antegrade arrest followed by coronary sinus blood cardioplegia at 37° C.

Coronary Artery Bypass

Two hundred and thirty-four consecutive patients underwent coronary artery bypass with continuous cold blood cardioplegia and 218 consecutive patients did so protected with warm blood cardioplegia (Table 2). Although they were sequential groups, patient demographics were comparable, with 90% in New York Heart Association class 3 and 4, 70% with left ventricular grade 3 and 4, and 35% requiring urgent operation. A subgroup of these patients have been reported already.[19] A spontaneous return to normal sinus rhythm following cross-clamp removal occurred in 99% of warm patients, and reperfusion time (i.e., time from removal of cross-clamp to discontinuation of bypass) was reduced significantly (not

TABLE 2.
Coronary Artery Bypass

Study Characteristic*	Cold	Warm
Number of patients	234	218
Male/female	176/58	174/44
Age (yr)	65 ± 9	64 ± 8
Urgent	35%	35%
Number of grafts	3.5 ± 0.7	3.8 ± 0.9
NSR	38 (16%)	215 (99%)‡
LOS	35 (15%)	11 (5%)†
IABP	22 (9%)	3 (1%)†
Perioperative MI	15 (6%)	5 (2%)†
Hospital mortality	7 (3%)	2 (1%)

*NSR = normal sinus rhythm; LOS = low output syndrome; IABP = intra-aortic balloon pump; MI = myocardial infarction.
†$P < .05$.
‡$P < .01$.

shown). A significantly lower requirement for intra-aortic balloon pump, and a reduced incidence of low output syndrome and perioperative myocardial infarction were found in patients undergoing warm heart surgery. Although it was lower in the warm group, mortality did not reach statistical significance (see Table 2).

Long Cross-Clamp Times

Myocardial protection has evolved to such an extent that excellent results may be achieved now using many techniques in the elective coronary artery bypass patient. Patient subgroups with acute ischemic syndromes and ventricular hypertrophy, and those requiring longer cross-clamp times may be expected to pose greater challenges to myocardial preservation. To demonstrate the potency of this method of myocardial protection, we have

TABLE 3.
Long Cross-Clamp Times*

Demographics	
Number of patients	22
Male/female	13/9
Age (yr)	68 ± 10
New York Heart Association class III and IV	86%
Left ventricular grade 3 and 4	86%
Operative Data	
Antegrade cardioplegia	20
Retrograde cardioplegia	2
Cross-clamp time (min)	Mean 204 ± 46 SD (range 180–393)
Reperfusion time (min)	Mean 17 ± 6 SD (range 7–31)
Pump time (min)	Mean 239 ± 58.4 SD (range 195–458)
Outcome Data	
Spontaneous return of normal sinus rhythm	22 (100%)
Low output syndrome	1 (4.5%)
Intra-aortic balloon pump	1 (4.5%)
Hospital mortality	1 (4.5%)
Stroke	0 (0%)

*From Lichtenstein SV, Abel JG, Slutsky AS, et al: *Ann Thorac Surg* 1991, in press. Used by permission.

reviewed the results in a complex group of 22 patients, out of a total of 308 consecutive operations, with cross-clamp times in excess of 3 hours[63] (Table 3). Eighty-six percent of patients had poor left ventricular function (left ventricular grade 3 and 4) and were in New York Heart Association class 3 and 4. Twenty patients were protected with antegrade and 2 with retrograde warm blood cardioplegia. The mean cross-clamp time was 204 minutes, and ranged from 180 to 393 minutes. Six patients underwent single-valve or coronary bypass surgery; the remainder had single- or multiple-valve surgery with or without coronary bypass and aortic outflow reconstructive procedures. Nine were repeat procedures and 6 patients were operated on urgently because of hemodynamic compromise. All patients returned spontaneously to normal sinus rhythm. Only 1 patient had low output syndrome and required intra-aortic balloon pump support. One of these patients, with a cross-clamp time in excess of 6½ hours, was the subject of a case report.[16] This same patient died postoperatively from recurrent atrioventricular dissociation, without ever exhibiting any clinical evidence of myocardial compromise. These clinical results are certainly respectable, and would be difficult to attain with any method of myocardial protection in clinical use today.

Conclusions

Although cold blood cardioplegia has been investigated extensively, until recently[16, 19] there have been no reports in the literature suggesting the sole use of warm blood cardioplegia for myocardial protection. The fundamental concept underlying our philosophy toward myocardial protection is that if electromechanical arrrest can be achieved easily chemically with potassium, and if ischemia can be kept to a minimum by blood perfusion, then hypothermia is not required or even desirable. Warm blood as a vehicle for potassium arrest promotes aerobic metabolism and may provide better recovery of myocardial function, maintenance of metabolic homeostasis, and sparing of energy supply than cold blood cardioplegia. This may prove to be true even if warm blood cardioplegia is delivered intermittently.

Despite advancements in both theory and practice, cardiac surgery still poses a significant risk. Of all the factors contributing to the success of open heart surgery, the most vital to postoperative recovery is the protection and preservation of the heart muscle itself. Improvement in myocardial protection during such procedures in which blood flow to the heart is stopped would permit extended safe operating times and allow for surgical intervention in high-risk cases previously considered inoperable.

References

1. Bigelow WG, Lindsay WK, Greenwood WF: Hypothermia: Its possible role in cardiac surgery. Ann Surg 1950; 132:849–866.

2. Gibbon JH: Application of a mechanical heart and lung apparatus to cardiac surgery. *Minn Med* 1954; 37:171–180.
3. Melrose DG, Dieger DB, Bentall HH, et al: Elective cardiac arrest: Preliminary communications. *Lancet* 1955; 2:21–22.
4. Tyers GFO, Todd GT, Niebauer IM, et al: The mechanism of myocardial damage following potassium citrate (Melrose) cardioplegia. *Surgery* 1975; 78:45–53.
5. Fremes SE, Christakis GT, Weisel RD, et al: A clinical trial of blood and crystalloid cardioplegia. *J Thorac Cardiovasc Surg* 1984; 88:726–741.
6. Feindel CM, Tait GA, Wilson GJ, et al: Multidose blood versus crystalloid cardioplegia. *J Thorac Cardiovasc Surg* 1984; 87:585–595.
7. Novick RJ, Stefaniszyn HJ, Michel RP, et al: Protection of the hypertrophied pig myocardium. *J Thorac Cardiovasc Surg* 1985; 89:547–566.
8. Warner KG, Josa M, Marston W, et al: Reduction in myocardial acidosis using blood cardioplegia. *J Surg Res* 1987; 42:247–256.
9. Khuri SF, Warner KG, Josa M, et al: The superiority of continuous cold blood cardioplegia in the metabolic protection of the hypertrophied human heart. *J Thorac Cardiovasc Surg* 1988; 95:442–454.
10. Neely JR, Whitmer JT, Rovetto MJ: Effect of coronary blood flow on glycolytic flux and intracellular pH in isolated rat hearts. *Circ Res* 1975; 37:733–741.
11. Kaijser L, Jansson E, Schmidt W, et al: Myocardial energy depletion during profound hypothermic cardioplegia for cardiac operations. *J Thorac Cardiovasc Surg* 1985; 90:896–900.
12. Macknight AC, Leaf A: Regulation of cellular volume. *Physiol Rev* 1977; 57:510–573.
13. Leaf A: Cell swelling. A factor in ischemic tissue injury. *Circulation* 1973; 48:455–458.
14. Cossins AR, Prosser CI: Evolutionary adaptation of membranes to temperature. *Proc Natl Acad Sci U S A* 1978; 75:2040–2043.
15. Flaherty JT, Schaff HV, Goldman RA, et al: Metabolic and functional effects of progressive degrees of hypothermia during global ischemia. *Am J Physiol* 1979; 236:H839–H845.
16. Lichtenstein SV, El Dalati H, Panos A, et al: Long cross-clamp times with warm heart surgery. *Lancet* 1989; 1:1443.
17. McGoon DW, Pestana C, Moffit EA: Decreased risk of aortic valve surgery. *Arch Surg* 1965; 91:779–787.
18. Cooley DA, Reul GJ, Wukasch DC: Ischemic contracture of the heart: "Stone heart." *Am J Cardiol* 1972; 29:575–577.
19. Lichtenstein SV, Ashe KA, El Dalati H, et al: Warm heart surgery. *J Thorac Cardiovasc Surg,* 1991; 101:269–274.
20. Lewis FJ, Taufic M: Closure of atrial septal defects with the aid of hypothermia: Experimental accomplishments and the report of one successful case. *Surgery* 1953; 33:52–59.
21. Swan H, Zeavin I, Blount SG Jr, et al: Surgery by direct vision in the open heart during hypothermia. *JAMA* 1953; 153:1081–1085.
22. Griepp RB, Stinson EB, Shumway NE: Profound local hypothermia for myocardial protection during open-heart surgery. *J Thorac Cardiovasc Surg* 1973; 66:731–741.
23. Conti VR, Bertranou EG, Blackstone EH, et al: Cold cardioplegia versus hypothermia for myocardial protection. *J Thorac Cardiovasc Surg* 1978; 76:577–589.
24. Engleman RM, Rousou JH, Lemeshow S: High-volume crystalloid cardioplegia. *J Thorac Cardiovasc Surg* 1983; 86:87–96.

25. Bolling SF, Flaherty JT, Bulkley BH, et al: Improved myocardial preservation during global ischemia by continuous retrograde coronary sinus perfusion. *J Thorac Cardiovasc Surg* 1983; 86:659–666.
26. Buckberg GD: A proposed "solution" to the cardioplegic controversy. *J Thorac Cardiovasc Surg* 1979; 77:803–815.
27. Buckberg GD: Strategies and logic of cardioplegic delivery to prevent, avoid, and reverse ischemic and reperfusion damage. *J Thorac Cardiovasc Surg* 1987; 93:127–139.
28. Martin DR, Scott DF, Downes GL, et al: Primary cause of unsuccessful liver and heart preservation. Cold sensitivity of the ATP-ase system. *Ann Surg* 1972; 175:111–117.
29. McMurchie EJ, Raison JK, Cairncross KD: Temperature-induced phase changes in membranes of heart: A contrast between the thermal response of poikilotherms and homeotherms. *Comp Biochem Physiol [B]*1973; 44B: 1017–1026.
30. Kurihara S, Sakai T: Effects of rapid cooling on mechanical and electrical responses in ventricular muscle of the guinea pig. *J Physiol (Lond)* 1985; 361:361–378.
31. Rahn H, Reeves RB, Howell BJ: Hydrogen ion regulation, temperature and evolution. *Am Rev Respir Dis* 1975; 112:165–172.
32. Braunwald E: The determinants of myocardial oxygen consumption. *Physiologist* 1979; 12:65–93.
33. Gibbs CL, Chapman JB: Cardiac energetics, in Berne RM (ed): *Handbook of Physiology—The Cardiovascular System.* Bethesda, Md, American Physiological Society, 1979, p 797.
34. Bernhard WF, Schwarz HF, Malick NP: Selective hypothermic cardiac arrest in normothermic animals. *Ann Surg* 1961; 153:43–51.
35. Buckberg GD, Brazier JR, Nelson RL, et al: Studies of the effects of hypothermia on regional myocardial blood flow and metabolism during cardiopulmonary bypass. *J Thorac Cardiovasc Surg* 1977; 73:87–94.
36. Chitwood WR, Sink JD, Hill RC, et al: The effects of hypothermia on myocardial oxygen consumption and transmural coronary blood flow in the potassium-arrested heart. *Ann Surg* 1979; 190:106–116.
37. Gibbs CL, Papadoyannis DE, Drake AJ, et al: Oxygen consumption of the nonworking and potassium chloride-arrested dog heart. *Circ Res* 1980; 47:408–417.
38. Digerness SB, Vanini V, Wideman FE: In vitro comparison of oxygen availability from asanguineous and sanguineous cardioplegic media. *Circulation* 1981; 60(suppl II):80–83.
39. Klocke FJ, Braunwald E, Ross J: Oxygen cost of electrical activation of the heart. *Circ Res* 1966; 18:357–365.
40. Nozawa T, Yasamura Y, Futaki S, et al: No significant increase in O_2 consumption of KCl-arrested dog heart with filling and dobutamine. *Am J Physiol* 1988; 255:H807–H812.
41. Krukenkamp I, Silverman N, Sorlic D, et al: Myocardial energetics after thermally graded hyperkalemic crystalloid cardioplegic arrest. *J Thorac Cardiovasc Surg* 1986; 91:259–269.
42. Suga H, Goto Y, Igarashi Y, et al: Cardiac cooling increases E_{max} without affecting relation between O_2 consumption and systolic pressure-volume area in dog left ventricle. *Circ Res* 1988; 63:61–71.
43. Coetzee A, Kotze J, Louw J, et al: Effect of oxygenated crystalloid cardioplegia

on the functional and metabolic recovery of the isolated perfused rat heart. *J Thorac Cardiovasc Surg* 1986; 91:259–269.

44. Guyton RA, Dorsey LMA, Craver JM, et al: Improved myocardial recovery after cardioplegic arrest with an oxygenated crystalloid solution. *J Thorac Cardiovasc Surg* 1985; 89:877–887.

45. Severinghaus JW: Blood gas calculator. *J Appl Physiol* 1966; 21:1108–1116.

46. Flaherty JT, Schaff HV, Goldman RA, et al: Metabolic and functional effects of progressive degrees of hypothermia during global ischemia. *Am J Physiol* 1979; 236:H839–H845.

47. Magovern GJ, Flaherty JT, Gott VL, et al: Failure of blood cardioplegia to protect myocardium at lower temperatures. *Circulation* 1982; 66(suppl I):I60–67.

48. McGregor DC, Wilson GJ, Holness DE, et al: Intramyocardial carbon dioxide tension. A guide to the safe period of anoxic arrest of the heart. *J Thorac Cardiovasc Surg* 1974; 68:101–107.

49. Follette DM, Mulder DG, Maloney JV, et al: Advantages of blood cardioplegia over continuous coronary perfusion or intermittent ischemia. *J Thorac Cardiovasc Surg* 1978; 76:604–619.

50. Buckberg GD, Follette DM, Steed DL, et al: Reduction of post-ischemic myocardial damage by maintaining arrest during initial reperfusion. *Surg Forum* 1977; 28:281–283.

51. Teoh KH, Christakis GT, Fremes SE, et al: Accelerated myocardial metabolic recovery with terminal warm blood cardioplegia (hot shot). *J Thorac Cardiovasc Surg* 1986; 91:888–895.

52. Hearse DJ, Stewart DA, Chain EB: Recovery from cardiac bypass and elective cardiac arrest. *Circ Res* 1974; 35:448–457.

53. Rosenkranz ER, Vinten-Johansen J, Buckberg GD, et al: Benefits of normothermic induction of cardioplegia in energy-depleted hearts, with maintenance of arrest by multi-dose cold blood cardioplegic infusions. *J Thorac Cardiovasc Surg* 1982; 84:667–676.

54. Peyton RB, van Tright P, Pellom GL, et al: Improved tolerance to ischemia in hypertrophied myocardium by preischemic enhancement of adenosine triphosphate. *J Thorac Cardiovasc Surg* 1982; 84:11–15.

55. Baim DS, Rothman MT, Harrison DC: Simultaneous measurement of coronary venous blood flow and oxygen saturation during transient alterations in myocardial oxygen supply and demand. *Am J Cardiol* 1982; 49: 743–752.

56. Opie LH: Importance of glycolytically produced ATP for the integrity of the threatened myocardial cell, in Piper HM (ed): *Pathophysiology of Severe Ischemic Myocardial Injury*. Dordrecht, Kluwer Academic Publishers, 1990, pp 41–65.

57. Weiss JN, Lamp ST: Glycolysis preferentially inhibits ATP-sensitive K^+ channels in isolated guinea pig cardiac myocytes. *Science* 1987; 238:67–69.

58. Schaper W, Binz K, Sass S, et al: Influence of collateral blood flow and of variations in MVO_2 on tissue-ATP content in ischemic and infarcted myocardium. *J Mol Cell Cardiol* 1987; 19:19–37.

59. Hoffmeister HM, Mauser M, Schaper W: Protective effects of short periods of ischemia on myocardial high energy phosphates. *Circulation* 1984; 70(suppl II):325.

60. Murry CE, Vincent RJ, Reimer KA, et al: Ischemic preconditioning slows energy metabolism and delays ultrastructural damage during a sustained ischemic episode. *Circ Res* 1990; 66:913–931.

61. Schott RJ, Rohmann S, Braun ER, et al: Ischemic preconditioning reduces infarct size in swine myocardium. *Circ Res* 1990; 66:1133–1142.
62. Buckberg GD: Studies of controlled reperfusion after ischemia. *J Thorac Cardiovasc Surg* 1986; 92:483–648.
63. Lichtenstein SV, Abel JG, Slutsky AS, et al: Warm heart surgery: Experience with long cross clamp times. *Ann Thorac Surg,* in press.
64. Pavos A, Salerno TA, Lichtenstein SV: Continuous retrograde warm blood cardioplegia in surgery for acute post-infarction mitral insufficiency. *J Molec Cell Cardiol* 1990; 22 (Suppl V): 531 (abstr).
65. Salerno TA: Single aortic cross-clamping for distal and proximal anastomoses in coronary surgery. An alternative to conventional techniques. *Ann Thorac Surg* 1982; 33:518–520.
66. Weisel RD, Hoy FBY, Baird RJ, et al: Comparison of alternative cardioplegic techniques. *J Thorac Cardiovasc Surg* 1983; 86:97–107.
67. Partington MT, Acar C, Buckberg GD, et al: Studies of retrograde cardioplegia. *J Thorac Cardiovasc Surg* 1989; 97:605–612.

Heart Transplantation in Children

Mario Chiavarelli, M.D.

Clinical Fellow in Cardiothoracic Surgery, Loma Linda University School of Medicine, Loma Linda University Medical Center, Loma Linda International Heart Institute, Loma Linda, California

Javier Alonso De Begoña, M.D.

Research Fellow in Cardiothoracic Surgery, Loma Linda University School of Medicine, Loma Linda University Medical Center, Loma Linda International Heart Institute, Loma Linda, California

Robert E. Vigesaa, M.D.

Chief Resident in Cardiothoracic Surgery, Loma Linda University School of Medicine, Loma Linda University Medical Center, Loma Linda International Heart Institute, Loma Linda, California

Steven R. Gundry, M.D.

Associate Professor of Surgery, Loma Linda University School of Medicine, Loma Linda University Medical Center, Loma Linda International Heart Institute, Loma Linda, California

Leonard L. Bailey, M.D.

Professor of Surgery, Loma Linda University School of Medicine, Loma Linda University Medical Center, Loma Linda International Heart Institute, Loma Linda, California

The Loma Linda University Pediatric Heart Transplant Group

Heart transplantation continues to evolve into an effective and rational therapy for infants and children with uncorrectable congenital and myopathic heart diseases. Heart transplant procedures were accomplished rarely in children prior to 1980 and were performed only occasionally before 1985. Even then, with few exceptions, recipients were not really children, but in most cases teenagers and young adults. Centers reporting experience with children included Stanford, Columbia, Pittsburgh, and Ann Arbor in the United States, and Harefield Hospital in London. The Ann Arbor group reported some of the earliest experience in toddlers.

Adrian Kantrowitz et al.[1] attempted heart transplantation unsuccessfully in a newborn baby dying of Ebstein's malformation in 1967. This clinical effort was based on laboratory experience in puppies. Early the next year, Denton Cooley and his associates[2] attempted heart-lung transplantation in a 3-month-old baby dying of complete atrioventricular canal. In the summer of 1984, Yacoub of Harefield Hospital in London (Yacoub, personal communication, 1990) and his associates attempted heart transplantation in a newborn baby dying of hypoplastic left heart syndrome. Despite an initial favorable response, his patient died 2½ weeks later of complications. The newborn's heart graft was functioning well at the time of her death. Later that same year, the Loma Linda group attempted cardiac xenotransplantation in a preterm newborn with the same syndrome. This child survived the operation, yet died 3 weeks later of graft/host ABO incompatibility.[3] At about the same time, Cooley and associates successfully transplanted a heart into an 8-month-old girl who continues to thrive. The first successful neonatal heart transplant operation was accomplished in November 1985 at Loma Linda University, in Loma Linda, California.[4] Subsequently, heart transplantation has proven to be effective therapy over a very broad age span, extending from birth to 70 years. However, within this chapter, we will limit discussion of this form of therapy as it applies to pediatric heart disease treated during the first 12 years of life.

Indications for Pediatric Heart Transplantation

Myocardial Diseases

Idiopathic and "burned-out" viral cardiomyopathy with its resultant chronic congestive heart failure has provided the major indication for heart transplantation in older children and young adults in every published series. A few infants have had heart transplant procedures for "congenital" cardiomyopathy, but this has been unusual. Additionally, cardiac tumors such as multiple obstructive fibromas or rhabdomyomas have been appropriate indications for transplantation.

Timing of transplantation in infants and children with myocardial disease is an unresolved issue. Dilated cardiomyopathy, particularly in children over the age of 2 years, has a very poor prognosis. The outlook is even worse if congestive failure is accompanied by significant arrhythmia. These youngsters should be referred for transplantation at the earliest signs of decompensation. Occasionally, heart transplantation may salvage an infant or child with unmanageable hemodynamic deterioration from acute myocarditis. However, experience is very limited in this setting. Hypertrophic cardiomyopathy in infants and young children may improve and even resolve over time. Consideration of transplantation for these infants remains problematic.

Structural Heart Diseases

Of the 25,000 to 30,000 babies born each year in North America with congenital heart disease, perhaps as many as 2,500 to 3,000 have malformations of such grave complexity that corrective surgery is impossible. Conventional palliative operations may benefit these infants temporarily, but a very large number are lost to operative mortality and natural attrition during and after serial palliative efforts. Newborns with hypoplastic left heart syndrome make up one large category of infants who fit this description. In addition, there are a large number of infants with complex univentricular hearts who might be better served with transplantation as a primary definitive operation. A few may require heart and lung transplantation as that therapeutic avenue develops. Transplantation is donor-dependent therapy and, although the availability of pediatric donor organs is increasing, supply in no way presently matches potential demand. Hence, a strategy that combines effective palliation when necessary (absence of an available donor organ) with transplantation is likely to provide the greatest salvage.

In addition to new instances of congenital heart disease, a very large number of children and young adults have had several palliative operations from which they are no longer realizing sufficient well-being. Additional palliative surgery may be quite risky and of marginal utility. These children ought to be referred for cardiac transplantation. In summary, a large number of pediatric patients potentially could benefit from heart transplant procedures. As confidence in this type of therapy increases, more of them will be salvaged.

Donor Dependency and Organ Procurement

A significant amount of skepticism persists among pediatricians about the efficacy of heart transplant therapy. It is thought by some to be too exotic, too capricious, and/or too expensive. It is true that heart transplantations are not elective procedures. They are donor-dependent and usually take place at night and on weekends. They usually are arranged in such a way as to be least disruptive at the donor facility and yet still be timely and efficient. Because of current graft ischemic time constraints, transplant operations are given priority in the operating rooms of transplant centers. Beyond that, there is nothing exotic about heart transplantation in busy centers. On the contrary, these operations are (arguably) remarkably conservative therapy *when they can be accomplished.* Society is still unable to produce enough organ donations to meet the current demand, to say nothing of the potential demand. Barriers to organ donation have to do mostly with unwillingness of medical professionals to encourage parents and loved ones to decide for this incredible act of altruistic love in an hour of intense grief. Bedside health professionals are sometimes inept at facilitating organ donation and, hence, very frequently avoid the issue. Coroners all too frequently are unwilling to permit heart, liver, and kidney procurement following traumatic or crib death for excuses that can be categorized only as "policy" in most instances.

There are literally dozens of "potential" organ donors of all ages every day across North America. There are clearly enough "potential" organ donors to meet the finite needs of pediatric patients, if only those organs were made available. Organ procurement agencies, distributed effectively throughout North America, are willing and very adept at facilitating organ procurement. All most agencies require is a telephone call and they will do virtually all the rest.

When an appropriate donor is identified and stabilized, procurement teams converge on the donor facility and discuss strategy for multiorgan retrieval. There is a current thrust toward standardization of organ removal based upon cold flush en bloc removal, and back table dissection of target organs. Actual heart removal is usually the final step in preparation for additional organ procurement. The heart graft is obtained by inflow exclusion, cold cardioplegia preservation, and en bloc excision. All veins and arteries necessary for subsequent reconstruction in the recipient are removed and carefully dissected in a cold bath on the back bench. Hearts are sealed in a cold bath and transported as efficiently as possible to the recipient transplant center. Cold ischemic times of 8 hours or more have been well tolerated. Very frequently, lung or heart-lung removal also will be a part of the process, but we shall consider only heart procurement here.

Pediatric Heart Transplantation Methods

The methods of pediatric heart transplantation are best considered when applied to the three most common conditions requiring this operation: (1) cardiomyopathies with normal cardiac and great vessel anatomy, (2) variants of hypoplastic left heart syndrome with atresia or hypoplasia of the left heart/aortic tract, and (3) congenital heart lesions previously treated by palliation with absence or alteration of one or more cardiac/great vessel structures. Each lesion produces its own constraints on the operative donor and recipient teams.

Heart transplantation in infants and children with cardiomyopathy closely mimics the now standardized methods set forth for adult cardiac transplantation. Donor hearts are procured with adequate lengths of ascending aorta and pulmonary arteries, but extensive vessel length is not necessary. All four pulmonary venous openings are routinely incised to produce a single, large left atrial opening posteriorly. Similarly, except in older children, a single cut is made from the divided inferior vena cava to the superior vena cava close to the interatrial groove to produce a larger right atrial opening. Any patent foramen ovale is closed at this time as well. In older children, as in adults, the superior vena cava is ligated and the atrial incisions are extended from the inferior vena cava into the right atrial appendage.

The recipient is cannulated high on the ascending aorta, usually opposite the innominate artery for arterial inflow. In young infants and children, a single venous cannula is placed in the right atrial appendage, while in older children, two venous cannulas are placed through right atrial pursestrings into both cava and controlled with separate caval snares. The latter technique is useful whenever the surgeon wishes to avoid profound hypothermic circulatory arrest.

The patient is cooled on cardiopulmonary bypass, the aorta is cross-clamped as high as possible, and, if a single venous cannula has been used, the patient is drained and circulatory arrest is instituted. Using dual venous cannulas, the caval snares are secured. Circulation is reduced, but not interrupted. The right atrium is opened parallel to the atrioventricular groove and angled toward the coronary sinus inferiorly. The apex of the heart then is retracted out of the pericardium and the atrial incision is carried around onto the left atrium, usually passing beneath the atrial appendage and behind the aorta and pulmonary artery. The atrial septum is incised in its midportion, thereby leaving generous cuffs of left and right atria. The aorta and pulmonary arteries are divided just above their commissural posts.

The donor heart is brought into the pericardial well and suturing is begun at the base of the atrial septum and extended superiorly, including both right and left atrial portions of the donor septum in a single layer. Upon reaching the superior margin of the septum, the suturing process continues along the free wall of the right atrium, completing the right atrial anastomosis. A second suture is started at the base of the septum/left atrial junction and, retracting the cardiac apex out of the pericardium, the free wall of the left atrium is anastomosed. As the suture line passes the donor appendage, the cardiac apex is replaced into the pericardium, allowing the roof of the left atrium to be closed easily. If circulatory arrest has been used, this point marks a convenient time to place the patient back on bypass. A new pursestring is placed around the right atrial appendage, the atrium is filled with cold saline, and the cannula is reintroduced. A small pursestring suture is placed around the left atrial appendage and the tip of the appendage is opened to decompress the left side of the heart.

The aorta then is trimmed and anastomosed in an end-to-end fashion. A previously placed pursestring can be used as a vent site; the cross-clamp is removed and rewarming commenced. During rewarming, the pulmonary artery is trimmed and anastomosed end-to-end to the recipient. Before the end of cardiopulmonary bypass, the left atrial and aortic vent sites are closed. Weaning from bypass follows an adequate period of graft reperfusion. Low-dose dopamine or isoproterenol may be added for hemodynamic support.

Heart transplantation for variants of hypoplastic left heart syndrome is accomplished as previously discussed, with several exceptions. Since the aorta is hypoplastic, donor aorta must be secured to make up this deficiency. This is accomplished during procurement by ligating and dividing the head and arm vessels in the superior mediastinum. The descending aorta is dissected down to the first intercostals, where division is accomplished. After graft excision, the superior margin of the arch is opened up to, and sometimes including, the orifice of the left subclavian artery. This wide opening will be used to reconstruct the aortic arch and isthmus of the recipient.

As a period of hypothermic arrest is needed to reconstruct the hypoplastic aorta, only a single venous cannula is used. The arterial inflow cannula is introduced through a pursestring in the main pulmonary artery and positioned through the patent ductus arteriosus. After cardiopulmonary bypass is begun, a snare is placed around the ductus, diverting blood flow solely into the aorta. During cooling, snares are placed loosely around the head and neck vessels arising from the arch, and the descending aorta is isolated beyond the ductus to the level of the intercostal arteries.

During circulatory arrest, the arterial and venous lines are clamped and the head vessel snares are tightened. Cannulas are withdrawn and the ductus is ligated. The heart is excised, taking care to preserve as much left atrial tissue as possible, sometimes including the appendage, which can be opened to increase the left atrial circumference. The ascending aorta is ligated and divided in its midportion, and its ligating suture is retracted toward the right shoulder. The ductus is cut from its insertion on the descending aorta, and all visible ductal tissue is excised from the aorta. The arch is incised along its undersurface and well into normal-caliber descending aorta.

After completion of the right and left atrial anastomoses, the distal donor arch is sutured down to the opened recipient's descending aorta, beginning the anastomosis distally and advancing along the undersurface of the recipient's aortic arch. Additional incisions on the donor or recipient's aorta may be needed to make up for any size mismatch. Cardiopulmonary by-

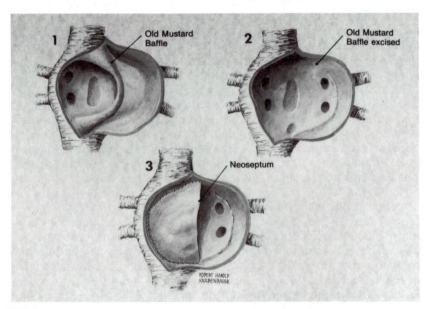

FIG 1.
Artist's view of surgical technique for septal reconstruction after Mustard procedure in preparation to graft insertion.

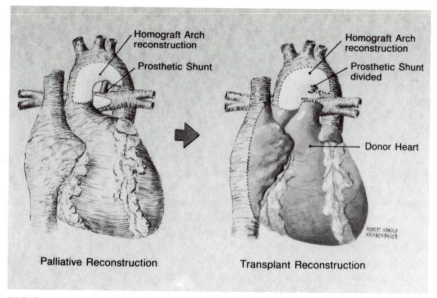

FIG 2.
Artist's view of surgical technique for transplantation after Norwood palliative reconstruction.

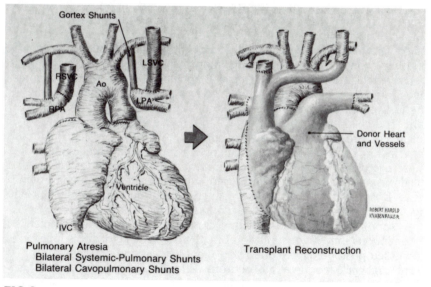

FIG 3.
Artist's view of surgical technique for transplantation after bilateral systemic-pulmonary shunts and bilateral cavopulmonary shunts. RSVC = right superior vena cava; LSVC = left superior vena cava; IVC = inferior vena cava; Ao = aorta; RPA = right pulmonary artery; LPA = left pulmonary artery.

pass is then reinstituted. It is convenient to use the cut stump of the innominate artery as the site for arterial inflow. The neck vessel snares are removed after deairing the aorta. During rewarming, the pulmonary artery is anastomosed.

Heart transplantation following palliative operations such as systemic-pulmonary shunts or reconstructions such as the Norwood or Fontan procedures is accomplished in much the same way as outlined above (Figs 1 to 3). However, the surgical team must consider the need to replace or augment surgically altered structures. The donor harvest team may need to return with extended portions of systemic veins, pulmonary arteries, and/or aorta with which to accomplish the transplantation and reconstructions. Depending upon the anticipated ischemic time, the recipient surgical team should be prepared to start the "redo" dissection long before the expected arrival of the harvest team. As with any reoperation, alternative sites for arterial and venous cannulation should be available.

Finally, retransplantation may become as commonplace in children as it has become in adults. It has been accomplished successfully for both salvage during irreversible acute rejection and advanced ischemic graft disease. Dissection and replacement of a diseased graft follow well-established principles of reoperation.

Immune Modulation

The success of any form of transplantation depends upon modulating the immune system's response to the graft, balancing tolerance to the graft with continued intolerance to a variety of pathogens. The steps and pharmacological agents used to achieve such modulation continue to evolve, and vary considerably, depending upon the age at which the patient is transplanted (Table 1). For example, it appears that the immunosuppressive requirements for an infant who receives a heart transplantation during the first month or so of life may be significantly different from those of infants and children beyond this age.[5] The exact mechanisms for this "graft tolerance" are poorly understood, but may relate to persistent maternal-fetal factors that allow engraftment of the fetus within the mother. The more aggressive immune response experienced among older infants and children may relate to their increased exposure to environmental pathogens. Despite these differences, maintenance immunosuppression at any age is the mainstay for achieving continuing engraftment.

As soon as a donor is identified, cyclosporine is given to the recipient as a continuous intravenous infusion of 0.1 to 0.5 mg/kg/hr. This infusion is continued postoperatively until the patient is tolerating oral intake. At that point, oral cyclosporine at a dose from 12 to 20 mg/kg/day is started (usually on a twice- or three-times-a-day schedule). Trough levels (by monoclonal antibody testing) of 200 to 300 ng/mL are maintained. Trough levels of cyclosporine are tapered over the first year to 100 to 150 ng/mL. These levels have correlated with excellent engraftment and minimal, if any, hypertension or renal impairment.

TABLE 1.
Pediatric Heart Transplantation: Recipient Immunomodulation
Protocol at Loma Linda University

I. Immunosuppression.
  A. Cyclosporine.
    1. First year whole blood levels: 200–300 ng/dL.
    2. After first year: 100–150 ng/dL
  B. Azathioprine.
    1. Newborn.
      a. First year: 3 mg/kg tapered to 0.
      b. Not administered after first year.
    2. Infant and child.
      a. First year: 3 mg/kg adjusted to maintain leukocytes >4,000.
      b. Tapered to 1 mg/kg after first year.
II. Rejection protocol.
  A. Patient condition.
    1. No symptoms (outpatient).
    2. Mild symptoms (inpatient).
    3. Moderate/severe symptoms (inpatient).
  B. Medications.
    1. Intravenous methylprednisolone.
    2. Intravenous methylprednisolone with or without antithymocyte serum.
    3. Intravenous methylprednisolone and antithymocyte serum with or
       without methotrexate and with or without mechanical assistance.
III. Immunoprotection.
  A. Gamma globulin.
    1. Dose of 400–600 mg/kg/day perioperatively and during rejection
       protocol.
  B. Acyclovir.
    1. Dose of 20–30 mg/kg/day in the first 3 months.

Azathioprine is started intravenously on a daily basis perioperatively at a dose of 3 mg/kg. This dose is adjusted to keep the white blood cell count greater than 4,000. It is changed to the same oral dosage after the patient begins eating and is continued for at least the first postoperative year. It has been Loma Linda policy to taper the dosage but to continue azathioprine indefinitely in children who undergo transplantation at an age greater than 1 month. Azathioprine is discontinued after the first year for neonatal transplant recipients.

Despite adequate levels of maintenance immunosuppression, rejection can and does occur in most infant and child transplant recipients. Rejection episodes are more frequent in older infants and children, such that additional agents are currently under evaluation as induction therapy to reduce or potentially eliminate rejection. Although highly successful in some adult transplant centers, OKT3, a monoclonal antibody directed against a specific T cell lymphocyte subgroup, has been less effective in the pediatric age range. Recent Loma Linda experience with Vanderbilt rabbit antithymocyte serum has been gratifying as rejection therapy. Its efficacy as induction therapy in older infants is currently being evaluated by randomized trials.

Rejection episodes that cannot be prevented are treated according to their severity. For the most part, rejection episodes in infants, particularly neonates, are mild and can be treated on an outpatient basis with intravenous steroids, utilizing more frequent daily surveillance until they are resolved. Symptomatic rejection episodes are handled on an inpatient basis with 125 mg of methylprednisolone twice daily for 6 to 8 doses. Rejection that responds slowly to intravenous steroids, has produced hemodynamic compromise, or does not respond appropriately to two courses of intravenous steroids is treated additionally with antithymocyte serum or occasionally with methotrexate. Rarely, hemodynamic decompensation is so sudden or intense that temporary extracorporeal circulation is required for several days to allow the antirejection drugs to take effect.

Infection of the transplanted recipient is a potentially lethal complication and has accounted for a significant percentage of early and late mortality among older children and adults. The incidence of lethal infection may very well reflect the more intense immune suppression utilized in most centers for these older recipients. Infection, while quite common, has been a very unusual cause of death following pediatric heart transplantation in the Loma Linda experience, perhaps because immunosuppressive maintenance is considerably less for the younger age group. Moreover, the absence of routine steroid therapy may contribute to the extremely low incidence of serious infection in these patients. Recipients with specific infections are managed with specific antimicrobial agents. Cytomegalovirus infection is so ubiquitous among immunosuppressed patients that Loma Linda current protocol includes the routine prophylactic use of gamma globulin infusions (400 to 600 mg/kg/day) perioperatively and oral acyclovir (20 to 30 mg/kg/day) during the first 3 postoperative months. Patients with symptomatic cytomegalovirus infection are given a 2-week course of intravenous ganciclovir (3 to 5 mg/kg/day) and supplemental gamma globulin.

Transplanted infants and children continue to receive most of the common childhood immunizations, including diphtheria, pertussis, tetanus, polio (Salk), pneumococcus, *Haemophilus influenzae* B, and influenza A and B. However, vaccination for measles, mumps, and rubella are deferred, owing to the live viruses involved. Opportunistic infections and infestations such as *Pneumocystis carinii, Nocardia,* tuberculosis, and fungus have been very unusual among pediatric recipients whose immune modulation follows the protocol described.

Early and Late Surveillance

Requirements of the immediate perioperative period focus on maintaining hemodynamic stability, pulmonary hygiene, and fluid balance. Nutritional

TABLE 2.
Pediatric Heart Transplantation: Early and Late Surveillance at Loma Linda University*

I. Inpatient testing.
   A. Spontaneous blastogenesis.
   B. Blood levels of cyclosporine.
   C. Roentgenogram.
   D. Electrocardiogram.
   E. Echocardiogram.
   F. Electrolytes, BUN, creatinine.
   G. Infectious disease surveillance.
      1. Bacteriologic.
         a. CBC and differential, platelet count.
         b. Endotracheal tube aspirate for gram stain.
         c. Urinalysis and urine and throat cultures.
         d. Wound exudate gram stain/culture.
      2. Virologic.
         a. Urine, throat swab for CMV on 14th post-transplant day.
II. Outpatient follow-up.
   A. Serial screening once or twice per week (tapered over time).
      1. Routine physician visit.
      2. Echocardiogram, electrocardiogram, and voltage plotting.
      3. Roentgenogram.
      4. Blood levels of cyclosporine.
      5. CBC and differential.
      6. Basic electrolytes.
   B. Serial screening by protocol.
      1. TORCH titer.
      2. CMV urine culture.
      3. CMV throat culture.
      4. EBV surveillance: EBV-IgM, EBV-IgG.
      5. Pre- and post-polio antibody titer.
      6. Pre- and post-DPT antibody titer.
      7. Neurologic assessment.
      8. Language and speech evaluation.
      9. Developmental assessment.
      10. Standard psychometric testing.
      11. Isotopic glomerular filtration rate.
      12. Twenty-four-hour Holter monitor
III. Invasive follow-up.
   A. Endomyocardial biopsies not routinely done during the first 12 months (optional for older children).
   B. Complete heart catheterization at ages 1, 4, 6, 8, 10, and 20 years (including selective coronary arteriography and endomyocardial biopsy).

*BUN = blood urea nitrogen; CBC = complete blood count; CMV = cytomegalovirus; TORCH = toxoplasmosis, rubella, cytomegalovirus, herpes; EBV = Epstein-Barr virus; DPT = diphtheria, pertussis, tetanus.

restoration with oral feeding, particularly in newborns, is an important management milestone. Acid peptic disease is prevented by the intravenous use of a histomineyic H_2 receptor-blockade until infants are taking full oral nutrition. The administration of immune regulatory drugs is converted to the oral route. Prophylactic antibiotics are given until central vascular lines are removed. Baseline graft surveillance data are obtained noninvasively, and include an electrocardiogram, a chest roentgenogram, an m-mode and two-dimensional echocardiogram, a complete blood count, and an assay of host immune reactivity labelled spontaneous blastogenesis. The first 10 to 14 postoperative days frequently are referred to as the "honeymoon" period.

Noninvasive graft surveillance (Table 2), which includes important bedside data such as a sustained increase in resting heart rate, tachypnea, irritability, poor feeding and/or vomiting, is performed twice per week initially. Data gathering then becomes less frequent as the rejection-free interval lengthens. Surveillance goes to once per week, once per month, and so on. Since most rejection episodes are confined to the first 6 post-transplant months, families that have relocated for transplantation frequently may return to their places of origin after this surveillance period. Family members are taught to monitor clinical signs at home and they learn important information about the medications that the transplant recipients must take. If rejection or infection do not present postoperatively, the life of the infant or child who has received a transplant is remarkably normal. Even if families must endure one or two rejection or infection episodes, life approximates normality usually within the first 6 months and beyond. Late acute rejection episodes are unusual, but experience has taught us that noncompliance may result in grave penalties. The surveillance learning curve is never easy for the transplant team. Heart graft surveillance in the pediatric population is an exercise in detail and attentiveness. At Loma Linda, outpatient follow-up is accomplished by a group of pediatricians and nurse coordinators.

Endocardial biopsy plays a limited role in graft surveillance in the pediatric age groups. However, it is a vital confirmatory adjunct in the unusual situation in which clinical diagnosis of graft rejection cannot be ruled out with confidence. Biopsy is used infrequently in the pediatric heart transplant program at Loma Linda, although other centers rely much more heavily on invasive diagnosis for graft surveillance in children.[6]

Complications in Pediatric Heart Transplantation

The twin threats of graft rejection and host infection, which together account for the majority of early and late deaths following heart transplantation, have been mentioned already. Table 3 illustrates the complications in pediatric heart transplantation.

Systemic hypertension complicates post-transplant treatment in virtually every adult patient and, despite the aggressive use of various combinations

TABLE 3.
Complications of Pediatric Heart Transplantation (Loma Linda University)

Cardiovascular
  Rejection
  Graft failure without rejection
  Hypertension
  Residual or recurrent aortic coarctation
  Bradyarrhythmias
Pulmonary
  Pneumonia
  Atelectasis
  Bronchospasm
  Pleural effusion
  Pulmonary vascular hypertensive crisis
Renal
  Acute and/or chronic failure
Neurologic
  Seizures
  Cerebrovascular accident
Gastrointestinal
  Gastroesophageal reflux
  Feeding disorders
  Peptic ulceration
Integumentary
  Hirsutism
  Gingival hyperplasia

of diuretics, vasodilators, and sympatholytic drugs, it remains a difficult problem to manage. Experience in children has been mixed. The Stanford University group[7] reported significant hypertension in 96% of their pediatric population. At the University of Pittsburgh,[8] hypertension was present in more than half of the long-term survivors. Hypertension occurred in 40% of the children operated on at Columbia-Presbyterian Medical Center.[9] In contrast, the University of Montreal group observed normal blood pressure in seven children, 2 months to 4 years after the procedure.[10] In the Loma Linda experience, very few survivors have required chronic antihypertensive treatment. This paucity of systemic hypertension is attributed to the continuous search for an individualized minimal immunosuppressive regimen.

Renal dysfunction is the most common and troublesome adverse effect of chronic cyclosporine therapy after heart transplantation in adults.[11] In children, a plasma creatinine rise to a mean level of 2 mg/dL was observed at 2 years by the Stanford group,[7] without further deterioration between 2 and 4 years. Several institutions[8-10] have reported normal late renal function. At Loma Linda University, some patients had perioperative renal dysfunction, but any recipient who was severely oliguric or anuric before or during the immediate perioperative hours was treated aggressively with peritoneal dialysis.[12] Very few survivors have shown evidence of chronic renal dysfunction.

Coronary artery disease represents the main impediment to long-term survival of adult heart transplant patients, since it has been the major complication responsible for graft failures in both the precyclosporine and cyclosporine eras.[13, 14] Accelerated coronary artery disease in adults occurs with an incidence of 18% at 1 year, 27% at 2 years, and 44% at 3 years.[14] Rejection-related coronary artery disease has been described in 6 children representing 28% of patients surviving 6 months to 6 years at the University of Pittsburgh.[8] Eight of 29 (26%) pediatric transplantations at Columbia University showed coronary artery disease either at pathologic examination or by angiography.[9] The Harefield Hospital group[15] reported no coronary artery disease in 57 children with heart or heart-lung transplantation after a mean follow-up of 21 months. The longest follow-up of a newborn heart transplant recipient in the Loma Linda series is over 5 years, and the patient has no evidence of atherosclerosis on a recent coronary angiogram. Interestingly, both the Harefield and the Loma Linda groups avoid chronic steroid immunosuppression in the pediatric population because of concern that steroids accelerate coronary artery disease. Coronary vasculitis and occlusion have played a role in the late results from chronic rejection in several infants in the Loma Linda series, each of whom had prolonged steroid therapy.

Residual or recurrent coarctation in patients with hypoplastic left heart syndrome or similar aortic arch anomalies developed in several infants early in the Loma Linda experience. Four such patients were treated successfully with balloon aortoplasty, and three underwent surgical coarctectomy. The distal aortic arch should always be completely and widely reconstructed to obtain a durable late result.

Malignancy is more common in transplanted patients as a consequence of impairment of intrinsic host immunosurveillance, direct action of immunosuppressive drugs, chronic antigenic stimulation by the allograft, and activation of oncogenic viruses. The incidence of lymphoproliferative disorders, usually non-Hodgkin's lymphoma, is less than 1%.[11] Malignancy following organ transplantation usually responds poorly to conventional anticancer treatment. The best therapeutic approach has been reduction of immunosuppressive treatment. Two heart-transplanted children with malignancy 33 and 19 months after operation have been reported.[9] As yet, there has been no neoplasia among Loma Linda pediatric cardiac recipients.

Liver dysfunction and cholecystitis have not been observed. Two surviving patients have severe cerebral palsy, but most transplanted infants have normal neurologic development.

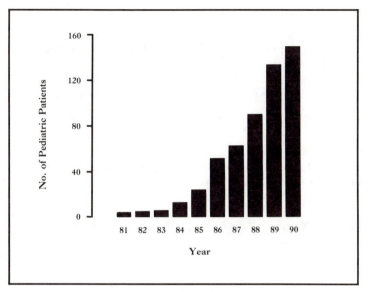

FIG 4.
Pediatric heart transplantation world experience reported to the International Society for Heart Transplantation Registry among recipients aged 0 to 12 years.

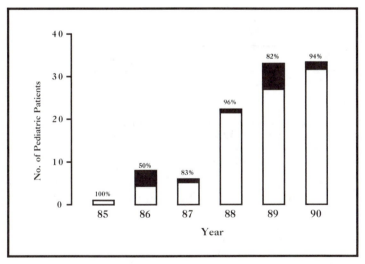

FIG 5.
Pediatric heart transplantation activity at Loma Linda University among recipients aged 0 to 12 years. The bars indicate the number of patients operated on; the black segment of the bar shows operative deaths. Percent survival is indicated atop each bar.

Results

Five hundred and fifty pediatric patients aged 0 to 12 years have been entered into the registry of the International Society for Heart Transplantation in the 10-year period from 1981 to December 1990 (M. P. Kaye, personal communication, 1991). The increasing frequency of pediatric heart trans-

TABLE 4.
Hospital and Late Mortality After Pediatric Heart
Transplantation (up to 12 Years Old) at Loma Linda University

Year	Number	Hospital Deaths			Late Deaths		
		Number	Percent	CL70*	Number	Percent	CL70*
1985	1	0	0	0%–86%	0	0	0%–86%
1986	8	4	50	27%–73%	1	25	3%–63%
1987	6	1	17	2%–46%	0	0	0%–31%
1988	23	1	4	1%–14%	6	27	17%–40%
1989	34	6	18	11%–27%	2	7	2%–16%
1990	35	2	6	2%–13%	1	3	0%–10%
Total	107	14	13	10%–17%	10	11	7%–15%

*CL70 = 70% confidence limits.

TABLE 5.
Hospital and Late Mortality After Neonatal Heart
Transplantation (1 to 30 Days Old) at Loma Linda University

Year	Number	Hospital Deaths			Late Deaths		
		Number	Percent	CL70*	Number	Percent	CL70*
1985	1	0	0	0%–86%	0	0	0%–86%
1986	3	1	33	4%–76%	0	0	0%–61%
1987	3	1	33	4%–76%	0	0	0%–61%
1988	10	0	0	0%–17%	1	10	1%–30%
1989	17	3	18	8%–32%	0	0	0%–13%
1990	13	0	0	0%–14%	1	8	1%–24%
Total	47	5	11	6%–17%	2	5	2%–11%

*CL70 = 70% confidence limits.

TABLE 6.
Hospital and Late Mortality After Infant Heart Transplantation
(1 to 12 Months Old) at Loma Linda University

Year	Number	Hospital Deaths			Late Deaths		
		Number	Percent	CL70*	Number	Percent	CL70*
1986	2	1	50	7%–93%	0	0	0%–86%
1987	2	0	0	0%–61%	0	0	0%–61%
1988	10	1	10	1%–30%	4	44	24%–66%
1989	13	3	23	10%–41%	1	10	1%–30%
1990	15	1	7	1%–21%	0	0	0%–13%
Total	42	6	14	9%–22%	5	14	8%–22%

*CL70 = 70% confidence limits.

plantation during the past decade is shown in Figure 4. Transplantations in the pediatric age group currently account for 10% of all cardiac transplantations annually. This percentage will increase, since the annual number of adult cardiac transplantations has leveled off in the past 4 years, while the number of pediatric recipients continues to rise. This increase is due primarily to growth in the field of neonatal and infant transplantation.

At Loma Linda University, 107 pediatric patients under 12 years of age

TABLE 7.
Hospital and Late Mortality After Heart Transplantation in
Children (1 to 12 Years Old) at Loma Linda University

Year	Number	Hospital Deaths			Late Deaths		
		Number	Percent	CL70*	Number	Percent	CL70*
1986	3	2	67	24%–95%	1	100	14%–100%
1987	1	0	0	0%–86%	0	0	0%–86%
1988	3	0	0	0%–46%	1	33	4%–76%
1989	4	0	0	0%–38%	1	25	3%–63%
1990	7	1	14	2%–41%	0	0	0%–27%
Total	18	3	17	7%–31%	3	20	9%–36%

*CL70 = 70% confidence limits.

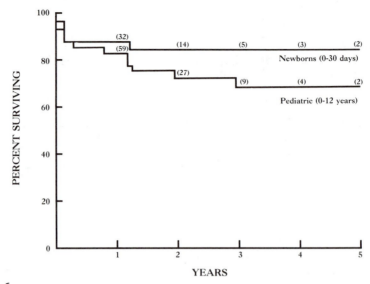

FIG 6.
Actuarial curves at 5 years of follow-up for the total pediatric transplant population
at Loma Linda University and for the newborns.

have been transplanted between 1985 and December 1990. Operative
mortality, including hospital and early (<30 days) mortality, has been 13%
(Fig 5 and Table 4). However, in 1990, 33 patients out of 35 (96%) survived the operation. Interestingly, all 13 newborn infants (Table 5) operated
on in 1990 survived the surgery. Similar early mortality was found among
older infants and children (Tables 6 and 7), but late mortality appears to
be higher. Actuarial survival associated with pediatric cardiac transplantation is 82% at 1 year and 67% at 5 years. The neonatal subgroup has a
1-year survival of 87% and a 5-year survival of 84% (Fig 6).

Future Outlook

More than 100 infants die daily in the United States. A small percentage of
this population, if referred for organ donation, would fulfill infant allograft
requirements in North America. Effective professional and public education
is the basis of adequate referral of potential donors to organ procurement
agencies.

Several congenital heart anomalies, other than hypoplastic left heart
syndrome, require multiple palliative operations to meet conventional criteria for "definitive" palliation in the form of atriopulmonary connection.
Results of this surgical strategy, however, continue to be disappointing. Although life is prolonged beyond infancy and palliation is superb for some
individuals, survival at 5 years does not compare with the survival that is

possible today with transplantation. If the long-term results of neonatal transplantation are favorable, this technique will become the initial therapeutic procedure for infants with complex malformations.

Despite recent improvement in the preoperative care of infants with complex uncorrectable heart disease, a small percentage will deteriorate while waiting for a suitable allograft. This subgroup eventually may be selected for xenotransplantation "bridging" to alloengraftment,[16] or for initial palliative intervention en route to transplantation.

Recent advances in transplant immunotherapy appear extremely promising. Clinical investigation of agents such as FK-506, rapamycin, and deoxyspergualin is in progress. Donor-specific chronic tolerance to cardiac alloengraftment was induced with the administration of anti-CD4 antibodies.[17] Similar strategies to obtain life-long engraftment other than long-term post-transplant immunosuppression will expand the indications for heart replacement further.

References

1. Kantrowitz A, Haller SD, Joos H, et al: Transplantation of the heart in an infant and an adult. *Am J Cardiol* 1968; 22:782–790.
2. Cooley DA, Bloodwell RD, Hallman GL, et al: Organ transplantation for advanced cardiopulmonary disease. *Ann Thorac Surg* 1969; 8:30–46.
3. Bailey LL, Nehlsen-Cannarella SL, Concepcion W, et al: Baboon-to-human cardiac xenotransplantation in a neonate. *JAMA* 1985; 254:3321–3329.
4. Bailey LL, Nehlsen-Cannarella SL, Doroshow RW, et al: Cardiac allotransplantation in newborns as therapy for hypoplastic left heart syndrome. *N Engl J Med* 1986; 315:949–951.
5. Nehlsen-Cannarella SL, Buckert L, Seltman K, et al: Unique newborn immune response. *J Heart Transplant,* in press.
6. Bhargava H, Donner RM, Sanchez G, et al: Endomyocardial biopsy after heart transplantation in children. *J Heart Transplant* 1987; 6:298–302.
7. Starnes VA, Stinson EB, Oyer PE, et al: Cardiac transplantation in children and adolescents. *Circulation* 1987; 76(suppl V):V-43–V-47.
8. Pahl E, Fricker J, Armitage J, et al: Coronary arteriosclerosis in pediatric heart transplant survivors: Limitation of long-term survival. *J Pediatr* 1990; 116:177–183.
9. Addonizio LJ, Hsu DT, Smith CR, et al: Late complications in pediatric cardiac transplant recipients. *Circulation* 1990; 82(suppl IV):IV-295–IV-301.
10. Chartrand C, Dumont L, Stanley P: Pediatric cardiac transplantation. *Transplant Proc* 1989; 21:3349–3350.
11. Kahan BD: Immunosuppressive therapy with cyclosporine for cardiac transplantation. *Circulation* 1987; 75:40–56.
12. Vricella L, Alonso de Begoña J, Gundry S, et al: Aggressive peritoneal dialysis for treatment of renal failure after neonatal cardiac transplant. *J Heart Lung Transplant* 1991; 10:183.
13. Pennock JL, Oyer PE, Reitz BA, et al: Cardiac transplantation in perspective for the future: Survival, complication, rehabilitation, and cost. *J Thorac Cardiovasc Surg* 1982; 83:168–177.
14. Uretsky BF, Murali S, Reddy PS, et al: Development of coronary artery dis-

ease in cardiac transplant patients receiving immunosuppressive therapy with cyclosporine and prednisone. *Circulation* 1987; 76:827–834.
15. Radley-Smith R, Yacoub MH: Heart and heart-lung transplantation in children. *Circulation* 1987; 76(suppl IV):IV-24.
16. Bailey LL: Another look at cardiac xenotransplantation. *J Cardiac Surg* 1990; 5:210–218.
17. Shizuru JA, Seydel KB, Flavin TF, et al: Induction of donor-specific unresponsiveness to cardiac allografts in rats by pretransplant anti-CD4 monoclonal antibody therapy. *Transplantation* 1990; 50:366–373.

Tetralogy of Fallot With Pulmonary Stenosis

Lynn B. McGrath, M.D.

Department of Surgery, Deborah Heart and Lung Center; Department of
Surgery, University of Medicine and Dentistry of New Jersey, Robert Wood
Johnson Medical School, New Brunswick, New Jersey

Although the tetralogy of Fallot is a relatively common form of complex
congenital heart disease, and much information is available regarding its diagnosis, repair, and surgical results, there still remains major controversy in
the literature regarding optimum methods to treat these patients. These controversies include questions regarding optimal timing of primary repair, with
some authors recommending routine early and even neonatal repair,[1-6] and
other groups proposing a conservative two-stage approach with initial shunting in younger patients and delayed secondary repair.[7-13] There are reports
that support the liberal, almost routine use of a ventriculotomy and transannular patching in order to reduce the risk of residual right ventricular outflow
tract obstruction,[14] while others maintain that up to 90% of patients can be
repaired routinely without the need to resort to a ventriculotomy. There has
been an evolution reported in the surgical literature in relation to the risk of
transannular patching, with an apparent trend toward neutralization of this
technique as a risk factor for hospital death in the modern era.[15, 16] However, the long-term effects on patients with the tetralogy of a right ventriculotomy plus iatrogenically induced chronic pulmonary valve incompetence secondary to transannular patching remain unresolved. In this review, we will attempt to examine these and other issues and to report recent advances and
the current state of the art regarding the diagnosis and repair of the tetralogy
of Fallot with pulmonary stenosis.

Historical Perspective

The tetralogy of Fallot was first repaired by Lillehei at the University of
Minnesota in 1954 and reported in 1955.[17] This clinical trial employed
controlled cross-circulation using another human as the oxygenator. The
first successful repair utilizing cardiopulmonary bypass was performed by
Kirklin et al. in 1955.[18] The evolution of surgical methods proceeded, as
reported by Warden in 1957,[19] who described a right ventricular approach
to the repair with patch enlargement of the outflow tract. Kirklin in 1959
reported the first use of infundibular and transannular patching to relieve
the pulmonary stenosis.[20]

Initially, repair of the tetralogy in infants was associated with important surgical risk and this led to the recommendation of protocols calling for a two-stage repair, with shunting performed at presentation and repair delayed for 1 to 2 years. However, reports from Greenlane Hospital supported an aggressive approach (for that era) of routine primary repair.[21, 22] Nonetheless, because of sometimes unsatisfactory results with primary repair in younger subjects, many groups continued to utilize, and were proponents of, a two-stage approach, and the controversy regarding optimal management endures to the modern era.

Definition

The tetralogy of Fallot is a congenital cardiac anomaly with the hallmark of mild, moderate, or severe degrees of underdevelopment of the right ventricular infundibulum plus anterior, superior, and leftward displacement of the infundibular septum.[23] This migration of the infundibular septum creates right ventricular outflow tract obstruction, produces a malalignment-type interventricular communication, and leaves the aortic valve partially connected to the morphological right ventricle. Depending on the age at which the child is diagnosed and repaired, varying degrees of right ventricular hypertrophy develop secondarily.

Right Ventricular Outflow Tract Obstruction

As indicated, the infundibular stenosis occurring in the tetralogy of Fallot is due to a congenital malformation of the infundibular septum. As noted by Bharati et al., the septal and parietal extensions of the infundibular septum may develop unusually prominent muscle bands that attach on either side of the anterior right ventricular free wall, thus encircling the outflow tract of the right ventricle.[24] The stenosis of the right ventricular outflow tract, which is related to the migration of the infundibular septum, may be contributed to also by hypertrophy of multiple septal and trabecular muscle bands located on the anterior wall of the right ventricle. In addition, in some patients a fibrous tissue rim develops in the inferior portion of the infundibular septum, which may form an obstructive discrete os infundibulum.[25–27]

Two basic types of surgical pathology may be encountered, either of which can cause the right ventricular outflow tract obstruction. The first is due to tubular hypoplasia and underdevelopment of the outflow tract, and the second is related to hypertrophy of the infundibular septum. Recognition of these two basic anatomic variations is important to surgical decision-making, and determines whether ventriculotomy should be used to repair the tetralogy.[28] Of course, a spectrum of anatomic arrangements may be found, with varying degrees of hypoplasia and hypertrophy.

A report by Pacifico diagramatically outlined these features of the infundibular anatomy in classical tetralogy of Fallot.[29] He indicated that ideal anatomy for a nonventricular approach existed when there was a well-developed infundibular chamber, localized low-lying infundibular obstruction, and normal-sized pulmonary valve annulus and pulmonary arteries; he called this "type A." This entity has an anatomic arrangement somewhat analogous to that found in a double-chambered right ventricle with low-lying infundibular stenosis,[30] and a patient possessing it is the ideal candidate for a transatrial repair.

Pacifico's types B and C outflow tract obstruction are closely related morphological variations. Type B denotes severe hypertrophy of the infundibular septum, but with length, and therefore a tunnel nature; type C reflects a high-lying, localized, hypertrophic infundibular stenosis located just beneath the pulmonary valve. Pacifico's types D and E consist of a tubular hypoplastic infundibulum not amenable to direct attack by dissection and resection of obstructing infundibular muscle and mandating the use of an infundibular patch. Often in these latter two groups a transannular patch is also required, as usually the degree of pulmonary valve annulus hypoplasia parallels that of the infundibulum.

Isolated infundibular stenosis (Pacifico's type A) occurs in about 25% of patients. As noted, these cases are ideal for transatrial repair. The combination of tunnel-type infundibular hypertrophy plus valvular stenosis occurs in about 50% of patients and generally constitutes favorable anatomy for combined transatrial and transpulmonary repair. Infundibular hypertrophy with valvular plus annular stenosis is found in approximately 15% of patients and may require a limited transannular patch. Severe right ventricular outflow tract hypoplasia occurs in about 10% of cases, and generally necessitates at least an infundibular patch. Complete repair in the latter group may carry increased surgical risk. A report by Kirklin[31] indicated a hospital mortality rate of 19% in this subset (10 out of 52 patients died), which may reflect earlier age at repair, more severe degrees of cyanosis, smaller pulmonary arterial size, and an increased use of transannular patching.

Other variations on the infundibular anatomy also may occur. Although the interventricular communication in the tetralogy of Fallot is almost always large and subaortic in location, occasionally the defect excavates from the perimembranous area into the infundibular septum, in which case the ventricular septal defect is subpulmonary as well. In this group (Neirotti's Syndrome),[32] an infundibular patch is almost always required since the right ventricular outflow tract is invariably hypoplastic. At the Deborah Heart and Lung Center from 1985 through 1990, 11 of 145 patients (8%) had a subpulmonary ventricular septal defect, and in each case an infundibular patch was required, with all but 3 also requiring a transannular patch.

The diameter of the pulmonary valve annulus in the tetralogy of Fallot determines whether or not a transannular patch is required. There is, of course, a tendency in the tetralogy for this structure to be narrower than in normal individuals. Intraoperative decision-making with regard to its enlargement will be described later in this review. For some authors, however, maintenance of the integrity of this structure, and therefore of the competency of the pulmonary valve, is an important criterion in the definition of a successful repair with the best chance for a good long-term result. Other groups have balanced concern for the induction of pulmonary valve incompetence against the desire to avoid late residual right ventricular outflow tract obstruction by adopting protocols for the very liberal use of combined infundibular and transannular patching.

Although there is information available, it has not been determined absolutely at this time whether or not it is worthwhile always to avoid, if possible, the use of a classical right ventriculotomy in the relief of right ventricular outflow tract obstruction during the repair of the tetralogy of Fallot. In 1980, Harken reported that mapping and excision of the right ventriculotomy scar abolished ventricular ectopic activity in some patients who had developed ventricular arrhythmias in the late phase following repair of the tetralogy.[33] Kawashima also noted enhanced ventricular performance with an improved stroke volume index when the transatrial repair was used, as

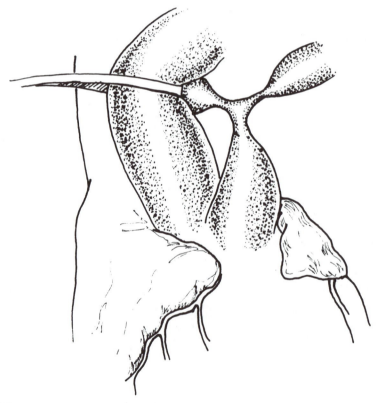

FIG 1.
Severe bifurcational pulmonary stenosis. (From McGrath LB: *Semin Thorac Cardiovasc Surg* 1990; 2:83–92. Used by permission.)

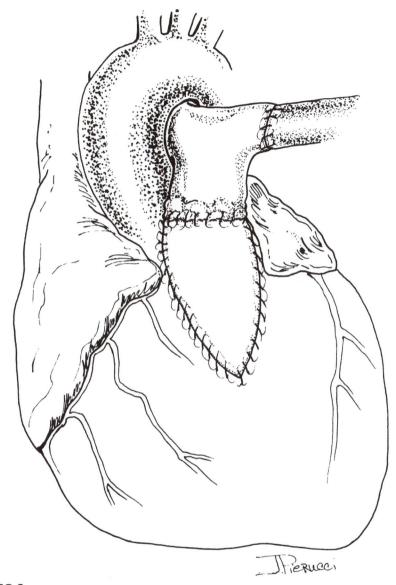

FIG 2.
Repair of bifurcational pulmonary stenosis utilizing a pulmonary valve homograft for reimplantation of the reconstructed left and right central pulmonary arteries, and completion of the repair utilizing a triangulated pericardial patch to close the right ventriculotomy. (From McGrath LB: *Semin Thorac Cardiovasc Surg* 1990; 2:83–92. Used by permission.)

opposed to the transventricular repair.[34, 35] As right ventriculotomy incision with transannular patching is reported to be an incremental risk factor for hospital death,[36-38] it is possible that if it could be determined preoperatively that a ventriculotomy incision would not be required in order to accomplish the repair, then complete repair could be performed earlier in life in these patients with favorable anatomy, without the need for a preliminary shunt. There is evidence available that this decision often can be made successfully based on preoperative angiography.[29]

In a high percentage of patients with the tetralogy (60% to 75%), there also may be important narrowing of the pulmonary valve leaflets. This obstruction may be due to a bicuspid valve with somewhat dysplastic leaflets, either secondary to commissural fusion or, occasionally, located at the supracommissural level. Usually the valve can be repaired; however, in some cases the pulmonary valve leaflets may be so dysplastic that they require partial or total valvulectomy.

Patients with tetralogy of Fallot may develop associated narrowings of the bifurcation of the ostia of the left or right central pulmonary arteries, or indeed of the entire bifurcation (Fig 1). The cause of these stenoses is not known. However, Hislop and Reid did note the presence of increased arterial wall thickness with muscularization and thickening of the media of the pulmonary arteries in these patients.[39] This, perhaps, may be causally related to the development of these ostial obstructions. Although it is not entirely clear what the influence of residual stenoses at this level is following repair in classical tetralogy, LeCompte reported that residual bifurcational pulmonary stenosis following repair of the tetralogy of Fallot with pulmonary atresia resulted in right ventricular hypertension with worse early and late results.[40] Recent reports have indicated that simple patching across these areas may not give a good long-term functional result, as residual stenoses may develop following somatic growth. Alternative methods of repair have been described, including transection and reimplantation for isolated right or left central pulmonary artery stenosis[31] and the placement of a pulmonary valve homograft bifurcation graft for patients with bilateral ostial pulmonary arterial stenoses (Fig 2).[41]

Interventricular Communication

The interventricular communication in the tetralogy of Fallot is usually located in the subaortic position and is perimembranous. The defect is related to malalignment of the infundibular septum and is usually unrestrictive. The penetrating and branching positions of the His bundle are located on the posteroinferior edge of the defect, as is the case for a usual isolated perimembranous ventricular septal defect.[42] Because of the anterosuperior and leftward movement of the infundibular septum, when the interventricular communication is examined through the tricuspid valve, the defect is often located much more craniad than is found in the usual isolated perimembranous ventricular septal defect approached through the same ex-

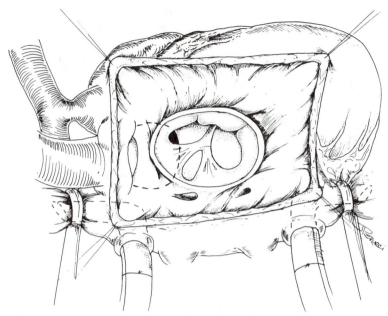

FIG 3.
Transatrial exposure of a large perimembranous ventricular septal defect in the tetralogy of Fallot. Note the more cephalad position of the defect.

posure (Fig 3). This may make exposure of the superior rim of the defect a little more difficult to visualize than in the usual perimembranous defect, and repair using a transatrial approach may be more challenging. Excessive traction on the tricuspid valve leaflets to arrange the exposure may result in damage to the tricuspid valve structure. Alternatively, the base of the septal leaflet of the tricuspid valve may be detached to permit the superior part of the ventricular septal defect patch suture line to be inserted.

Approximately 10% of patients with tetralogy of Fallot will have a subpulmonary interventricular communication. As indicated earlier, this generally means that an infundibular patch will be required, as the outflow tract is likely to be hypoplastic already, due to absence of part of the infundibular septum.[32]

Coronary Artery Anatomy

In 5% to 8% of patients with tetralogy of Fallot, the left anterior descending coronary artery arises from the right coronary artery and traverses the right ventricular outflow tract on its course to the interventricular groove.[43-46] This anomaly may be diagnosed by aortography or on a long-axis left ventriculogram performed preoperatively.[47] Although generally this coronary artery arrangement has been considered an indication for placement of a valved extracardiac conduit in order to accomplish repair, it is possible to perform primary repair on some of these patients using a transatrial approach.

At the Deborah Heart and Lung Center from 1985 through 1990, of 145 patients repaired with the tetralogy, 8 had an anomalous left anterior descending artery arising from the right coronary artery (6%). Based on preoperative angiographic assessment of the right ventricular anatomy, it was determined that 5 patients could be repaired utilizing a transatrial approach, and indeed all 5 had primary repair without a ventriculotomy. Three patients required the placement of a valved extracardiac conduit to accomplish the repair, 2 of whom had an initial shunt with delayed repair.

Occasionally, a very large right coronary artery conus branch may cross the right ventricular outflow tract of the right ventricle. In general, if a transventricular repair is made, these are sacrificed. However, if a transatrial approach is utilized, these branches may be salvaged, perhaps for the long-term benefit of the patient.

Clinical

Tetralogy patients usually present with cyanosis at an early age and, in general, its severity and the degree of polycythemia present are directly proportional to the severity of the pulmonary stenosis, which may include main and branch artery hypoplasia. Those infants who present with severe cyanosis early in life are more likely to have a diffuse hypoplastic type of right ventricular outflow tract obstruction. There may be severe infundibular, valvular, and annular pulmonary stenosis present. In regard to timing repair in younger patients presenting with severe cyanosis, Castaneda advocates early repair in neonates,[14] although this may be associated with increased risk since these patients may have unfavorable anatomy.

Other patients with the tetralogy present later in infancy with less severe forms of infundibular stenosis, which may gradually increase in severity and result in cyanotic spells. In this group, it is more likely that the stenosis can be resected directly, without the need for a patch. Overall, a patient's clinical presentation provides clues regarding the method of repair required.

Metabolic

An analysis of levels of adrenergic receptor activity of the myocytes of the septal extension of the infundibular septum in a group of patients with tetralogy of Fallot, compared to a control group of patients with isolated ventricular septal defect, revealed a marked elevation in α-adrenergic receptor activity in the former.[48] This may have important consequences for the development of treatment protocols. Although β-adrenergic blocking agents are known to palliate patients with tetralogy of Fallot,[49] perhaps α-adrenergic blockers might be useful also, both in the preoperative period for patients with cyanotic spells and in the perioperative period for those with residual right ventricular systolic hypertension. A current protocol is analyzing the clinical potential of α-adrenergic blockade in treating patients with evidence of dynamic right ventricular outflow tract obstruction in the tetralogy.

Diagnosis

The single most valuable tool for diagnosing the anatomy of right ventricular outflow tract obstruction in the tetralogy of Fallot is biplane cineangiography.[50, 51] Lateral, angled, and craniocaudal views are optimal for demonstrating not only the anatomy of the infundibular septum but also that of the bifurcation of the pulmonary arteries, which otherwise may go undiagnosed. All patients at the Deborah Heart and Lung Center undergo

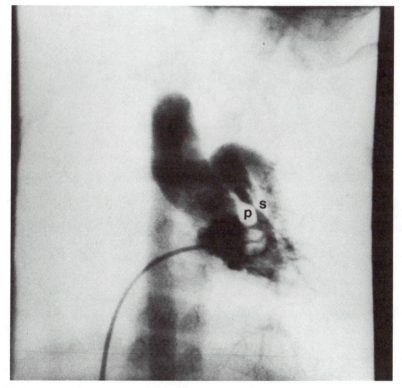

FIG 4.
Right ventricular angiocardiogram in systole of an 11-month-old patient with a craniocaudal view, indicating severe obstructive hypertrophy of the parietal *(p)* and septal *(s)* extensions of the infundibular septum. Repair was performed using a transpulmonary and transatrial approach. (From McGrath LB, Gonzalez-Lavin L: *J Thorac Cardiovasc Surg* 1988; 96:947–951. Used by permission.)

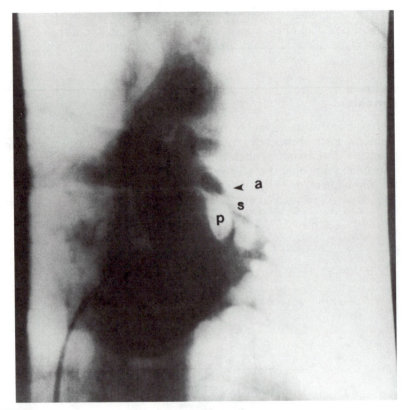

FIG 5.
Right ventricular angiocardiogram in diastole of a 3-year-old patient with a cranio-caudal view. Severe obstructive hypertrophy of the parietal *(p)* and septal *(s)* extensions of the infundibular septum is seen and annular hypoplasia is demonstrated *(a)*. Repair was performed with a transpulmonary and transatrial approach, plus a limited ventriculotomy. The pulmonary valve annulus was a Z value of -3.0, as measured with a Hegar dilator. (From McGrath LB, Gonzalez-Lavin L: *J Thorac Cardiovasc Surg* 1988; 96:947–951. Used by permission.)

detailed angiographic assessment of the infundibular septal anatomy, including cranial, caudal, and axial views. In previously published reports, cineangiocardiograms were reviewed retrospectively in a series of 52 patients with the tetralogy to define the angiographic characteristics of the right ventricular outflow tract obstruction.[28] Analysis revealed that it was possible for a blinded reviewer to predict accurately, on the basis of the angiocardiographic anatomy, the method of repair that had been utilized in each case, i.e., either transatrial plus transpulmonary or transventricular. In that study, 32 patients (62%) were found angiographically to have severe muscular hypertrophy of the infundibular septum as a predominant cause of the right ventricular outflow tract obstruction. Each of these patients underwent repair without a ventriculotomy, and in each case the approach was predicted by the reviewer. The other 20 patients (38%) had transventricular repair mandated by hypoplasia of the outflow tract. The angiocardiograms may reveal severe obstructive hypertrophic lesions of the parietal and septal extensions of the infundibular septum (Fig 4), obstructive lesions of the infundibular septum plus annular hypoplasia (Fig 5), or outflow tract hypoplasia (Fig 6).

Angiocardiography is also useful for examining the pulmonary arteries. Assessment of the anatomy and calibration of the size of the pulmonary valve annulus and the left and right central pulmonary artery diameters, and nor-

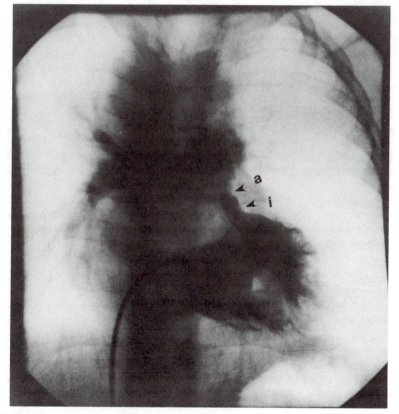

FIG 6.
Right ventricular angiocardiogram in diastole of a 4-year-old patient with a craniocaudal view. Severe hypoplasia of the right ventricular outflow tract, including the infundibulum *(i)* and the pulmonary valve annulus *(a)* is demonstrated. The diameter of the right ventricular outflow tract was a Z value of −3.5. Repair was performed utilizing a formal ventriculotomy plus infundibular and transannular patching. (From McGrath LB, Gonzalez-Lavin L: *J Thorac Cardiovasc Surg* 1988; 96:947–951. Used by permission.)

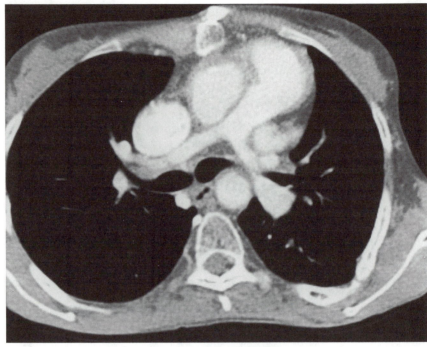

FIG 7.
Rapid computed tomographic scan demonstrating bifurcation of the pulmonary arteries in a patient with severe infundibular stenosis in whom the pulmonary arteries could not be well visualized angiographically. (From McGrath LB: *Semin Thorac Cardiovasc Surg* 1990; 2:83–92. Used by permission.)

malization of their ratio to the diameter of the descending aorta at the diaphragm (McGoon ratio) may produce a reliable prediction of the ratio between the right and left ventricular systolic pressures following repair.[52] There is information suggesting that utilization of the McGoon ratio enables an accurate estimation of the post repair right ventricular to left ventricular systolic pressure (PRV/LV) ratio. Some authors have recommended that when the McGoon ratio is less than 2.0, the creation of a shunt should be considered in order to promote pulmonary arterial growth and decrease the risk of later repair.[53–59]

In those patients in whom the central or bifurcational portion of the pulmonary arteries is not well visualized using conventional and axial angiography, rapid computed tomographic scanning with the Imatron (Imatron, Inc., San Francisco, California) device is often useful (Fig 7). This methodology permits three-dimensional visualization of the pulmonary arterial tree, measurement of pulmonary artery diameters, calculation of the cross-sectional area, and volumetric analysis of the pulmonary arteries.[60, 61]

Transatrial Repair

When there is isolated infundibular stenosis, either of the low-lying variety or with tunnel-type hypertrophy of the right ventricular outflow tract, the anatomy is generally amenable to repair using an atrial approach, without a right ventriculotomy.[62–66]

A median sternotomy incision is utilized, the thymus is excised, and the pericardium is opened rightward. If a limited or formal transannular patch is required, the leftward portion of the pericardium will be harvested and utilized later. The ascending aorta is dissected free from the main pulmonary artery in order to facilitate aortic cross-clamping without impingement on the pulmonary artery. Any systemic-to-pulmonary arterial shunts are dissected free from the surrounding tissues and encircled with number 2 silk. The patient is systemically heparinized and cardiopulmonary bypass is established at a flow rate of 2.2 L/min/m^2 up to a maximum flow of 4 L/min. The venous return is accomplished by direct caval vein cannulation using thin-walled, right-angle, metal-tipped venous cannulas (DLP, Inc., Grand Rapids, Michigan). Arterial inflow is to the ascending aorta. Bypass initially is established at 25° C and when it has been accomplished successfully and the shunts are secured, the patient is cooled. The cardiac activity becomes ineffective, the caval tapes are snugged, and the aorta is cross-clamped. Cold blood cardioplegia is infused into the aortic root and reinfused at 30-minute intervals, if necessary. A standard oblique right atriotomy incision is made, another incision is made in the fossa ovalis, and the vent is placed into the left atrium. If it is believed that the repair can be accomplished completely working through the right atrium, then stay sutures are placed on the right atrial wall and on the septal, anterior, and posterior leaflets of the tricuspid valve, in order to arrange the exposure. A completely transatrial approach may be accomplished when there is low-lying infundibular stenosis or occasionally when there is tunnel-type stenosis. Working through the right atrium, a pulmonary valvotomy also may be performed and ventricular septal defect closure accomplished.

If the narrowing is tunnel-like, often an initial longitudinal incision is made on the main pulmonary artery. The pulmonary valve is examined and a commissurotomy is performed, if required. If there is supravalvular tethering at the level of the leaflet commissures, they are released. If the valve is dysplastic, one or both leaflets may require excision.

The next step in the repair is to decide the fate of the pulmonary valve annulus based on normal pulmonary valve diameters, according to the work of Rowlatt, Rimoldi, and Lev,[67] and the nomogram generated by Pacifico, Blackstone, and colleagues.[53] Utilizing Hegar dilators, the diameter of the pulmonary valve annulus is calibrated. If the annular diameter is ≤2 SD smaller than normal, transannular patching will be necessary. This incision is limited, with extension of the pulmonary arteriotomy onto the infundibular portion of the right ventricle for a distance of only 5 to 10 mm, merely enough to release the pulmonary annulus. When this maneu-

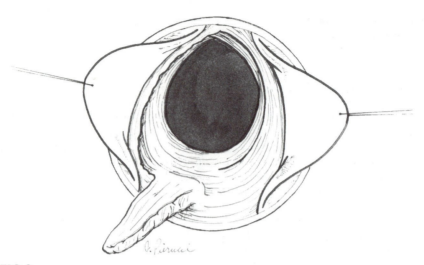

FIG 8.
The infundibular dissection is initiated working through the pulmonary artery and pulmonary valve. The septal extension of the infundibular septum is detached from the free wall of the right ventricle and completely excised. (From McGrath LB, Gonzalez-Lavin L: *J Cardiac Surg* 1987; 2:41. Used by permission.)

ver is required, the pulmonary valve is excised totally, since leaving it may result in late calcification of the leaflets and recurrent pulmonary stenosis.

Whether or not a limited transannular patch is required after the pulmonary valvotomy has been performed, the first portion of the infundibular dissection is begun from above, working through the pulmonary valve. Initial positioning of the patient is important; the child should be situated on the right side of the operating table, toward the operating surgeon, in reverse Trendelenburg position. The dissection is performed entirely using sharp dissection with a number 15 scalpel. It is begun anteriorly at the anterior wall of the right ventricle. Once the proper plane is developed, the incision is carried leftward to envelop and include the septal extension of the infundibular septum (Fig 8). Care is taken not to excavate too deeply at the base of the septal extension where it arises from the interventricular septum, as to do so may result in injury to the first septal branch of the left anterior descending coronary artery. Indeed, it is possible to create a ventricular septal defect and to injure the left anterior descending coronary artery itself during this leftward portion of the dissection. Multiple septal bands that may be contributing to tunnel-type stenosis are resected at this time.

The rightward portion of the dissection is performed by initially detaching the parietal extension of the infundibular septum from the anterior wall of the right ventricle. The dissection plane is developed around the parietal extension, and this is excised completely down to the ventriculo-infundibular fold (Fig 9). The aortic sinuses are at risk during this part of the dissection, as are the tricuspid valve chordal attachments.

After working from above, the remainder of the infundibular dissection is performed looking through the tricuspid valve. When assessing the infundibular stenosis from this angle, one must recognize that the anatomy is rotated in a clockwise fashion compared to the transventricular exposure, with the septal extension now located posteroinferiorly and the parietal extension lying in an almost anterior plane. It is advantageous to deal with the moderator band first, if necessary. In tetralogy, the moderator band may be severely hypertrophied and possibly contributing to low-lying infundibular stenosis. The band is divided and the base excised, with care taken to avoid injury to the chordal attachments of the anterior papillary muscle of the tricuspid valve. Next, the remnant of the septal extension of the infundibular septum is excised completely (Fig 10). Next, the remnant of the parietal extension of the infundibular septum is excised (Fig 11). Again, the risk of creating an inadvertent anterior right ventriculotomy or entering the aortic root is present when resecting the parietal extension. Nonetheless, complete resection is absolutely essential in order to accomplish successful transatrial repair and eliminate the risk of residual infundibular stenosis.

Having completed the infundibular dissection, the Hegar dilator appropriate for the patient's body surface area is passed through the right ventricular outflow tract from below. Calibrating the outflow tract in this manner enables one to determine the adequacy of the repair. At this point, a planned nonventricular approach may have to be converted to a formal ventriculotomy if the outflow tract repair is not satisfactory. However, from 1985 through 1990 at the Deborah Heart and Lung Center, only 1 of the 66 patients who underwent attempted nonventricular repair (1.5%) re-

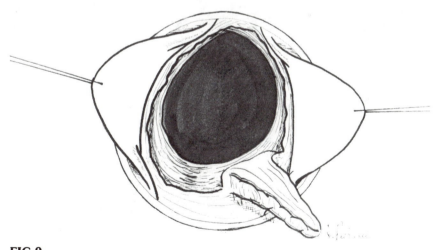

FIG 9.
Transpulmonary resection of the parietal extension of the infundibular septum is illustrated. (From McGrath LB, Gonzalez-Lavin L: *J Cardiac Surg* 1987; 2:41. Used by permission.)

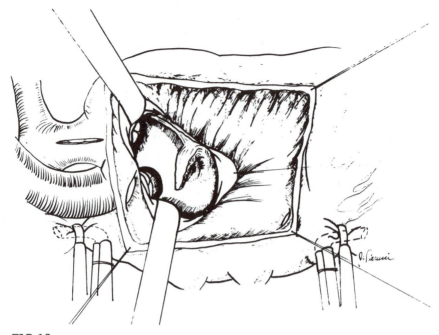

FIG 10.
Working through the right atrium and tricuspid valve, the remnant of the septal extension is completely excised. (From McGrath LB, Gonzalez-Lavin L: *J Cardiac Surg* 1987; 2:43. Used by permission.)

quired a formal ventriculotomy at this point. Therefore, utilizing preoperative angiographic information and intraoperative examination of the right ventricular outflow tract through the pulmonary artery via the tricuspid valve, it is almost always possible to determine whether a ventriculotomy will be necessary.

The next step is to close the interventricular communication utilizing a Sauvage (Bard Cardio Surgery Division, Billerica, Massachusetts) Dacron patch and continuous 4-0 monofilament suture. The interventricular communication generally is closed working through the tricuspid valve, whether or not a ventriculotomy is planned. Even when a ventriculotomy is required, this approach prevents excessive traction on the right ventricular free wall and avoids any unnecessary ventriculotomy retraction or enlargement, which sometimes is needed to enhance exposure of the ventricular septal defect when working through the right ventricle.

The suture line for the defect closure is started on the infundibular septum and carried leftward and superiorly completely around the annulus of the aortic valve. Once the patch is sewn onto the ventriculo-infundibular fold, the suture is brought out through the base of the anterior leaflet of the tricuspid valve. The other limb of the suture line is then completed, attaching the patch consecutively to the remainder of the infundibular septum and the trabecular and inflow portions of the muscular septum. Inferiorly, the suture line is carried 1 cm below the edge of the ventricular septal defect in order to avoid the branching portion of the His bundle. The suture is then brought out through the base of the septal leaflet of the tricuspid valve and a running horizontal mattress stitch is used between the edge of the ventricular septal defect patch and the base of the septal leaflet of the tricuspid valve. With the defect closure complete, the interatrial communication is closed, the patient is rewarmed, high suction is placed on the aortic needle vent, and the aortic cross-clamp is removed.

Any questions regarding ostial pulmonary stenoses are addressed at this point in the procedure. Normally, the ostia should be at least 75% of the diameter of the main pulmonary artery. They are both calibrated using Hegar dilators, and if one or both are noted to be hypoplastic, then an appropriate repair is performed. Repair may consist of pericardial patching, excision of the ostia, and reimplantation, or, occasionally, pulmonary homograft reconstruction, as described earlier.[41, 68]

Next, the pulmonary arteriotomy incision is closed primarily using continuous 6−0 monofilament suture if a limited transannular patch is not required. If the incision has been carried across the pulmonary valve annu-

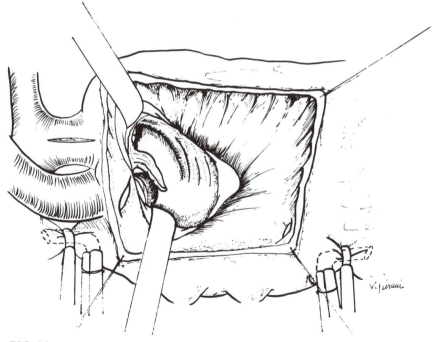

FIG 11.
Completion of the infundibular dissection is performed by resecting the remnant of the parietal extension of the infundibular septum. (From McGrath LB, Gonzalez-Lavin L: *J Cardiac Surg* 1987; 2:43. Used by permission.)

lus, then the pericardial patch is inserted using continuous 6-0 monofila-ment suture. After closing the pulmonary artery, the right atriotomy inci-sion is secured, the vent is removed from the right atrium, and the caval tapes are released.

For those patients in whom it is clear that a transatrial approach to the infundibulum is not appropriate and that formal infundibular patching will be required in order to relieve the stenosis, in general we will still close the interventricular communication working through the right atrium, as indi-cated earlier. Having performed a ventriculotomy with as limited an exten-sion onto the sinus portion of the right ventricle as possible, it is important, even when an infundibular patch is planned, that the parietal and septal extensions of the infundibular septum at least be transected, if not re-sected. This is necessary when simple ventricular patching is performed without resection of the infundibular stenosis;[14, 69] otherwise, late reopera-tions may be necessary.

Deciding whether to carry the infundibular incision superiorly across the pulmonary valve annulus is the same whether a ventriculotomy is per-formed or not. As described previously, if the pulmonary ring diameter is a Z value ≤ -2, then the ventriculotomy should be carried superiorly onto the main pulmonary artery.

Whenever a patch is placed on the right ventricle, the one with the smallest diameter compatible with an adequate repair should be em-ployed. Too large a patch may increase the risk for early- and late-phase ven-tricular dilatation and dysfunction with elevation in the right ventricular end-diastolic pressure, and late aneurysmal transformation of the patch.[70-73]

Management of right ventricular outflow tract obstruction is a complex process. The morphology of the obstruction and the individual surgeon's experience with individual management techniques will affect decision-making. Too liberal (some would say unnecessary) use of infundibular and transannular patching in an attempt to assure complete early- and late-phase relief of the infundibular stenosis may increase the risk of pulmonary valve incompetence,[74-78] ventricular arrhythmias,[79, 80] and ventricular dysfunction.[81-86] If the repair is performed directly with no retreat to patching, it seems intuitively as if the risk for residual right ventricular out-flow tract obstruction would be increased, lessening the chance for a good result. However, in our experience with 66 patients who did not undergo formal ventriculotomy, there have been no instances of early- or interme-diate-phase reoperation for residual right ventricular outflow tract obstruc-tion, and no echocardiographic, Doppler, or perioperative PRV/LV ratio data that have indicated that reoperation is necessary.

Right Ventricular/Left Ventricular Systolic Pressure Ratio

An assessment of the adequacy of the surgical repair is performed by mea-suring the PRV/LV ratio immediately after discontinuing cardiopulmonary bypass, again just prior to sternal closure, and in the intensive care unit at

18 hours postoperatively.[52, 53] A PRV/LV ratio of less than 0.85 is generally accepted to be satisfactory intraoperatively if a transannular patch has not been placed and particularly if a transatrial repair has been performed. Between the discontinuation of bypass and the time of sternal closure, the ratio declines more if an infundibular and transannular patch has not been placed (unpublished Deborah data, 1990, P[paired *t*-test] = .01). However, Coles[87] reported no difference in the change in PRV/LV ratio from perioperatively to 18 hours postoperatively, according to type of repair. It has been shown that, in general, if the PRV/LV ratio intraoperatively is 0.85 or less, then by 18 hours postoperatively the right ventricular/left ventricular ratio will be in the range of 0.50 to 0.60; this reflects what the right ventricular/left ventricular ratio will be if measured 2 years later and is consistent with a good late-phase result.[52]

It is useful to review the factors that constitute an increased postrepair PRV/LV ratio: incomplete closure of the ventricular septal defect, the presence and severity of any residual or recurrent right ventricular outflow tract obstruction, the size of the right and left central pulmonary arteries, and the presence and severity of any localized stenoses or arborization anomalies in the central or peripheral pulmonary arteries and arterioles. Realistically, the surgeon is responsible for relieving obstruction occurring between the infundibular septum and hilar portions of the pulmonary arteries. If the right and left central pulmonary arteries are somewhat small (McGoon's ratio less than 1.5), this may result in a worse early- or late-phase result. However, although shunting could be considered when the McGoon ratio is 1.5 or less, our policy is to make a repair regardless of the ratio (unless the pulmonary arteries are diminutive), with the intent to perforate the ventricular septal defect patch, if required. Using this protocol, only once out of 145 cases repaired (0.6%) have we had to perforate the ventricular septal defect patch. Among the 145 patients, the McGoon ratio was less than 1.5 in 27 (17%), and none of those died in the hospital (70% confidence limits = 0.5% to 12.1%).

It has been demonstrated previously that a higher postrepair right ventricular/left ventricular systolic pressure ratio is a significant risk factor for late death following repair of the tetralogy of Fallot. Wessel found that a right ventricular systolic pressure greater than 70 mm Hg had a negative effect on late functional status after tetralogy repair, and also claimed that important elevation of this pressure postoperatively is associated with an increased incidence of late events, including death.[88, 89]

One-Stage vs. Two-Stage Repair

The justification for early primary repair of the tetralogy of Fallot, including that of neonates, is based partly on the premise that early repair of congenital cardiac defects, particularly those associated with cyanotic conditions, would ameliorate secondary cardiac, pulmonary, and cerebral changes. In addition, eliminating right ventricular outflow tract obstruction early in life might minimize the development of secondary right ventricular hypertrophy and avoid hypertrophic cardiomyopathy, thereby preserving right ventricular function and the chance for a better late result.[90] Reportedly, establishing early antegrade pulmonary blood flow during the development of pulmonary arterioles and alveoli may normalize the structural integrity in these patients.[14] This is the basis upon which treatment protocols for routine primary repair of symptomatic patients with the tetralogy of Fallot, irrespective of body surface area or age, were developed.

Castaneda recently reported the results of 250 infants between 1 and 365 days of age who underwent primary repair between 1973 and 1988.[14] Eight of these patients had had a prior shunt procedure. There was a high incidence of transannular patching in this group (90%). The mortality rate was 4.4% overall, but 14.8% in neonates. Twenty-one patients (8%) required reoperations, 12 because of residual right ventricular outflow tract obstruction and 4 for re-resection of a residual infundibular obstruction.

A report by Gustafson in 1988 of the results of early primary repair of 40 patients with tetralogy of Fallot, following a protocol of early complete repair, found good results, with no hospital deaths (70% confidence limits 0% to 5%).[90] However, in an accompanying editorial, Kirklin indicated that there was no evidence that deferring repair in the tetralogy of Fallot from 6 or 12 weeks of age until 2 years of age (which is frequently possible) is detrimental to later ventricular performance, exercise capacity, or survival.[91]

Disadvantages of following a two-stage approach to tetralogy of Fallot repair include the socioeconomic and medical drawbacks of two hospitalizations and two operations, the potential morbidity and mortality associated with the shunting operation, and the chance for intervening events to occur between the shunting operation and the subsequent repair.[92-96] In a report of a large series of patients covering the entire spectrum of tetralogy of Fallot, Kirklin reported no deaths among 53 patients with tetralogy plus pulmonary stenosis who received a primary classical or modified Blalock-Taussig shunt.[37] Serious interim complications after these shunts occurred in 2 patients (sudden death, brain abscess) and no iatrogenic pulmonary arterial problems were recognized. However, it was postulated that although there was an important increase in hospital death among patients who required an infundibular and transannular patch, many of the selective recommendations regarding two-stage repair perhaps ultimately would be revised if improved methods of cardiopulmonary bypass and myocardial preservation were to develop.

Transannular Patching

It appears that the controversy that has continued over the use of transannular patching in the tetralogy of Fallot with pulmonary stenosis is related to conflicting information and differing philosophies regarding its effects on early- and late-phase results. There have been many reports indicating that transannular patching is an incremental risk factor for hospital death following repair of the tetralogy.[37, 38] However, recent reports by Kirklin[16, 17] indicate that this risk factor has weakened in the current era, with a trend toward neutralization. This evolution may reflect advances in postoperative care, improved methods of myocardial protection, and changes in the conduct of cardiopulmonary bypass in the modern era. Kirklin's report[17] also indicated that hazard function analysis discovered that transannular patching was not an instantaneous risk factor for premature late death. However, transannular patching, not unexpectedly, was a risk factor for reoperation for pulmonary regurgitation late postoperatively. Reportedly, reoperation for important pulmonary valve incompetence usually is required when the incompetence is associated with residual pulmonary stenosis, often occurring peripherally.

Although transannular patching ultimately may be completely neutralized as a risk factor for hospital death, there remain residual concerns regarding late events. With regard to the importance of iatrogenically induced pulmonary valvular incompetence, some inferences can be made from Shimazaki's experience with congenital pulmonary valve incompetence;[97] he reported that right ventricular failure ultimately developed in a high proportion of these patients. Therefore, not just late, but very late, results will have to be assessed in order to decide what the ultimate negative effects of routine transannular patching will be. Because of the potential for late detrimental effects, continued attempts to preserve the function of the pulmonary valve appear to be worthwhile.[98]

Although there have been recent reports of satisfactory early-phase results with primary orthotopic valve implantation, there is no late-phase information available regarding primary insertion of a homograft valve or single cusp valve repair. As a result, routine utilization of these techniques in patients with a transannular patch is probably not supportable at this time, since these patients almost certainly will require reoperation due to biodegeneration of the prosthesis.[99-101]

Deborah Heart and Lung Center Data

From 1985 through 1990, 145 consecutive patients underwent repair of the tetralogy of Fallot with pulmonary stenosis at the Deborah Heart and Lung Center. There were 84 males (58%) and 61 females (42%). Mean age at repair was 2.6 years, with a range of 0.3 to 45.8 years. Mean body surface area was 0.72 m^2, with a range of 0.32 to 2.05 m^2. The mean hematocrit was 46.5% with a range of 27 to 88 g%. One hundred thirty-six patients (94%) were in New York Heart Association functional class III or IV. Fifty-four patients (37%) had had a prior operation. The PRV/LV ratio intraoperatively at 30 minutes after cardiopulmonary bypass was a mean of 0.45 with a range of 0.18 to 1.00. There were 4 hospital deaths (2.7%, 70% confidence limits = 1.4% to 4.9%). Two patients died of acute cardiac failure and 2 of subacute cardiac failure. Among the 80 patients who

TABLE 1.
Tetralogy of Fallot Repaired at the Deborah Heart and Lung Center Between 1985 and 1990 (145 cases)

Methods of Repair	Number of Patients	Percentage of Patients
Transventricular plus transannular patch	75	52%
Transatrial plus transpulmonary plus limited transannular patch	32	22%
Transatrial	17	12%
Transatrial plus transpulmonary	16	11%
Transventricular with no transannular patch	6	4%
Transpulmonary	1	0.7%

underwent transventricular repair, there were 3 deaths (3.7%); among the 65 who underwent transatrial repair, there was 1 death (1.5%, P(Fisher) = .42). The methods of repair utilized and concomitant procedures performed are indicated in Tables 1 and 2, respectively.

An extensive list of incremental risk factors for hospital death was analyzed univariately and multivariately. This included age, height, weight, body surface area, preoperative right ventricular pressure, preoperative left

TABLE 2.
Tetralogy of Fallot Repaired at the Deborah Heart and Lung Center Between 1985 and 1990 (145 Cases)

Concomitant Procedures Performed*	Number of Patients	Percentage of Patients
Pulmonary valvotomy	82	54.3%
Closure of Blalock-Taussig shunt	39	25.8%
Repair of peripheral pulmonary stenosis	31	20.5%
Closure of atrial septal defect	13	8.6%
Closure of Potts Shunt	7	4.6%
Closure of patent ductus arteriosus	5	3.3%
Orthotopic valve insertion	4	2.6%
Valved extracardiac conduit	3	1.9%
Nonvalved extracardiac conduit	2	1.3%
Reopening of ventricular septal defect	1	0.6%

*One hundred eighty-seven procedures performed in 105 patients.

ventricular pressure, preoperative hematocrit, preoperative New York Heart Association functional class, preoperative severity of cyanosis, total cardiopulmonary bypass time, total aortic occlusion time, early and late intraoperative PRV/LV ratio, 18-hour postoperative PRV/LV ratio, earlier date of surgery, gender, previous cardiac operation, method of repair, and associated procedures, but no significant risk factors were noted. However, a discriminant analysis that combined decreasing body surface area with increasing intraoperative PRV/LV ratio indicated a tendency toward an increasing risk of hospital death (P[student's t-test] = .07). Similarly, a discriminant analysis of decreasing body surface area plus increasing total cardiopulmonary bypass time indicated an increased risk for hospital death as well (P[student's t-test] = .0011). This method of analysis perhaps indicates the presence of weak incremental risk factors (smaller size, increasing bypass time) in the process of neutralization.

All patients underwent postoperative echocardiographic and Doppler examination. Five patients had mild residual right ventricular outflow tract obstruction (3%). There were no significant residual interventricular communications. Mild to moderate pulmonary insufficiency was present in 58 patients (40%). One late death of unknown cause occurred at 4 years post-repair (0.7%, 70% confidence limits = 0.1% -2%), and no reoperations have been required.

Conclusions

Our present treatment protocols for patients with tetralogy of Fallot and pulmonary stenosis indicate that primary repair is recommended at any age or body surface area in patients in whom angiography indicates that the repair can be performed using a transatrial and transpulmonary approach. However, if the patient is less than 6 months of age and a ventricular patch appears to be required, then an initial shunt should be made with delayed repair performed at about 2 years of age. In any patient over 6 months of age, the repair is made at the time of presentation, regardless of the surgical approach required. Regarding McGoon's ratio, the pulmonary arterial size presently is not a factor in the decision-making process unless the pulmonary arteries are diminutive. Although there is evidence that the pulmonary arteries and pulmonary valve annulus may grow in response to a systemic-pulmonary arterial shunt, we have found that the amount of growth that occurs generally will not be sufficient to influence the type of repair that ultimately will be required.

Presently, every attempt is made to avoid the use of a right ventriculotomy incision and to spare the pulmonary valve annulus and valve in the repair of the tetralogy of Fallot. Although as a risk factor for hospital death, the use of an infundibular and transannular patch apparently is becoming neutralized in the modern era due to advances in the conduct of myocardial preservation and cardiopulmonary bypass, very late results following tetralogy of Fallot repair undoubtedly will be enhanced if right ventricular and pulmonary valve functions are preserved.

References

1. Starr A, Bonchek L, Sunderland CO: Total correction of tetralogy of Fallot in infancy. *J Thorac Cardiovasc Surg* 1973; 65:45–57.
2. Castaneda AR, Freed MD, Williams RG, et al: Repair of tetralogy of Fallot in infancy. *J Thorac Cardiovasc Surg* 1977; 74:372–381.
3. Tucker WY, Turley K, Ullyot DJ, et al: Management of symptomatic tetralogy of Fallot in the first year of life. *J Thorac Cardiovasc Surg* 1979; 78:494–501.
4. Castaneda AR, Norwood WI: Repair of Fallot's tetralogy in infancy. Modern Technics in Surgery Cardiac/Thoracic Surgery 1981; 42-1–42-7.
5. Walsh EP, Rockenmacher S, Keane JF, et al: Late results in patients with tetralogy of Fallot repaired during infancy. *Circulation* 1988; 77:1062–1067.
6. Touati GD, Vouhe PR, Amodeo A, et al: Primary repair of tetralogy of Fallot in infancy. *J Thorac Cardiovasc Surg* 1990; 99:396–403.
7. Bender HW Jr, Fisher RD, Conkle DM, et al: Selective operative treatment for tetralogy of Fallot: Rationale and results. *Ann Surg* 1976; 183:685–690.
8. Stephenson LW, Friedman S, Edmunds LH Jr: Staged surgical management of tetralogy of Fallot in infants. *Circulation* 1978; 58:837–841.
9. Kirklin JW, Blackstone EH, Pacifico AD, et al: Routine primary repair vs. two-stage repair of tetralogy of Fallot. *Circulation* 1979; 60:373–386.
10. Arciniegas E, Farooki ZQ, Hakimi M, et al: Results of two-stage surgical treatment of tetralogy of Fallot. *J Thorac Cardiovasc Surg* 1980; 79:876–883.
11. Garson A Jr, Gorry GA, McNamara DG, et al: The surgical decision in tetralogy of Fallot: Weighing risks and benefits with decision analysis. *Am J Cardiol* 1980; 45:108–116.
12. Rittenhouse EA, Mansfield PB, Hall DG, et al: Tetralogy of Fallot: Selective staged management. *J Thorac Cardiovasc Surg* 1985; 89:772–779.
13. Hammon JW Jr, Henry CL Jr, Merrill WH, et al: Tetralogy of Fallot: Selective surgical management can minimize operative mortality. *Ann Thorac Surg* 1985; 40:280–284.
14. Castaneda AR: Classical repair of tetralogy of Fallot: Timing, technique, and results. *Semin Thorac Cardiovasc Surg* 1990; 2:70–75.
15. Kirklin JK, Kirklin JW, Blackstone EH, et al: Effect of transannular patching on outcome after repair of tetralogy of Fallot. *Ann Thorac Surg* 1989; 48:783–791.
16. Kirklin JK, Kirklin JW, Pacifico AD: Transannular outflow tract patching for tetralogy: Indications and results. *Semin Thorac Cardiovasc Surg* 1990; 2:61–69.
17. Lillehei CW, Cohen M, Warden HE, et al: Direct vision intracardiac surgical correction of the tetralogy of Fallot, pentalogy of Fallot, and pulmonary atresia defects: Report of first ten cases. *Ann Surg* 1955; 142:418–442.
18. Kirklin JW, DuShane JW, Patrick RT, et al: Intracardiac surgery with the aid of a mechanical pump-oxygenator system (Gibbon type): Report of eight cases. *Proc Staff Meet Mayo Clin* 1955; 30:201.
19. Warden HE, DeWall RA, Cohen M, et al: A surgical-pathologic classification for isolated ventricular septal defects and for those in Fallot's tetralogy based on observations made on 120 patients during repair under direct vision. *J Thorac Surg* 1957; 33:21–44.
20. Kirklin JW, Ellis FH Jr, McGoon DC, et al: Surgical treatment for the tetral-

ogy of Fallot by open intracardiac repair. *J Thorac Surg* 1959; 37:22–46.

21. Barratt-Boyes BG, Simpson M, Neutze JM: Intracardiac surgery in neonates and infants using deep hypothermia with surface cooling and limited cardiopulmonary bypass. *Circulation* 1971; 63–64(suppl I):I25–I30.

22. Barratt-Boyes BG, Neutze JM: Primary repair of tetralogy of Fallot in infancy using a profound hypothermia with circulatory arrest and limited cardiopulmonary bypass: A comparison with conventional two-stage management. *Ann Surg* 1973; 178:406–411.

23. Van Praagh R, Van Praagh S, Nebesar RA, et al: Tetralogy of Fallot: Underdevelopment of the pulmonary infundibulum and its sequelae. *Am J Cardiol* 1970; 26:25–33.

24. Bharati S, Paul MH, Idriss FS, et al: The surgical anatomy of pulmonary atresia with ventricular septal defect: Pseudotruncus. *J Thorac Cardiovasc Surg* 1975; 69:713–721.

25. Becker AE, Connor M, Anderson RH: Tetralogy of Fallot: A morphometric and geometric study. *Am J Cardiol* 1975; 35:402–412.

26. Anderson RH, Allwork SP, Yen Ho S, et al: Surgical anatomy of tetralogy of Fallot. *J Thorac Cardiovasc Surg* 1981; 81:887–896.

27. Soto B, McConnell ME: Tetralogy of Fallot: Angiographic and pathological correlation. *Semin Thorac Cardiovasc Surg* 1990; 2:12–26.

28. McGrath LB, Gonzalez-Lavin L: Determination of the need for a ventriculotomy in the repair of tetralogy of Fallot. *J Thorac Cardiovasc Surg* 1988; 96:947–951.

29. Pacifico AD, Kirklin JK, Colvin EV, et al: Transatrial-transpulmonary repair of tetralogy of Fallot. *Semin Thorac Cardiovasc Surg* 1990; 2:76–82.

30. McGrath LB, Joyce DH: Transatrial repair of double-chambered right ventricle. *J Cardiac Surg* 1989; 4:291–298.

31. Kirklin JW, Barratt-Boyes BG: *Cardiac Surgery.* New York, John Wiley & Sons, 1986.

32. Neirotti R, Galindez E, Kreutzer G, et al: Tetralogy of Fallot with subpulmonary ventricular septal defect. *Ann Thorac Surg* 1978; 25:51–56.

33. Harken AH, Horowitz LN, Josephson ME: Surgical correction of recurrent sustained ventricular tachycardia following complete repair of tetralogy of Fallot. *J Thorac Cardiovasc Surg* 1980; 80:779.

34. Kawashima Y, Kitamura S, Nakano S, et al: Corrective surgery for tetralogy of Fallot without or with minimal right ventriculotomy and with repair of the pulmonary valve. *Circulation* 1981; 64(suppl II):II147–II153.

35. Kawashima Y, Matsuda H, Hirose H, et al: Ninety consecutive corrective operations for tetralogy of Fallot with or without minimal right ventriculotomy. *J Thorac Cardiovasc Surg* 1985; 90:856–863.

36. Piccoli GP, Dickinson DF, Musumeci F, et al: A changing policy for the surgical treatment of tetralogy of Fallot: Early and late results in 235 consecutive patients. *Ann Thorac Surg* 1982; 33:365–373.

37. Kirklin JW, Blackstone EH, Kirklin JK, et al: Surgical results and protocols in the spectrum of tetralogy of Fallot. *Ann Surg* 1983; 198:251–265.

38. Kirklin JW, Blackstone EH, Pacifico AD, et al: Risk factors for early and late failure after repair of tetralogy of Fallot, and their neutralization. *Thorac Cardiovasc Surg* 1984; 32:207–214.

39. Hislop A, Reid L: Structural changes in the pulmonary arteries and veins in tetralogy of Fallot. *Br Heart J* 1973; 35:1178–1183.

40. LeCompte Y, Hazan E, Baillot F, et al: La reparation chirugicale de la voie

pulmonaire dans la tetralogic de Fallot. *Couer* 1977; 8:739–747.

41. McGrath LB: Management of pulmonary bifurcation obstruction in classical tetralogy of Fallot. *Semin Thorac Cardiovasc Surg* 1990; 2:83–92.

42. Lev M: The architecture of the conduction system in congenital heart disease: Tetralogy of Fallot. *Arch Pathol* 1959; 67:114/572–129/587.

43. Bonchek LI: A method of outflow tract reconstruction in tetralogy of Fallot with anomalous anterior descending coronary artery. *Ann Thorac Surg* 1976; 21:451–453.

44. Shaffer CW, Berman W Jr, Waldhausen JA: Repair of divided anomalous anterior descending coronary artery in tetralogy of Fallot. *Ann Thorac Surg* 1979; 27:250–253.

45. Dabizzi RP, Caprioli G, Aiazzi L, et al: Distribution and anomalies of coronary arteries in tetralogy of Fallot. *Circulation* 1980; 61:95–102.

46. Di Carlo D, De Nardo D, Ballerini L, et al: Injury to the left coronary artery during repair of tetralogy of Fallot: Successful aorta-coronary polytetrafluoroethylene graft. *J Thorac Cardiovasc Surg* 1987; 93:468–470.

47. Fellows KE, Freed MD, Keane JF, et al: Results of routine preoperative coronary angiography in tetralogy of Fallot. *Circulation* 1975; 51:561–566.

48. McGrath LB, Gu J, Bianchi J, et al: Determination of infundibular innervation and amine receptor content in cyanotic and acyanotic myocardium: Relation to clinical events in the tetralogy of Fallot. *Pediatric Cardiology,* 1991; 12:155–160..

49. Wensley DF, Karl T, Deanfield JE, et al: Assessment of residual right ventricular outflow tract obstruction following surgery using the response to intravenous propranolol. *Ann Thorac Surg* 1987; 44:633–636.

50. Bargeron LM Jr, Elliott LP, Soto B, et al: Axial cineangiography in congenital heart disease: Section I. Concept, technical and anatomic considerations. *Circulation* 1977; 56:1075–1083.

51. Soto G, Pacifico AD, Ceballos R, et al: Tetralogy of Fallot: An angiographic-pathologic correlative study. *Circulation* 1981; 64:558–566.

52. Blackstone EH, Kirklin JW, Bertranou EG, et al: Preoperative prediction from cineangiograms of postrepair right ventricular pressure in tetralogy of Fallot. *J Thorac Cardiovasc Surg* 1979; 78:542–552.

53. Pacifico AD, Kirklin JW, Blackstone EH: Surgical management of pulmonary stenosis in tetralogy of Fallot. *J Thorac Cardiovasc Surg* 1977; 74:382–395.

54. Kirklin JW, Bargeron LM Jr, Pacifico AD: The enlargement of small pulmonary arteries by preliminary palliative operations. *Circulation* 1977; 56:612–617.

55. Arciniegas E, Blackstone EH, Pacifico AD, et al: Classic shunting operations as part of two-stage repair for tetralogy of Fallot. *Ann Thorac Surg* 1979; 27:514–518.

56. Gale AW, Arciniegas E, Green EW, et al: Growth of the pulmonary annulus and pulmonary arteries after the Blalock-Taussig shunt. *J Thorac Cardiovasc Surg* 1979; 77:459–465.

57. Guyton RA, Owens EJ, Waumett JD, et al: The Blalock-Taussig shunt: Low risk, effective palliation, and pulmonary artery growth. *J Thorac Cardiovasc Surg* 1983; 85:917–922.

58. Rosenberg HG, Williams WG, Trusler GA, et al: Structural composition of central pulmonary arteries: Growth potential after surgical shunts. *J Thorac Cardiovasc Surg* 1987; 94:498–503.

59. Brandt B III, Camacho JA, Mahoney LT, et al: Growth of the pulmonary arteries following Blalock-Taussig shunt. *Ann Thorac Surg* 1986; 42(suppl):S1–S4.
60. Eldredge WJ, Flicker S: Evaluation of congenital heart disease using cine-CT. *American Journal of Cardiac Imaging* 1987; 1:38–50.
61. Eldredge WJ, Flicker S, Steiner RM: Cine-CT in the anatomical evaluation of congenital heart disease. *New Concepts in Cardiac Imaging* 1987; 3:265–285.
62. Hudspeth AS, Cordell AR, Johnston FR: Transatrial approach to total correction of tetralogy of Fallot. *Circulation* 1963; 27:796–800.
63. Edmunds H Jr, Saxena NC, Friedman S, et al: Transatrial resection of the obstructed right ventricular infundibulum. *Circulation* 1976; 54:117–122.
64. Binet JP: Correction of tetralogy of Fallot with combined transatrial and pulmonary approach. *Surgical Rounds* 1986; 9:33–50.
65. McGrath LB, Gonzalez-Lavin L: Tetralogy of Fallot repair with minimal or no ventriculotomy. *J Cardiac Surg* 1987; 2:37–47.
66. Dietl CA, Torres AR, Cazzaniga ME, et al: Right atrial approach for surgical correction of tetralogy of Fallot. *Ann Thorac Surg* 1989; 47:546–552.
67. Rowlatt UF, Rimoldi HJA, Lev M: The quantitative anatomy of the normal child's heart. *Pediatr Clin North Am* 1963; 10:499.
68. McGrath LB, Gonzalez-Lavin L, Graf D: Pulmonary homograft implantation for ventricular outflow tract reconstruction: Early phase results. *Ann Thorac Surg* 1988; 45:273–277.
69. Pacifico AD, Kirklin JK, Colvin EV, et al: Tetralogy of Fallot: Late results and reoperations. *Semin Thorac Cardiovasc Surg* 1990; 2:108–116.
70. Rosenthal A, Gross RE, Pasternac A: Aneurysms of right ventricular outflow patches. *J Thorac Cardiovasc Surg* 1972; 63:735–740.
71. Furuse A, Mizuno A, Shindo G, et al: Optimal size of outflow patch in total correction of tetralogy of Fallot. *Jpn Heart J* 1977; 18:629–637.
72. Seybold-Epting W, Chiariello L, Hallman GL, et al: Aneurysm of pericardial right ventricular outflow tract patches. *Ann Thorac Surg* 1977; 24:237–240.
73. Oku H, Shirotani H, Yokoyama T, et al: Right ventricular outflow tract prosthesis in total correction of tetralogy of Fallot. *Circulation* 1980; 62:604–610.
74. Furuse A, Mizuno A, Shindo G, et al: Pulmonary regurgitation following total correction of tetralogy of Fallot. *Jpn Heart J* 1977; 18:621–628.
75. Calder AL, Barratt-Boyes BG, Brandt PWT, et al: Postoperative evaluation of patients with tetralogy of Fallot repaired in infancy: Including criteria for use of outflow patching and radiologic assessment of pulmonary regurgitation. *J Thorac Cardiovasc Surg* 1979; 17:705–720.
76. Misbach GA, Turley K, Ebert PA: Pulmonary valve replacement for regurgitation after repair of tetralogy of Fallot. *Ann Thorac Surg* 1983; 36:684–691.
77. Guo-Wei H, Chia-Chiang K, Mee RBB: Pulmonic regurgitation and reconstruction of right ventricular outflow tract with patch. *J Thorac Cardiovasc Surg* 1986; 92:128–137.
78. Ilbawi MN, Idriss FS, DeLeon SY, et al: Long-term results of porcine valve insertion for pulmonary regurgitation following repair of tetralogy of Fallot. *Ann Thorac Surg* 1986; 41:478–482.
79. Zahka KG, Horneffer PJ, Rowe SA, et al: Long-term valvular function after total repair of tetralogy of Fallot: Relation to ventricular arrhythmias. *Circulation* 1988; 78(suppl III):III14–III19.

80. Vaksmann G, Fournier A, Davignon A, et al: Frequency and prognosis of arrhythmias after operative "correction" of tetralogy of Fallot. *Am J Cardiol* 1990; 66:346–349.
81. Graham TP Jr, Cordell D, Atwood GF, et al: Right ventricular volume characteristics before and after palliative and reparative operation in tetralogy of Fallot. *Circulation* 1976; 54:417–423.
82. Borow KM, Green LH, Castaneda AR, et al: Left ventricular function after repair of tetralogy of Fallot and its relationship to age at surgery. *Circulation* 1980; 61:1150–1158.
83. Reduto LA, Berger HJ, Johnstone DE, et al: Radionuclide assessment of right and left ventricular exercise reserve after total correction of tetralogy of Fallot. *Am J Cardiol* 1980; 45:1013–1018.
84. Lange PE, Onnasch DGW, Bernhard A, et al: Left and right ventricular adaptation to right ventricular overload before and after surgical repair of tetralogy of Fallot. *Am J Cardiol* 1982; 50:786–794.
85. Bove EL, Byrum CJ, Thomas FD, et al: The influence of pulmonary insufficiency on ventricular function following repair of tetralogy of Fallot. *J Thorac Cardiovasc Surg* 1983; 85:691–696.
86. Klinner W, Reichart B, Pfaller M, et al: Late results after correction of tetralogy of Fallot necessitating outflow tract reconstruction. *Thorac Cardiovasc Surg* 1984; 32:244–247.
87. Coles JG, Kirklin JW, Pacifico AD, et al: The relief of pulmonary stenosis by a transatrial versus a transventricular approach to the repair of tetralogy of Fallot. *Ann Thorac Surg* 1988; 45:7–10.
88. Wessel HU, Cunningham WJ, Paul MH, et al: Exercise performance in tetralogy of Fallot after intracardiac repair. *J Thorac Cardiovasc Surg* 1980; 80:582–593.
89. Kirklin JW, Blackstone EH: Editorial on papers by Naito, Wessel, and their colleagues. *J Thorac Cardiovasc Surg* 1980; 80:594–599.
90. Gustafson RA, Murray GF, Warden HE, et al: Early primary repair of tetralogy of Fallot. *Ann Thorac Surg* 1988; 45:235–241.
91. Kirklin JW, Blackstone EH, Colvin EV, et al: Early primary correction of tetralogy of Fallot. *Ann Thorac Surg* 1988; 45:231–233.
92. Folger GM Jr, Shah KD: Subclavian steal in patients with Blalock-Taussig anastomosis. *Circulation* 1965; 31:241–248.
93. Midgley FM, McClenathan JE: Subclavian steal syndrome in the pediatric age group. *Ann Thorac Surg* 1977; 24:252–257.
94. Newfeld EA, Waldman JD, Paul MH, et al: Pulmonary vascular disease after systemic-pulmonary arterial shunt operations. *Am J Cardiol* 1977; 39:715–720.
95. Geiss D, Williams WG, Lindsay WK, et al: Upper extremity gangrene: A complication of subclavian artery division. *Ann Thorac Surg* 1980; 30:487–489.
96. Lodge FA, Lamberti JJ, Goodman AH, et al: Vascular consequences of subclavian artery transection for the treatment of congenital heart disease. *J Thorac Cardiovasc Surg* 1983; 86:18–23.
97. Shimazaki Y, Blackstone EH, Kirklin JW: The natural history of isolated congenital pulmonary valve incompetence: Surgical implications. *Thorac Cardiovasc Surg* 1984; 32:257–259.
98. Delisle G, Olley PM: Epreuve d'effort sous-maximal chez les enfants atteints de tetralogie de Fallot: Avant et apres correction chirurgicale. *Union Med Can* 1974; 103:886.
99. Abdulali SA, Silverton NP, Yakirevich, et al: Right ventricular outflow tract

reconstruction with a bovine pericardial monocusp patch: Long-term clinical and hemodynamic evaluation. *J Thorac Cardiovasc Surg* 1985; 89:764–771.

100. Oku H, Shirotani H, Ohnishi H: Two-cusp plasty for the right ventricular outflow tract in complete repair of tetralogy of Fallot. *Ann Thorac Surg* 1988; 45:97–98.

101. Clarke DR, Campbell DN, Pappas G: Pulmonary allograft conduit repair of tetralogy of Fallot. *J Thorac Cardiovasc Surg* 1989; 98:730–737.

Arterial Switch for Transposition of the Great Arteries and Associated Malposition Anomalies

Constantine Mavroudis, M.D.

Division Head and A.C. Buehler Professor of Cardiovascular-Thoracic Surgery, Children's Memorial Hospital; Professor of Surgery, Northwestern University Medical School, Chicago, Illinois

Carl L. Backer, M.D.

Attending Surgeon, Division of Cardiovascular-Thoracic Surgery, Children's Memorial Hospital; Assitant Professor of Surgery, Northwestern University Medical School, Chicago, Illinois

Farouk S. Idriss, M.D.

Attending Surgeon, Division of Cardiovascular-Thoracic Surgery, Children's Memorial Hospital; Professor Emeritus of Surgery, Northwestern University Medical School, Chicago Illinois

The arterial switch operation for transposition of the great arteries (TGA) and related great-vessel malposition deformities has been made possible due to improved techniques of coronary transfer, myocardial protection, and neo–great-vessel reconstruction.[1–32] Presently, the perioperative death risk after the arterial switch operation is approaching that of the atrial baffle procedures.[2, 33–38] These results are perhaps more important since the arterial switch operation has not been associated with the atrial arrhythmias, baffle stenoses, tricuspid insufficiency, right ventricular failure, and sudden death that have been documented in patients with the atrial baffle operations. The most common midterm complication of the arterial switch operation has been supravalvular pulmonary stenosis.[22] Potential problems of semilunar valvular incompetence, coronary insufficiency, and supravalvular aortic stenosis have been infrequent.

This chapter summarizes multiple studies by the authors[2, 8–10, 17–21] and will highlight the evolutionary technical advancements of the arterial switch operation and its application to the more complex malposition anomalies. The principles of arterial switch for TGA with intact ventricular septum are basically the same as for the more complex anatomic variations, including TGA with ventricular septal defect, the Taussig-Bing type of double-outlet right ventricle, and staged conversion of the Mustard operation to anatomic repair. In the latter cases, arterial switch must be accompanied by ventricular septal defect closure, possible sub–semilunar-valve muscular resection, or atrial baffle conversion. We will review our results with the arterial switch operation along with those from other institutions.

Surgical Technique

Arterial switch for TGA can be divided into six stages consisting of (1) precannulation evaluation and dissection, (2) cannulation and cardiopulmonary bypass, (3) myocardial protection, (4) neoaortic reconstruction with coronary artery transfer, (5) neo–pulmonary-artery reconstruction, and (6) separation from extracorporeal circulation and postoperative support.

Precannulation Evaluation and Dissection

The precannulation phase includes the pericardial harvest for future reconstruction of the neo-pulmonary artery; coronary artery evaluation as related to the orientation of the great vessels; and extensive dissection of the great vessels, the ductus arteriosus, and the right and left pulmonary arteries to their respective hili. The pericardial harvest is performed with great care to avoid injury to the phrenic nerves, much like that described for the Mustard operation.[39, 40] The visceral side eventually will serve as the inner surface of the neo-pulmonary artery. Some authors have advocated glutaraldehyde pretreatment of the pericardium[3, 26] ostensibly to stiffen and shrink it, thereby enhancing the surgical technique and preventing any further pericardial shrinkage, which may result in supravalvular pulmonary stenosis. We have avoided this pretreatment method because of anecdotal experience with one patient referred to our institution for supravalvular pulmonary stenosis caused by continued pericardial shrinkage after glutaraldehyde pretreatment at the original corrective operation. Rather, we have instituted a technique employing a large redundant pantaloon pericardial patch that allows for shrinkage and pulmonry artery growth.

Coronary anatomy evaluation is the most important planning stage of the operation. Recognition of coronary patterns and flow distribution to the ventricles will allow the surgeon to project and visualize the coronary transfer to the pulmonary artery for the neoaortic reconstruction. In the early development of neonatal arterial switch, some authors speculated that some patterns of coronary anatomy were "unswitchable" based on poor results in selected patients. Other authors[8, 9, 26, 30–32] have felt that the greater majority of patients can be "switched" as long as the dissection and rotation of the coronary arteries is performed to avoid kinking and obstruction to flow. This issue has not been fully resolved, mostly due to the wide variety of coronary anatomy,[41–46] the operative conditions relating anatomic configurations at the time of surgery, and the widely divergent experience of surgeons with this operation. Increasing experience performing the arterial switch operation will lessen the incidence of resorting to the "bail-out" atrial baffle procedure, which has a high complication rate under these conditions.[5, 22]

Great-vessel and patent ductus arteriosus dissection usually can be accomplished before the start of cardiopulmonary bypass. Many authors[4, 9–15, 18–24, 30–32] have emphasized the necessity for meticulous dissection to free the patent ductus arteriosus and the pulmonary arteries from their attachments to facilitate ductal division and the maneuver of LeCompte.[15] Failure to perform this part of the operation effectively may result in excessive tension, bleeding, and supravalvular neo–pulmonary-artery stenosis.

Cannulation and Cardiopulmonary Bypass

Cannulation techniques employed for neonates and infants are dependent on the method of cardiopulmonary bypass employed and the surgeon's decision regarding the use of deep hypothermia and circulatory arrest for

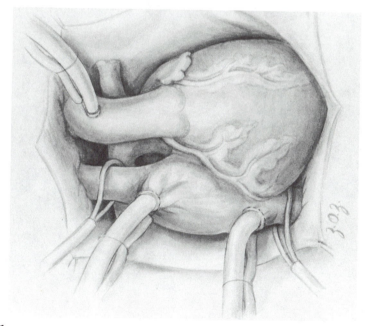

FIG 1.
Bicaval venous cannulation in preparation for cardiopulmonary bypass in a patient with TGA and intact ventricular septum. (From Mavroudis C, Backer CL, Idriss FG: Surgical techniques and intraoperative judgements to facilitate the arterial switch operation in transposition with intact ventricular septum, in Mavroudis C, Backer CL (eds): *Arterial Switch. Cardiac Surgery: State of the Art Review,* vol 5. Philadelphia, Hanley & Belfus, Inc, 1991, p 101. Used by permission.)

the neoaortic reconstruction. The aortic cannulation is placed just proximal to the origin of the innominate artery to preserve the aortic length and facilitate the maneuver of LeCompte. Bicaval cannulation (Fig 1) allows the surgeon the most versatility, since the atrial septal defect (patent foramen ovale or tear caused by Rashkind balloon septostomy) or ventricular septal defect can be closed through right atrial exposure with continuous cardiopulmonary bypass without subjecting the patient to the hazards of circulatory arrest. The disadvantages of bicaval cannulation are the size and fragility of the neonatal right atrium, possible tension on the coronary arteries, and the possibility of causing atrial arrhythmias.

Single right atrial cannulation (Fig 2) is simple, quick, and provides effective venous drainage during cardiopulmonary bypass. The surgeon may elect to use deep hypothermia and circulatory arrest or other forms of continuous cardiopulmonary bypass to perform the various stages of the operation. Circulatory arrest during the atrial septal defect repair and neoaortic reconstruction avoids operative hardware such as the left ventricular vent, two venous cannulas, and vena caval slings. Many authors[4, 13, 30–32] have had excellent results with this technique. However, we feel that long peri-

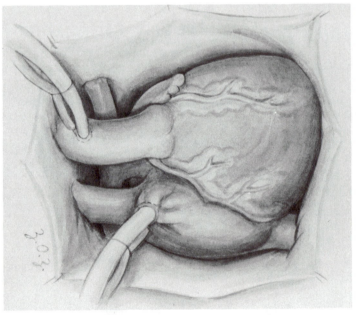

FIG 2.
Single right atrial venous cannulation in preparation for cardiopulmonary bypass in a patient with TGA with intact ventricular septum. (From Mavroudis C, Backer CL, Idriss FS: Surgical techniques and intraoperative judgements to facilitate the arterial switch operation in transposition with intact ventricular septum, in Mavroudis C, Backer CL (eds): *Arterial Switch. Cardiac Surgery: State of the Art Review*, vol 5. Philadelphia, Hanley & Belfus, Inc, 1991, p 102. Used by permission.)

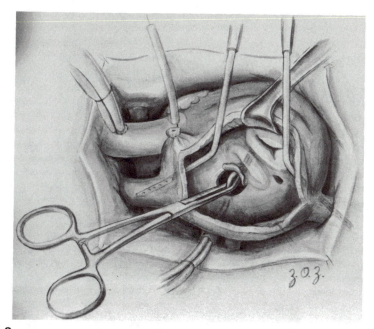

FIG 3.
After right atriotomy, sucker cardiopulmonary bypass is instituted and the 8-French drainage catheter is placed directly into the left atrium via the right superior pulmonary vein and then through the mitral valve into the left ventricle. (From Mavroudis C, Backer CL, Idriss FS: Surgical techniques and intraoperative judgements to facilitate the arterial switch operation in transposition with intact ventricular septum, in Mavroudis C, Backer CL (eds): *Arterial Switch. Cardiac Surgery: State of the Art Review,* vol 5, Philadelphia, Hanley & Belfus, Inc, 1991, p 103. Used by permission.)

ods of circulatory arrest (greater than 30 minutes) should be avoided if other reasonable means are available. More recent studies[47–52] have cautioned that the "safe" period of deep hypothermia and circulatory arrest may be shorter than originally thought. Ongoing studies eventually may clear this matter and standardize the approach to these infants.

Single venous cannulation does not necessarily demand deep hypothermia and circulatory arrest for arterial switch. Low flow state (0.2 to 0.4 L/min/m^2) with systemic hypothermia (22° C) can be initiated during cardiotomy sucker bypass to place the left ventricular vent (Fig 3) and close the atrial septal defect (Fig 4). After atriotomy closure, single venous cardiopulmonary bypass can be reinstituted for arterial switch. The three disadvantages with this technique are as follows: (1) air may enter the venous line during the neo–pulmonary-artery reconstruction, which will require attention; (2) undrained atrial blood will enter the right ventricle and outflow tract, which may cause local myocardial warming during cardioplegic cross-clamp time and poor myocardial preservation; and (3) the undrained

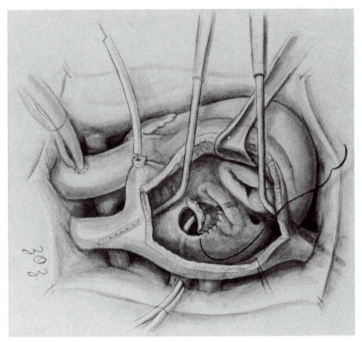

FIG 4.
The atrial septal defect is repaired with sucker cardiopulmonary bypass. Atriorrhaphy is then performed, followed by the reinstitution of single atrial venous drainage. (From Mavroudis C, Backer CL, Idriss FS: Surgical techniques and intraoperative judgements to facilitate the arterial switch operation in transposition with intact ventricular septum, in Mavroudis C, Backer CL (eds): *Arterial Switch, Cardiac Surgery: State of the Art Review*, vol 5. Philadelphia, Hanley & Belfus, Inc, 1991, p 104. Used by permission.)

blood may cause poor visibility and obscure the landmarks for accurate suturing. Recent experimental data have shown the superiority of the low flow state to deep hypothermia and circulatory arrest.[53, 54] We have always used the continuous flow technique with either single atrial or bicaval venous cannulation, recognizing that the potential complications of circulatory arrest far outweigh the inconveniences of the continuous flow technique. Recently, we have shown a bias toward bicaval venous cannulation. The initial extra technical steps required to establish bicaval drainage allow the surgeon uninterrupted time to perform the neoaortic reconstruction, free from the inconveniences of venous line and air, and their attendant problems.

Conduct of Cardiopulmonary Bypass

Cardiopulmonary bypass is commenced with a standard blood prime through a membrane oxygenator and a nonpulsatile roller pump. Flows are calculated at 2.0 to 2.5 L/min/m^2 and systemic hypothermia is employed to 22° C. The low flow state (0.2 to 0.4 L/min/m^2) is established to facilitate right atriotomy (sucker bypass) for left ventricular vent placement and atrial septal defect closure as well as neoaortic reconstruction to minimize venous blood return and venous-line air trapping and enhance myocardial preservation. After the neoaortic reconstruction and cross-clamp removal, the flow is increased to 2.0 L/min/m^2. Halfway through the neo–pulmonary-artery reconstruction the flow is increased further to 2.5 L/min/m^2 and the patient is rewarmed to 35° C in anticipation of separation from cardiopulmonary bypass.

Myocardial Protection

We have employed many techniques of myocardial protection. During the early experience, multidose crystalline cardioplegia was used via direct intracoronary ostial instillation after the first dose. Presumed coronary injury in one patient, myocardial swelling after reperfusion in others, and growing experimental evidence favoring blood cardioplegia[23, 55–58] resulted in the present technique of single-dose hypothermic blood cardioplegia.[56] In the event of an unforeseen long cross-clamp time, retrograde coronary sinus cardioplegia infusion may be preferable to direct coronary injection.[59] We also bathe the heart with iced saline slush to augment the benefits of blood cardioplegia.[60]

Neoaortic Reconstruction with Coronary Artery Transfer

The neoaortic reconstruction starts with the careful and accurate delivery of blood cardioplegia after the aortic cross-clamp is applied. The cardioplegia solution combines the cardiopulmonary bypass perfusate with 20 mEq of potassium chloride per liter, 3 g of mannitol per liter, 200 µg of nitroglycerin per liter, and 12.5 g of albumin per liter. Great-vessel transection, the maneuver of LeCompte, and neoaortic reconstruction then can proceed. Adjustments for great-vessel transection may need to be made at the time of surgery, based on the length of the great vessels and their anatomic relationship.

Excision of the coronary patches from their respective sinuses of Valsalva is performed close to the aortic commissures and top of the annulus, creating a liberal patch surrounding the coronary ostium that will facilitate transfer and suture reconstruction (Fig 5). Usually, fine-needle Bovie or scissor dissection will be necessary to dissect the coronary artery connective tissue attachments from the upper ventricular wall. Early in our series, Dr. Mavroudis performed coronary dissection before aortic cross-clamp and cardioplegic arrest.[19] Although no complications arose from this practice, it became increasingly clear that the coronary dissection could be accomplished extensively and carefully enough from inside the aorta. Extreme care is taken to avoid injury or denuding of the coronaries or their vasa vasorum during this part of the procedure. Rarely, a small conal branch of the left anterior descending artery may be ligated in order to create more length for the coronary transfer. We have found, however, that

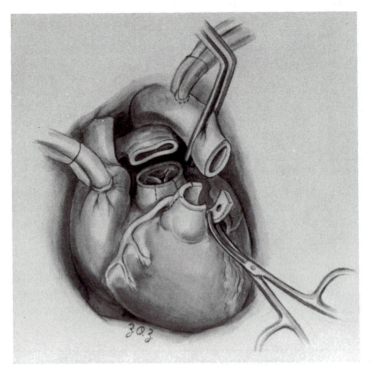

FIG 5.
Fine scissor excision of the left coronary artery patch from its sinus of Valsalva is shown. A liberal amount of aortic wall with the coronary artery is taken to facilitate the transfer to the neoaorta. Care is taken to avoid injury to coronary arteries and their vasa vasorum. (From Mavroudis C, Backer CL, Idriss FS: Surgical techniques and intraoperative judgements to facilitate the arterial switch operation in transposition with intact ventricular septum, in Mavroudis C, Backer CL (eds): *Arterial Switch. Cardiac Surgery: State of the Art Review*, vol 5. Philadelphia, Hanley & Belfus, Inc, 1991, p 106. Used by permission.)

ligation of this branch usually is not necessary with appropriate dissection. The maneuver of LeCompte now can be performed, after which time the aortic cross-clamp can be repositioned for pulmonary artery retraction (Fig 6). Some authors have advocated anatomic orientation of the reconstruction,[11, 12] but the majority employ the LeCompte maneuver, thereby avoiding tension on the neo–pulmonary-artery reconstruction.

Preparation of the proximal transected pulmonary artery facing the sinuses of Valsalva for coronary transfer has been accomplished by punch excision,[11–13, 15, 18, 23, 26] partial wall excision,[19] and linear incision[3, 8, 9] without overall agreement. Others have advocated initial neoaortic anastomosis without immediate concomitant coronary transfer. The coronary patches then can be aligned with the blood-filled neoaorta before anastomosis, presumably for a more accurate and anatomic reconstruction. The aortic clamp then is reapplied for the coronary patch transfer. We prefer

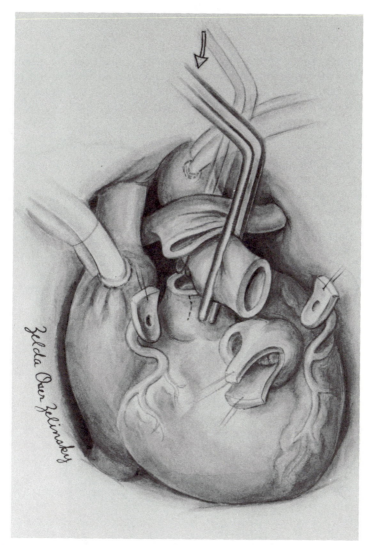

FIG 6.
The maneuver of LeCompte is shown with aortic cross-clamp repositioning to re-tract the pulmonary artery during the neoaortic reconstruction. The phantom clamp represents the initial position on the aorta just before the administration of blood cardioplegia. The real clamp represents the new position on the aorta in or-der to retract the pulmonary artery after the maneuver of Lecompte. (From Mavroudis C, Backer CL, Idriss FS: Surgical techniques and intraoperative judge-ments to facilitate the arterial switch operation in transposition with intact ventricu-lar septum, in Mavroudis C, Backer CL (eds): *Arterial Switch. Cardiac Surgery: State of the Art Review,* vol 5. Philadelphia, Hanley & Belfus, Inc, 1991, p 107. Used by permission.)

linear incisions for aortic tissue preservation, which allow more rotation and liberal excursion of the coronary patches, thereby minimizing the possibility of kinking or obstruction. This technique, however, creates a rather large circumference of the proximal neoaorta, which can be alleviated by coronary patch rotation and tapering techniques to narrow the proximal neoaorta and allow a more anatomic anastomosis to the distal aorta (Fig 7). To accomplish a "best-lie" coronary artery configuration, we may rotate the coronary patches at various stages between 30 degrees counterclockwise and 30 degrees clockwise referable to their original orientation depending upon their anatomic natural lie to avoid kinking and obstruction after the reconstruction. The anastomotic lines are performed with running 8–0 monofilament suture. The superior portions of the coronary patches can be evaluated for a "best-fit" configuration to facilitate the eventual end-to-end anastomosis. Usually the excess coronary patches can be sewn to ech other to accomplish this part of the operation (see Fig 7). As the aortic anastomosis is completed, the aortic cross-clamp is removed and the myocardium is reperfused.

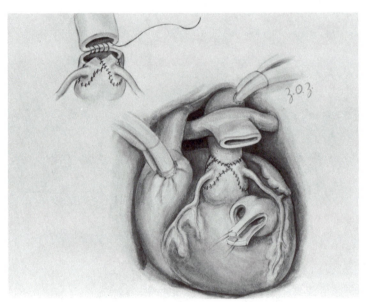

FIG 7.
After the coronary patches are rotated for a "best-fit" lie, they are sutured to the linearly incised facing sinuses of Valsalva at the old pulmonary artery (neoaorta). Oftentimes, the redundant aortic tissue of the coronary patches can be sutured together anteriorly to slightly narrow the neoaortic outflow in order to decrease the size discrepancy between the proximal and distal neoaorta, thereby facilitating the neoaortic reconstruction. (From Mavroudis C, Backer CL, Idriss FS: Surgical techniques and intraoperative judgements to facilitate the arterial switch operation in transposition with intact ventricular septum, in Mavroudis C, Backer CL (eds): *Arterial Switch. Cardiac Surgery: State of the Art Review*, vol 5. Philadelphia, Hanley & Belfus, Inc, 1991, p 108. Used by permission.)

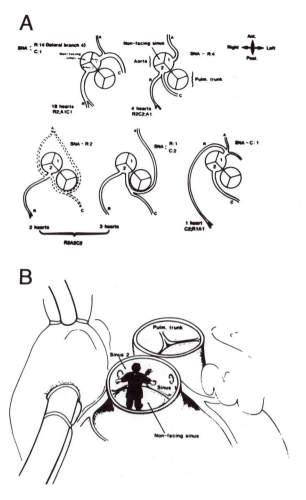

FIG 8.
These two drawings show the convention for naming the aortic sinuses by Gittenberger-de Groot and colleagues. **A,** the four patterns of coronary artery origin, including the origins of the sinus node *(SNA)* in each pattern are noted. In all, the sinus node artery arose from the right coronary artery *(R)* in 25 hearts and from the circumflex artery *(C)* in 3 hearts. The coronary artery patterns are described using a simple system that takes into account the origins of the right coronary artery, the circumflex artery, and the anterior descending coronary artery *(A)* from either sinus 1 or sinus 2. The designation R2; A1C1, for example, describes the origin of the right coronary artery from sinus 2 and the circumflex and anterior descending coronary arteries from sinus 1. **B,** the two sinuses of the aorta face two sinuses of the pulmonary trunk and the third sinus is nonfacing. The figure in the diagram is standing in the nonfacing sinus and looking toward the pulmonary trunk. The coronary sinus to the right is sinus 1 and that to the left is sinus 2. (From Rossi MB, Ho SY, Anderson RH, et al: *Ann Thorac Surg* 1986; 42:573–577). Used by permission.)

Special Coronary Problems

The variety and anomalies of the coronary circulation are many in patients with TGA.[41-46] In the greater percentage of cases, there are two coronary ostia independent of the arising arteries that favorably face the adjacent pulmonary artery sinuses of Valsalva (Fig 8). Special consideration must be given to coronary arteries arising from the nonfacing sinus; the single coronary artery; and the intramural coronary artery,[42] which oftentimes traverses a commissure before emerging from the aortic wall.

The artery that arises from the nonfacing cusp is basically nontransferable unless the surgeon elects to use prosthetic material or an internal mammary artery graft. Under these circumstances, the surgeon may choose to perform an atrial baffle operation. The single coronary artery, however, is transferable by a number of techniques,[25, 46] depending on the anatomic findings. Yacoub[46] and Planche[25] have advocated techniques for successful transfer by the "trap-door" technique to ensure optimal coronary flow by utilizing aortic wall flaps to avoid distortion and kinking. Occasionally, the coronary patch can be rotated for a "best-lie" configuration and transferred in the usual manner. The surgeon must be familiar with all these techniques in order to select the proper reconstruction to best serve optimal coronary flow.

The intramural coronary artery represents the greatest risk for the patient and challenge to the surgeon. Gittenberger-de Groot described the intramural course of these arteries with anatomic possibilities for transfer.[42] The main principles for transfer are (1) to identify the anatomy before coronary patch formation to avoid coronary transection, (2) to identify the coronary ostium and the exact downstream location where the coronary emerges from its intramural course, and (3) to sacrifice valvular and commissural tissue to benefit the coronary transfer since the neo-pulmonary valve (old aortic valve) can be resuspended and reconstructed with pericardium to minimize the well-tolerated resultant neo–pulmonary-valvular insufficiency. Methods for transfer have not been standardized due to the rarity of this anomaly. Our experience is limited to one patient in whom we successfully transferred an intramural right coronary artery that originated and exited within the same cusp. This transfer did not require any special consideration.

Neo–Pulmonary-Artery Reconstruction

The principles of neo–pulmonary-artery reconstruction are (1) to fill in the sinuses of Valsalva of the old aorta from which the coronary buttons were removed; (2) to perform the end-to-end anastomosis without tension, thereby minimizing the potential for stenosis; (3) to prevent right and left main pulmonary artery distortion using extensive dissection to their respective hili; and (4) to have direct continuity of native proximal and distal pulmonary artery for at least a portion of the anastomosis for eventual growth. Many methods have been described. Pacifico and others[23] have emphasized the posterior incision approach in which the distal pulmonary artery

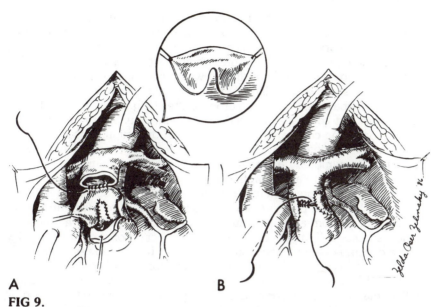

A   **B**

FIG 9.
A and B, a single pantaloon pericardial patch is shown filling out the dissected sinuses of Valsalva for neopulmonary artery reconstruction. We presently use this
technique for the added benefits of hemostasis and decreased incidence of supravalvular pulmonary stenosis. (From Idriss FS, Ilbawi MN, DeLeon SY, et al: *J Thorac Cardiovasc Surg* 1988; 95:255–262. Used by permission.)

provides for the tissue to primarily repair the neo-pulmonary artery,
thereby avoiding pericardial or prosthetic patches. Redundant double pericardial patches have been proposed by others[5, 19, 20] to fill out the respective sinuses of Valsalva. This method theoretically helps to minimize acquired supravalvular pulmonary stenosis and to avoid future reoperations.
After a series of trial periods, which included the posterior incision approach, Goretex patch augmentation, and single pericardial patches, we
have employed the single pantaloon pericardial patch technique[3, 8, 9] (Fig
9). Generous oversizing of the patch is recommended to avoid the possibility of supravalvular stenosis. Added benefits of the single patch include
better hemostasis and the ability to extend the length of the
neo–pulmonary-artery reconstruction. A portion of the neo-pulmonary artery proximally is always anastomosed to a portion of the distal pulmonary
artery directly to allow for growth of the anastomosis. Complete circumfer-
ential prosthetic material or pericardium should not be used.

Separation from Cardiopulmonary Bypass and Postoperative Care

Separation from cardiopulmonary bypass is the final stage toward successful repair. The surgeon must check all anastomotic suture lines for tension,

bleeding, and kinking. Regional wall motion is evaluated, qualitatively which may give some hint to regional malperfusion. If separation from cardiopulmonary bypass requires high doses of pressor agents or if ischemic electrocardiographic changes are present, immediate resumption of cardiopulmonary bypass should be instituted with a careful reevaluation of coronary flow. In some cases, filling of the heart with separation from cardiopulmonary bypass may result in coronary stretching, kinking, or occlusion. Other causes of coronary obstruction are pulmonary artery compression, malrotation of the coronary arteries, or intimal dissection. Corrective measures can be instituted that may include coronary pericardial patch augmentation,[20] pulmonary artery suspension to treat coronary compression, or internal mammary artery grafting to the affected coronary artery.[61]

Rarely, extracorporeal membrane oxygenation may become necessary to rest the "stunned myocardium" and allow time for recovery and eventual separation from assisted circulation. In general, this extreme measure is most successful if the affected patient has a period of circulatory stability before decompensation. Some successful cases have been reported.[62] We have used extracorporeal membrane oxygenation in two postoperative patients, with success in one who was presumed to have coronary artery kinking that, when relieved, resulted in improvement and eventual normal cardiac contractility and function. It is important to correct the original problem that led to hemodynamic instability if a successful outcome is to be achieved.

Most patients are separated from cardiopulmonary bypass with dobutamine (5 to 10 μg/kg/min), dopamine (5 to 10 μg/kg/min), and intravenous nitroglycerin (1 to 2 μg/min). Isoproterenol (0.02 to 0.1 μg/kg/min) is used in most cases and titrated to achieve a heart rate between 160 and 200 beats per minute. With this regimen, the blood pressure can be anticipated to range between 65 and 85 mm Hg systolic with a wide pulse pressure and excellent peripheral perfusion. Drug doses may vary to achieve the optimal level of cardiac output and afterload reduction. The patient is best evaluated by repeated physical examination, noting the fullness of the fontanelle, level of the liver edge, strength of the peripheral pulses, capillary filling time, and hourly urinary output.

Postoperative ventilatory support is adjusted to maintain adequate oxygenation and mild respiratory alkalosis (PCO_2 28, pH 7.50), optimize cardiac output, and avoid pulmonary hypertension. Eighteen to 24 hours postoperatively, paralysis and sedation can be tapered, thereby starting the weaning process from the ventilator.

Results and Analysis

Between October 1983 and July 1990, 30 neonates at Kosair Children's Hospital in Louisville, Kentucky and 49 at the Children's Memorial Hospital in Chicago, Illinois underwent the arterial switch operation for TGA and intact ventricular septum. These combined results revealed 8 early deaths in 79 patients for an operative mortality of 10%. The most common cause of death was myocardial dysfunction due to technical difficulties with the coronary implantation.[4] All of these deaths occurred early in the series. One patient died from severe cyanosis due to pulmonary hypertension and atrial shunt reversal, which prompted routine atrial septal defect closure. One patient with preoperative atrial tachycardia died of postoperative arrhythmia. Two patients appeared to have global cardiac dysfunction after bypass, 1 of whom died of sepsis 11 days after a 7-day period on extracorporeal membrane oxygenation. In this same group there have been 2 late deaths, 1 at 4 months postoperatively and 1 at 3 years postoperatively, both unexplained. Of the original group of 79 neonates, 69 are still alive for an overall survival rate of 87%. One patient has had successful reoperation for supravalvular pulmonary stenosis. All patients are in normal sinus rhythm, except 1 who was treated temporarily for premature ventricular contractions. In the latest communication from the Congenital Heart Surgeon's Society, 212 infants at 16 separate institutions underwent an arterial switch repair.[22] The 1-week, 1-year, and 2½-year survival rates were 82%, 79%, and 78%, respectively. At the six "low-risk" institutions, the 1-week, 1-year, and 2½-year survival rates were 96%, 91%, and 90%, respectively. Freedom from reoperation for pulmonary outflow obstruction at 1 week and 1 year was 99% and 89%, respectively.

Planche reported on 110 infants with TGA and intact ventricular septum who underwent the arterial switch operation with a 9% perioperative mortality. Two late deaths occurred from myocardial infarction, adjusting the overall survival to 89%. Two patients had reoperation for pulmonary stenosis caused by retraction of the heterologous pericardial patches. Two patients have trivial aortic insufficiency and all patients are in normal sinus rhythm.

Bove reported a 5% mortality in 61 patients with TGA and intact ventricular septum who had arterial switch.[3] In his early experience, supravalvar pulmonary stenosis occurred in 5 patients who required reoperation. His conversion to the autologous pantaloon-shaped pericardial patch has minimized the incidence of supravalvular pulmonary stenosis. Mild, nonprogressive aortic regurgitation was noted in 5 patients and all remain in normal sinus rhythm.

Quaegebeur reported on 23 neonates with TGA and intact ventricular septum in a group of 66 patients who have undergone the arterial switch repair since 1977.[26] There was 1 hospital death, resulting in a 4% operative mortality. Coronary artery morphology and position of the great arteries were not risk factors. Ninety-six percent of the surviving patients are in normal sinus rhythm.

Wernovsky and colleagues prospectively evaluated 49 consecutive survivors of the arterial switch operation for TGA and intact ventricular septum by clinical examination, echocardiography, cardiac catheterization, ambulatory electrocardiographic monitoring, and invasive electrophysiologic studies.[63] All children were asymptomatic and medication-free. Five children underwent reoperation for supravalvular pulmonary stenosis and

7 had trivial or mild aortic insufficiency (14%). Systemic ventricular function was normal, and only 1 patient had sinus node dysfunction. There were no late deaths.

At Children's Memorial Hospital in Chicago, we compared the results of the Mustard procedure vs. the arterial switch for infants operated on in the first 3 months of life.[2] Of 60 infants with TGA and intact ventricular septum, 23 had a Mustard procedure and 37 underwent an arterial switch. Operative mortality was 8.7% for the Mustard procedure and 8.1% for the arterial switch. There were 2 late deaths after Mustard operation and 1 after arterial switch. Fifty-seven percent of the Mustard patients had late arrhythmias compared with only 3% of the arterial switch patients. The ejection fraction of the systemic ventricle was 79% ± 15% of predicted normal after the Mustard operation and 98% ± 6% of predicted normal after the arterial switch ($P < .005$).

The arterial switch operation for neonates with TGA and intact ventricular septum now can be performed with a 5% to 10% operative mortality that has been established at many different institutions. Accomplishing both anatomic and physiologic connection appears to offer great potential for excellent long-term results. The postoperative complications associated with atrial baffle operations, such as atrial arrhythmias and ventricular dysfunction, have not emerged. Moreover, the incidence of anastomotic narrowing and neoaortic insufficiency are quite low. Preliminary intermediate results would indicate that the arterial switch operation is the procedure of choice for neonates with TGA and intact ventricular septum.

Arterial Switch and Ventricular Septal Defect Closure for Transposition of the Great Arteries and Ventricular Septal Defect

The early experience statistics with the arterial switch operation for TGA and intact ventricular septum did not compare favorably to the atrial baffle procedures.[31] In contrast, survival statistics with the arterial switch operation for patients with this condition were superior to those of the atrial baffle procedures, even in the early experience with arterial switch. Jatene reported, only 2 deaths among 12 patients undergoing ventricular septal defect closure and arterial switch (16% operative mortality) in 1982.[12] These results stood in stark contrast to the high mortality of the atrial baffle operations combined with ventricular septal defect closure due to right ventricular failure and tricuspid insufficiency.[64] Williams reported 62 patients undergoing ventricular septal defect repair and the Mustard procedure from 1973 to October 1980 with a 21% operative mortality and a 44% 5-year actuarial survival.[29] The subsequent experience with arterial switch and ventricular septal defect closure reported by Pacifico in 1983[23] showed no early or late deaths and provided a more optimistic future for these patients virtually free from the complications of arrhythmias, right ventricular failure, and late death.

Patient selection and timing of the operation has also evolved with increasing experience. Initially, arterial switch was delayed until 2 to 18 months of age, during which time the infants were treated medically for excessive pulmonary blood flow, or with pulmonary artery banding. Recently, the trend toward arterial switch and ventricular septal defect closure soon after birth has gained favor, since the death and complication rate appears to be the same as in the older infant group. Bove reported 12 infants with TGA and large ventricular septal defect who had arterial switch and ventricular septal defect closure at a mean age of 19 days, with 1 early death and no late deaths.[65] The only limiting factor appears to be patient size. The surgeon may elect to perform pulmonary artery banding with subsequent anatomic repair at a later appropriate time in low–birth weight neonates.

From 1983 to 1990, we have performed arterial switch and ventricular septal defect closure in 24 patients with TGA and ventricular septal defect. The average age at operation was 12 months (range 3 days to 9 years). With increasing experience, the mean age at operation has fallen to 2 months, allowing an earlier repair without the hazards of preliminary pulmonary artery banding. In the past 2 years, all patients with TGA and ventricular septal defect had neonatal primary repair except for those who had coarctation and were treated by subclavian flap aortoplasty with pulmonary artery banding. Early survival was 92%, with 2 late deaths (late intermediate survival 83%). Six patients had other major complications, which included postoperative pulmonary stenosis at the pulmonary artery banding site requiring successful pulmonary arterioplasty in 1 patient, heart block requiring pacemaker insertion in 2 patients, aortic valve replacement for aortic insufficiency 8 months following arterial switch in 1 patient, and successful extracorporeal membrane oxygenator support for 4 days starting 1 day after arterial switch in 1 patient.

The operative approach to these patients is similar to that previously described, with the obvious addition of ventricular septal defect closure. Bicaval venous cannulation is employed to allow right atrial, transpulmonary, or transaortic access to the ventricular septal defect. We recommend that the ventricular septal defect be closed at the beginning of the operation under blood cardioplegic arrest, with subsequent clamp removal during atrial septal defect repair and great-vessel preparation. This serves two purposes: (1) the neoaortic reconstruction cannot be disrupted by the retraction maneuvers necessary to visualize the ventricular septal defect since it has not been performed at this stage, and (2) the total cross-clamp time is lowered since myocardial reperfusion is allowed during the atrial septal defect closure and great-vessel preparation for arterial switch. The issue of cardioplegic arrest and reperfusion and subsequent cardioplegic arrest is supported by experimental studies[66, 67] when used under these clinical conditions.

Figure 10 shows the right atrial approach for ventricular septal defect closure. Occasionally, the ventricular septal defect is subpulmonic (Fig 11) and can be closed through the pulmonary artery. Under these conditions, the pulmonary artery is transected before aortic transection to visualize and

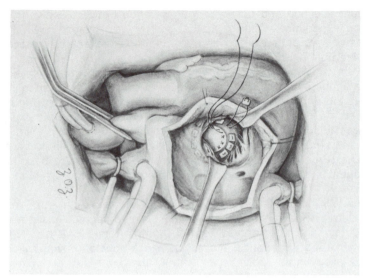

FIG 10.
After arterial and bicaval venous cannulation, the ventricular septal defect is approached and closed through the right atrium under blood cardioplegic arrest. Interrupted pledgeted sutures through a Dacron patch ensure accurate and complete closure. (From Mavroudis C, Backer CL, Idriss FS: Special considerations for and reoperations after the arterial switch operation, in Mavroudis C, Backer CL (eds): *Arterial Switch, Cardiac Surgery: State of the Art Review,* vol 5. Philadelphia, Hanley & Belfus, Inc, 1991, p 122. Used by permission.)

evaluate the ventricular septal defect for closure. If favorable, the ventricular septal defect can be closed under cardioplegic arrest. The cross-clamp is removed for the atrial septal defect closure and great-vessel preparation. The cross-clamp can be reapplied thereafter and the arterial switch operation can be performed under cardioplegic rearrest. In our series of 24 patients, 6 ventricular septal defects were closed through the pulmonary artery, 14 were closed through the right atrium, and none were closed through a right ventriculotomy.

Many authors have reported excellent results with arterial switch and ventricular septal defect closure. Quaegebeur reported on 33 infants and children with an operative mortality of 18% and 3 late deaths in 1986.[26] In the Congenital Heart Surgeon's Society report, there was a 17% mortality in 30 patients operated on at the group of low-risk institutions.[22] In a recent report from Japan, there was a 16% mortality in 103 patients undergoing arterial switch for TGA and ventricular septal defect.[68] Planche reported 106 patients having arterial switch for TGA and ventricular septal defect.[69] The mean age at operation was 2.8 months. Twenty-eight patients had aortic coarctation and 21 patients had prior pulmonary artery banding. The ventricular septal defect was approached through the right ventricle in 50% of the patients, through the right atrium in 40%, and

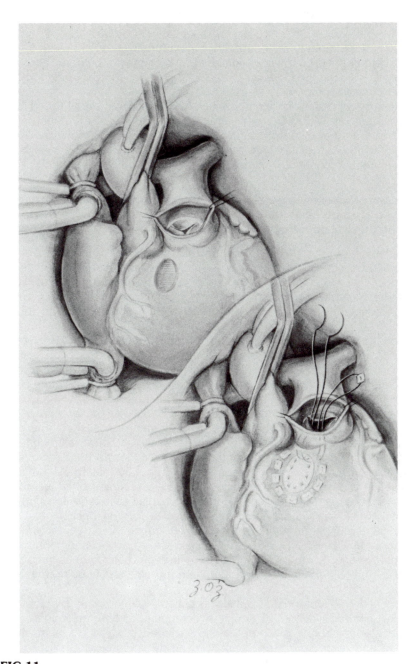

FIG 11.
Diagrammatic representation of TGA and subpulmonic ventricular septal defect. The ventricular septal defect is closed with a Dacron patch and interrupted pledgeted sutures through pulmonary artery exposure. (From Mavroudis C, Backer CL, Idriss FS: Special considerations for and reoperations after the arterial switch operation, in Mavroudis C, Backer CL (eds): *Arterial Switch. Cardiac Surgery: State of the Art Review,* vol 5. Philadelphia, Hanley & Belfus, Inc, 1991, p 123. Used by permission.)

through the pulmonary artery in 10%. Early mortality was 15%, with death related either to coronary artery kinking (8 patients) or to anatomy and size discrepancy of the great vessels (8 patients). There was 1 late death and 7 reoperations for pulmonary stenosis.

The survival results for arterial switch and ventricular septal defect closure in patients with TGA and ventricular septal defect are superior to those of the atrial baffle procedures both in the short- and intermediate-term. The fate of the neoaortic valve and the pulmonary artery reconstruction will require continuous surveillance for the long-term.

Staged Repair of Transposition of the Great Arteries With Intact Ventricular Septum

For infants who present late or after initial palliation for planned atrial baffle repair, left ventricular training must precede arterial switch for adequate postoperative systemic circulatory support.[70] This staged repair of TGA with intact ventricular septum consisting of pulmonary artery band, aorto-pulmonary shunt, and subsequent anatomic correction was first described in 1977 by Yacoub.[31] In our series of patients with arterial switch, this operation (pulmonary artery band and aortopulmonary shunt[71]) was relatively common in the early years. As more experience has been gained with neonatal arterial switch for TGA with intact ventricular septum during the first weeks of life, fewer and fewer patients are presenting late, and fewer patients in the series have required left ventricular preparation.

Surgical guidelines and techniques of left ventricular preparation at the Children's Memorial Hospital have been published previously.[10] The procedure generally is performed through a left thoracotomy, although the median sternotomy approach may be useful if the decision regarding arterial switch is to be made at operation (Fig 12). The initial postoperative evaluation is determined by echocardiographic assessment of left ventricular wall thickness. Most patients had repeat cardiac catheterization prior to arterial switch to measure ventricular volumes, ejection fraction, and left ventricular muscle mass. Patients were felt to be prepared for arterial switch when (1) left ventricular wall thickness by echocardiography was normal for age, (2) the left ventricular/right ventricular pressure ratio was >70%, and (3) left ventricular volume and muscle mass were normal predicted for age.

At Children's Memorial Hospital, 18 patients with TGA and intact ventricular septum have had the arterial switch operation after preliminary pulmonary artery banding. Complications included thoracic empyema in 1 patient and respiratory arrest leading to residual neurologic deficit in another. Following arterial switch, there was 1 operative death due to coronary complications and 3 late deaths due to pneumonia in 2 patients and complications of tracheostomy in the other. The operative death occurred in a child who underwent atrial septectomy at 3 days of age and pulmonary artery banding without systemic-to-pulmonary artery shunt at 21

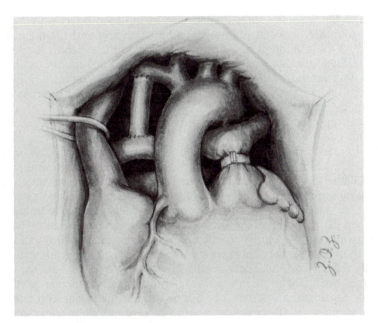

FIG 12.
Diagrammatic representation of pulmonary artery banding with a polytetrafluoro-ethylene systemic-to-pulmonary artery shunt for left ventricular training in preparation for arterial switch. With the band positioned but not tightened, a standard 5-mm modified Blalock-Taussig shunt (4 mm if the infant weighs <2.5 kg) is performed. The systemic blood pressure is monitored as the band is tightened sequentially until the proximal pulmonary artery approaches two-thirds of the systemic pressure or until the oxygen saturation drops below 85%. (From Mavroudis C, Backer CL, Idriss FS: Special considerations for and reoperations after the arterial switch operation, in Mavroudis C, Backer CL (eds): *Arterial Switch. Cardiac Surgery: State of the Art Review,* vol 5. Philadelphia, Hanley & Belfus, Inc, 1991, p 124. Used by permission.)

months of age. At the time of arterial switch, both the right and the left coronary artery arose from the same posterior sinus. The left coronary anastomosis had to be revised, and the child expired of low cardiac output, presumably from a combination of myocardial ischemia and small left ventricle. This child is an example of the importance of the size of the interatrial communication as a factor in preparing the left ventricle for arterial switch.[72] After pulmonary artery banding, the compliance of the left ventricle decreases dramatically, favoring increased left-to-right shunting at the atrial level. If the interatrial communication is too large, the left ventricle is deprived of an adequate preload and consequently may become underdeveloped. Infants who are candidates for the staged operation benefit from a small-to-moderate atrial septal defect as compared to those with a large, nonrestrictive atrial septal defect.

Both patients who died late from pneumonia had autopsy findings of left ventricular fibroelastosis, presumably due to the long interval (5 months and 15 months) between pulmonary artery banding and arterial switch. What effect these findings had on their subsequent late deaths is speculative. The final late death in this group occurred in a 4-month-old boy 3 months after arterial switch. The child had multiple congenital anomalies, including Goldenhar's syndrome, and died of complications of an indwelling tracheostomy.

Yacoub reported on 20 patients undergoing a first-stage operation for TGA with intact ventricular septum in 1980.[32] There were 3 early deaths (15%). Fourteen patients subsequently underwent arterial switch, with 4 early deaths (295) and no late deaths. Yasui and associates reported 18 patients with TGA with intact ventricular septum having arterial switch after prior pulmonary artery banding/shunt, with 2 deaths.[73] They concluded that arterial switch was safe to perform if the left ventricular mass was larger than 60% of normal the left ventricular pressure was greater than 65 mm Hg, and/or the left ventricular/right ventricular pressure ratio was greater than 0.8. Yamaguchi reported two-stage repair in 91 infants with a mortality rate of 7% and 3 late deaths.[68]

Optimal treatment of infants with TGA and intact ventricular septum is anatomic repair within the first 14 days of life. For the infant with this condition who presents after the first month of life or initially is considered for an atrial baffle procedure, preparation of the left ventricle for arterial switch with pulmonary artery banding and systemic-to-pulmonary artery shunt is a therapeutic alternative with excellent short-term and midterm results.

Arterial Switch Operation for Double-Outlet Right Ventricle and Subpulmonary Ventricular Septal Defect (Taussig-Bing Anomaly)

Taussig and Bing first described the catheterization and autopsy results of a 5-year-old girl with a complex congenital cardiac malformation in which the aorta arose entirely from the right ventricle and the pulmonary artery arose primarily from the right ventricle and overrode a ventricular septal defect.[74] This was redefined by Van Praagh as a double-outlet right ventricle with semilunar valves side by side, a bilateral conus, and a subpulmonic ventricular septal defect.[75] Lev expanded this definition to encompass a spectrum of four types of hearts,[76] including the right-sided type without an overriding pulmonary trunk, the right-sided type with an overriding pulmonary trunk, an intermediate type, and the left-sided type.

A variety of techniques have been employed to repair the Taussig-Bing anomaly. The initial attempts at repair centered on constructing an intraventricular tunneling from the left ventricle to the aorta, keeping right ventricle-to-pulmonary artery continuity. This was first described by McGoon in 1968.[77] This operation was refined by Kawashima in 1971,[78] who described a similar intraventricular repair but emphasized the need for resection of the conal septum to avoid subaortic stenosis. This technique may require enlargement of the ventricular septal defect, tricuspid papillary muscle transfer, and/or an external valved conduit.[79] Experience with this repair is somewhat limited. Harvey reported four patients with one survivor.[80] Kirklin reported nine patients, most of whom had external conduits, with no operative mortality and four late deaths.[81] Yacoub reported two successful cases.[82] We have used this intraventricular tunnel from the left ventricle to the aorta successfully in two patients. In both cases, the right ventricle-to-pulmonary artery continuity was restored without a conduit. Adequate conal septum resection was of paramount importance. Yacoub[82] and Van Praagh[83] have suggested that this repair should be limited to patients with side-by-side great vessels, and should not be used for those with anteroposterior relationship of the great arteries.

Another therapeutic alternative was first described by Hightower and Kirklin in 1969.[84] They created an intraventricular tunnel from the left ventricle through the ventricular septal defect into the pulmonary artery in 3 patients. The Mustard operation then was used to transpose the venous return. This accomplished physiologic but not anatomic correction while avoiding the use of a conduit. Wedemeyer reported successful application of this procedure to a patient who also had coarctation of the aorta in 1970.[85] Harvey reported 4 patients with this correction, with 3 survivors.[80] Kirklin reported 23 patients undergoing this procedure with 10 operative and 6 late deaths.[81] Luber reported 6 survivors out of 7 patients.[86] Ottino modified this repair by transpulmonary artery ventricular septal defect closure.[87] Abe described this type of repair using a Senning instead of a Mustard atrial baffle.[88] However successful the initial repair, these patients are left with only a physiologic repair and are subject to all the known complications of the atrial baffle procedures, including atrial arrhythmias, tricuspid insufficiency, right ventricular dysfunction, baffle leak, and superior vena caval obstruction.[2]

In patients with the Taussig-Bing anomaly, a very serious and important consideration is that of possible mitral valve straddling or abnormal valvular attachments to the crest of the ventricular septal defect. We previously reported this occurrence in five patients with the left-sided or intermediate type (according to Lev's definition) of the Taussig-Bing anomaly.[89] Under these circumstances, closure of the subpulmonic ventricular septal defect and either arterial switch or atrial baffle may lead to death from subvalvular neoaortic obstruction and left ventricular failure. Preoperative evaluation and intraoperative confirmation can determine accurately the anatomy of the mitral valve attachments and their relationship to the ventricular septal defect. If unfavorable anatomy is found, an atrial baffle operation, closure of the ventricular septal defect, and left ventricle-to-pulmonary artery conduit can be performed.

A third approach to the Taussig-Bing heart utilizes a modification of the technique described by Damus, Stansel, and Kaye.[90-92] In this procedure, the ventricular septal defect is closed to connect the left ventricle to the pulmonary artery. The pulmonary trunk is divided and the proximal pulmonary artery is connected end-to-side to the ascending aorta. A valved extracardiac conduit then is placed from the right ventricle to the distal pulmonary artery.[93, 94] Ceithaml reported four patients, with three survivors.[95] Although this procedure has the advantage of left ventricle-to-aorta continuity, it has the disadvantage of requiring an extracardiac conduit.

A fourth alternative for the Taussig-Bing heart is ventricular septal defect closure and arterial switch. Freedom and colleagues in 1981 were the first to report successful application of the arterial switch procedure to the Taussig-Bing heart.[96] In 1984, Yacoub reported successful arterial switch and ventricular septal defect closure in two patients with Taussig-Bing anatomy.[82] The ventricular septal defect is closed through the right atrium or pulmonary artery to direct left ventricular flow into the pulmonary artery. This is followed by arterial switch and the accomplishment of both anatomic and physiologic repair. We have operated on eight patients with Taussig-Bing anatomy with ventricular septal defect closure and arterial switch between 2 weeks and 39 months (mean 10 months) of age. Seven of the eight patients had prior pulmonary artery banding.

There was one operative death in a 3-month-old child who had undergone prior pulmonary artery banding from an apparent subendocardial myocardial infarction. One late death, from severe pulmonary hypertension (the first child in the series) occurred 5 years following arterial switch. This child underwent initial pulmonary artery banding and then arterial switch and ventricular septal defect closure at the age of 3 years. Two years later, a second ventricular septal defect was closed, and 3 years after this the child died.

Two of the eight patients had associated coarctation of the aorta repaired by subclavian flap aortoplasty at the time of pulmonary artery banding. An association between coarctation and Taussig-Bing anatomy has been noted previously by Parr and colleagues.[97] In their review of 105 Taussig-Bing heart specimens, coarctation and/or aortic outflow tract obstruction was noted in 56 (53%). Six of 9 patients treated surgically for Taussig-Bing heart also had coarctation of the aorta.

Our experience indicates that arterial switch can be performed successfully for patients with both side-by-side and anteroposterior orientation of the great vessels. This was supported by Quaegebeur, but he cautioned that the LeCompte maneuver may not be useful when the great arteries are side by side.[98] In some cases, it may be easier to slide the redundant pulmonary artery behind the new aorta for a direct anastomosis. He also emphasized that there is very little difference in coronary artery anatomy between hearts with the Taussig-Bing anomaly and those with classic TGA. Therefore, the same principles for coronary artery transfer can be applied.

Kanter recently reported 7 patients with Taussig-Bing anatomy who underwent ventricular septal defect closure and arterial switch with 1 operative and no late deaths.[99] The LeCompte maneuver was used in 3 patients. Quaegebeur reported 10 patients with Taussig-Bing anatomy who had arterial switch and ventricular septal defect closure with 1 operative and no late deaths.[26] Planche reported 16 patients with double-outlet right ventricle and subpulmonary ventricular septal defect who had arterial switch and ventricular septal defect closure with a 15% early mortality.[69]

Anatomic correction of double-outlet right ventricle and subpulmonary ventricular septal defect (Taussig-Bing heart) by ventricular septal defect closure and arterial switch has the advantages of acceptable operative mortality, left ventricular-to-aortic continuity, no need for extracardiac conduits, and applicability to patients with most variations of coronary and great artery anatomy.

Staged Arterial Switch Operation for the Failing Right Ventricle After the Atrial Baffle Procedures

One of the more serious complications of the atrial baffle procedure is TGA systemic right ventricular dysfunction. Review of 198 patients who underwent the Mustard operation for TGA at Children's Memorial Hospital in Chicago between 1968 and 1987 revealed 14 who died of severe systemic right ventricular dysfunction,[100] which was the most common cause of late death. Nearly all patients with right ventricular dysfunction have associated severe tricuspid insufficiency.[101] The surgical alternatives for patients with a failing right ventricle and tricuspid insufficiency after atrial repair of TGA include tricuspid valve replacement, staged conversion to the arterial switch operation, and orthotopic cardiac transplantation.

At our institution, tricuspid valve replacement was performed in six patients with right ventricular dysfunction and tricuspid insufficiency. Four of these patients died and one had further deterioration of ventricular function requiring heart transplantation. Only one had a good result following tricuspid valve replacement. These results would indicate that tricuspid insufficiency in these patients is a manifestation of severe right ventricular dysfunction. Tricuspid valve replacement does not appear to improve patients with systemic right ventricular dysfunction. The preferable alternatives appear to be staged conversion to arterial switch or orthotopic cardiac transplantation.

Staged conversion from the Mustard operation to arterial switch initially was presented and described by Mee.[102] Twelve patients underwent pulmonary artery banding to prepare the left ventricle for subsequent arterial switch, with two deaths from this procedure alone. Six patients subsequently underwent the arterial switch operation after pulmonary artery banding, with two deaths. Three patients underwent orthotopic cardiac transplantation, with one late death.

In the series of 198 patients from Children's Memorial Hospital, 5 patients have undergone pulmonary artery banding for staged conversion to arterial switch. The first patient underwent the Mustard procedure and ventricular septal defect closure at the age of 1 year. The child developed severe right ventricular dysfunction and underwent pulmonary artery banding at 2 years of age. After left ventricular improvement, arterial switch was performed at the age of 5 years. The child required subsequent aortic valve replacement due to severe neoaortic valve insufficiency, presumably caused by prolonged trauma from the pulmonary artery banding. The second patient had a Mustard procedure and ventricular septal defect closure at the age of 1½ years. This child underwent pulmonary artery banding at the age of 8 years for severe right ventricular dysfunction. Following the banding, the child developed biventricular failure and required urgent orthotopic cardiac transplantation. A third child underwent the Senning operation and ventricular septal defect closure at the age of 1 year. This child had pulmonary artery banding for severe right ventricular dysfunction after failed tricuspid valve replacement at the age of 4 years. At the age of 5 years, the child was explored for possible arterial switch procedure, but it was felt that the aortic valve was not of adequate size. Orthotopic cardiac transplantation was performed successfully shortly thereafter. The fourth patient underwent the Mustard procedure at the age of 2 months for simple TGA. This child underwent pulmonary artery banding at the age of 5 years and the arterial switch procedure at the age of 6 years. The child died of intraoperative myocardial infarction due to coronary insufficiency caused by misidentification of the coronary anatomy because of dense adhesions. The fifth patient had pulmonary artery banding for failing right ventricle after a Mustard procedure and is now awaiting arterial switch.

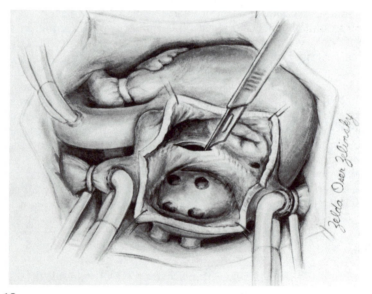

FIG 13.
Atrial view of the Mustard pericardial baffle. Lines of incision and scalpel show the technique at baffle excision. (From Mavroudis C, Backer CL, Idriss FS: Special considerations for and reoperations after the arterial switch operation, in Mavroudis C, Backer CL (eds): *Arterial Switch. Cardiac Surgery: State of the Art Review*, vol 5. Philadelphia, Hanley & Belfus, Inc, 1991, p 130. Used by permission.)

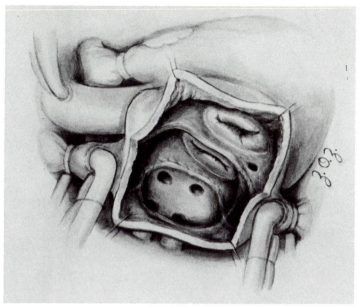

FIG 14.
Diagrammatic representation of the common atrium after pericardial baffle excision. (From Mavroudis C, Backer CL, Idriss FS: Special considerations for and reoperations after the arterial switch operation, in Mavroudis C, Backer CL (eds): *Arterial Switch. Cardiac Surgery: State of the Art Review*, vol 5. Philadelphia, Hanley & Belfus, Inc, 1991, p 131. Used by permission.)

The technique for staged conversion from atrial baffle to arterial switch begins with the pulmonary artery banding to retrain the left ventricle. The pulmonary artery band is constricted to achieve proximal pulmonary artery pressure equal to 75% of the aortic or right ventricular pressure. Dopamine pressor support and mechanical ventilation usually are required for the first few days. Postoperative surveillance is performed by serial echocardiography and cardiac catheterization to determine left ventricular volume, pressure, and muscle mass. When these parameters are close to normal for the child's age, the child undergoes arterial switch. This has required anywhere between 1 to 3 years following pulmonary artery banding. The technique of arterial switch is performed in the usual manner after atrial baffle takedown (Figs 13 through 15), pulmonary artery band removal, and proper coronary artery identification. In our series, a conduit has been used to provide continuity between the proximal neo-pulmonary artery and the distal pulmonary artery, because of inadequate pulmonary artery length caused by dense scarring from the multiple procedures. The overall results at the Children's Memorial Hospital of the patients with a failing right ventricle are tricuspid valve replacement in 7 patients, with 4 deaths; pulmonary artery banding in 4 patients, with no deaths; arterial switch in 2 pa-

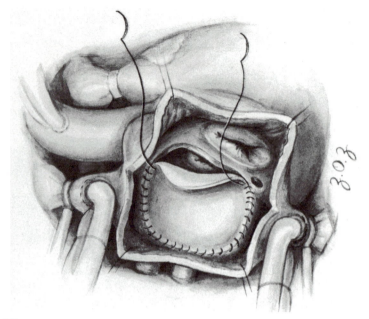

FIG 15.
Atrial septation with polytetrafluoroethylene to reconstruct the right and left atria anatomically and physiologically. (From Mavroudis C, Backer CL, Idriss FS: Special considerations for and reoperations after the arterial switch operation, in Mavroudis C, Backer CL (eds): *Arterial Switch. Cardiac Surgery: State of the Art Review,* vol 5. Philadelphia, Hanley & Belfus, Inc, 1991, p 131. Used by permission.)

tients, with 1 death; and orthotopic cardiac transplantation in 2 patients, with 1 late death (1½ years postoperatively) due to rejection.

In conclusion, tricuspid valve replacement does not improve right ventricular function in patients with a failing right ventricle following the Mustard or Senning procedure. Staged conversion to arterial switch can improve right ventricular function and provide anatomic repair with left ventricle-to-aorta continuity. Orthotopic cardiac transplantation may be the only alternative if the left ventricle does not respond to pulmonary artery banding.

Acquired Supravalvular Pulmonary Stenosis

The potential long-term complications after successful arterial switch center around great-vessel anastomotic constriction, neoaortic valvular insufficiency, and coronary insufficiency. The most common cause for reoperation in these patients has been supravalvular pulmonic stenosis. This problem was recognized as early as 1982 by Yacoub and his associates[32] and since has been confirmed by others.[26, 32, 103, 104] Several authors[26, 32, 104] have found residual right ventricle-to-pulmonary artery gradients in these patients by both invasive and noninvasive methods. The stenosis localization has been found at a number of anatomic sites, the greater proportion of which have been at the supravalvular anastomotic site caused by possible pericardial patch constriction, anastomotic tension, or suture purse-string. In other patients, the gradient was located more peripherally, perhaps caused by inadequate dissection or unfavorable anatomy as a result of the maneuver of LeCompte.[15] Paillole and his associates[103] found that the incidence of pulmonary artery stenosis is low (<10%) in contrast to that reported earlier.[46, 105] Distal pulmonary artery stenosis was infrequent and not affected by the LeCompte maneuver. Pulmonary artery growth is not impaired by current surgical techniques and pulmonic stenosis does not increase as a function of time after operation. A single patch of fresh autologous pericardium is the preferred method of neopulmonary artery reconstruction[9] and, in contrast to earlier reports,[26, 105] side-by-side great-vessel anatomic configuration did not affect coronary transfer or future incidence of pulmonary stenosis. The Congenital Heart Surgeons Society Transposition Study has underlined these findings, showing a low incidence of supravalvular pulmonary stenosis (6%).[22]

We have reoperated only 3 patients for pulmonary stenosis in our combined series of 135 patients. We attribute these results to the use of large pericardial patches (early in the series) and a single large pantaloon pericardial patch (later in the series) to fill out the dissected sinuses of Valsalva

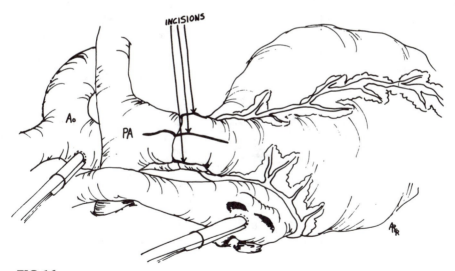

FIG 16.
The lines of incisions for reoperation to repair supravalvular pulmonary stenosis (Ao = aorta; PA = pulmonary artery). (From Mavroudis C: *Ann Thorac Surg* 1987; 43:495–501. Used by permission.)

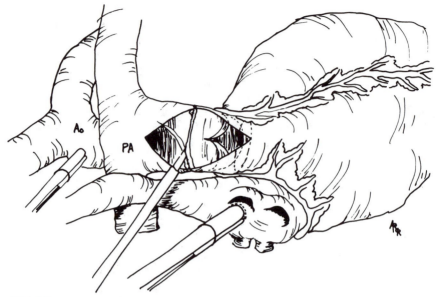

FIG 17.
Sharp dissection of the posterior ridge at the previous anastomotic site of the neo-pulmonary artery *(PA)*. Ao = aorta. (From Mavroudis C: *Ann Thorac Surg* 1987; 43:495–501. Used by permission.)

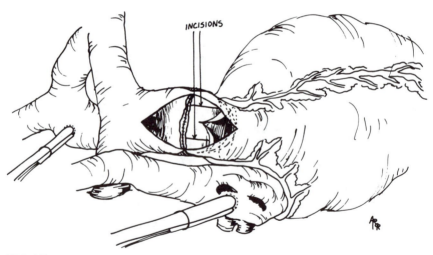

FIG 18.
The longitudinal incision across the stenosis into the anterior sinus of Valsalva of the neo-pulmonary artery. *Broken lines* represent the incisions into the other sinuses of Valsalva for adequate outflow augmentation. (From Mavroudis C: *Ann Thorac Surg* 1987; 43:495–501.)

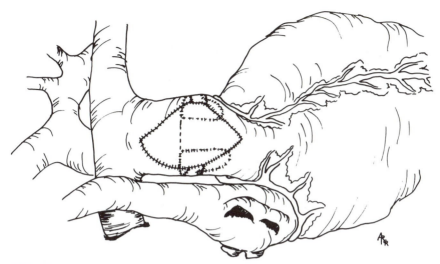

FIG 19.
The completed repair of supravalvular pulmonary stenosis in the neo-pulmonary artery. Outflow augmentation was achieved with three separate patches of polytetrafluoroethylene. (From Mavroudis C: *Ann Thorac Surg* 1987; 43:495–501. Used by permission.)

of the neo-pulmonary artery. When necessary, reoperation should be uncomplicated. Polytetrafluoroethylene supravalvular pulmonary arterioplasty can be performed as shown in Figures 16 through 19. Fortunately, the incidence of reoperation for pulmonary stenosis has been low in the midterm. The multiple refinements with neo-pulmonary artery reconstruction have fulfilled their theoretical expectations. More information will become available as these children grow into adulthood.

Neoaortic Insufficiency and Neoaortic Anastomotic Stenosis

Early angiographic and echocardiographic evaluation[41, 46, 104, 106] has not demonstrated significant supravalvular neoaortic stenosis. There is also a low incidence of neoaortic valvular insufficiency that, when present, does not progress.[2, 107] We also have found a low incidence of neoaortic valvular insufficiency in our patients, resulting in only two replacements. Both of these patients had a pulmonary artery band prior to arterial switch for staged conversion from a Mustard operation in one and staged palliation of TGA and ventricular septal defect in the other. The speculation is strong that pulmonary artery banding under these circumstances causes proximal pulmonary artery and annular dilatation that can lead to neoaortic insufficiency after arterial switch. The trend away from the use of pulmonary artery banding should help to minimize this problem in the future. Patients with TGA and intact ventricular septum or TGA with ventricular septal defect can be treated successfully by arterial switch and ventricular septal defect closure as appropriate in the first 2 weeks of life without pulmonary banding. However, there will be patients who require pulmonary artery banding such as those born with low birth weight, those with low left ventricular mass, and those with right ventricular failure after atrial baffle. Care must be taken to minimize the time between pulmonary artery banding and arterial switch to avoid the annular dilatation effects of the pulmonary artery band.

Summary

The arterial switch operation has taken its place in the treatment of most forms of TGA. Improved surgical techniques and optimal myocardial preservation have allowed surgeons to perform this operation in conjunction with other procedures to create left ventricular-to-aortic continuity. The midterm results have fully justified continued application of the arterial switch operation.

References

1. Abe T, Kuribayashi R, Sato M, et al: Successful Jatene operation for transposition of the great arteries with intact ventricular septum: A case report. J Thorac Cardiovasc Surg 1978; 75:64–67.
2. Backer CL, Ilbawi MN, Ohtake S, et al: Transposition of the great arteries: A comparison of results of the Mustard procedure versus the arterial switch. Ann Thorac Surg 1989; 48:10–14.
3. Bove EL: Current techniques of the arterial switch procedure for transposition of the great arteries. J Cardiovasc Surg (Torino) 1989; 4:193–199.
4. Castaneda AR, Norwood WI, Jonas RA, et al: Transposition of the great arteries and intact ventricular septum: Anatomical report in the neonate. Ann Thorac Surg 1984; 38:438–443.
5. Castaneda AR, Trusler GA, Paul MH, et al: Congenital Heart Surgeons Society: The early results of treatment of simple transposition in the current era. J Thorac Cardiovasc Surg 1988; 95:14–28.
6. Freedom RM, Culham JAG, Olley PM, et al: Anatomic correction of transposition of the great arteries: Pre- and post-operative cardiac catheterization, with angiocardiography in five patients. Circulation 1981; 63:905–914.
7. Harinck E, Van Mill GJ, Ross D, et al: Anatomical correction of transposition of great arteries with persistent ductus arteriosus. Br Heart J 1980; 43:95–98.
8. Idriss FS, Ilbawi MN, DeLeon SY, et al: Arterial switch in simple and complex transposition of the great arteries. J Thorac Cardiovasc Surg 1988; 95:29–36.
9. Idriss FS, Ilbawi MN, DeLeon SY, et al: Transposition of the great arteries with intact ventricular septum: Arterial switch in the first month of life. J Thorac Cardiovasc Surg 1988; 95:255–262.
10. Ilbawi MN, Idriss FS, DeLeon SY, et al: Preparation of the left ventricle for anatomical correction in patients with simple transposition of the great arteries: Surgical guidelines. J Thorac Cardiovasc Surg 1987; 94:87–94.

11. Jatene AD, Fontes VG, Paulista PP, et al: Anatomical correction of transposition of the great vessels. *J Thorac Cardiovasc Surg* 1976; 72:364–370.
12. Jatene AD, Fontes VF, Souza LCB, et al: Anatomical correction of transposition of the great vessels. *J Thorac Cardiovasc Surg* 1982; 83:20–26.
13. Kreutzer G, Neirotti R, Galindez E, et al: Anatomical correction of transposition of the great vessels. *J Thorac Cardiovasc Surg* 1977; 73:538–542.
14. Kurosawa H, Imai Y, Takanashi Y, et al: Infundibular septum and coronary anatomy in Jatene operation. *J Thorac Cardiovasc Surg* 1986; 91:572–583.
15. LeCompte Y, Zannini L, Hazan E, et al: Anatomic correction of transposition of the great arteries. *J Thorac Cardiovasc Surg* 1981; 82:629–631.
16. Mamiya RT, Moreno-Cabral RJ, Nakamura FT, et al: Retransposition of the great vessels for transposition with ventricular septal defect and pulmonary hypertension. *J Thorac Cardiovasc Surg* 1977; 73:340–344.
17. Mavroudis C, Backer CL, Idriss FS: Surgical techniques and intraoperative judgements to facilitate the arterial switch operation in transposition with intact ventricular septum, in Mavroudis C, Backer CL (eds): *Arterial Switch. Cardiac Surgery: State of the Art Review,* vol 5. Philadelphia, Hanley & Belfus, Inc, 1991, pp 99–118.
18. Mavroudis C, Backer CL, Idriss FS: Special considerations for and reoperations after the arterial switch operation, in Mavroudis C, Backer CL (eds): *Arterial Switch. Cardiac Surgery: State of the Art Review,* vol 5. Philadelphia, Hanley & Belfus, Inc, 1991, pp 119–140.
19. Mavroudis C: Anatomical repair of transposition of the great arteries with intact ventricular septum in the neonate: Guidelines to avoid complications. *Ann Thorac Surg* 1987; 43:495–501.
20. Mavroudis C, Arensman FW, Rees AH: Anatomical repair of transposition of the great arteries with intact ventricular septum in the neonate, in Kron IL, Mavroudis C (eds): *Innovations in Congenital Heart Surgery. Cardiac Surgery: State of the Art Review,* vol 3. Philadelphia, Hanley & Belfus, 1989, pp 331–354.
21. Muster AJ, Berry TE, Ilbawi MN, et al: Development of neo-coarctation in patients with transposed great arteries and hypoplastic aortic arch after LeCompte modification of anatomical correction. *J Thorac Cardiovasc Surg* 1987; 93:276–280.
22. Norwood WI, Dobell AR, Freed MD, et al: Congenital Heart Surgeons Society: Intermediate results of the arterial switch repair: A 20-institution study. *J Thorac Cardiovasc Surg* 1988; 96:854–863.
23. Pacifico AD, Stewart RW, Bargeron LM: Repair of transposition of the great arteries with ventricular septal defect by an arterial switch operation. *Circulation* 1983; 68:49–55.
24. Pigott JD, Chin AJ, Weinberg PM, et al: Transposition of the great arteries with aortic arch obstruction: Anatomical review and report of surgical management. *J Thorac Cardiovasc Surg* 1987; 94:82–86.
25. Planche C, Bruniaux J, Lacour-Gayet F, et al: Switch operation for transposition of the great arteries in neonates: A study of 120 patients. *J Thorac Cardiovasc Surg* 1988; 96:354–363.
26. Quaegebeur JM, Rohmer J, Ottenkamp J, et al: The arterial switch operation: An eight-year experience. *J Thorac Cardiovasc Surg* 1986; 92:361–384.
27. Ross D, Rickards A, Somerville J: Transposition of the great arteries: Logical anatomical arterial correction. *Br Med J [Clin Res]* 1976; 1:1109–1111.
28. Sidi D, Heurtematte Y, Kachaner J, et al: Problemes poses par la preparation du ventricule gauche a la correction anatomique de la transposition simple des gros vaisseaux. *Arch Mal Coeur* 1983; 76:575–583.

29. Williams WG, Freedom RM, Culham G, et al: Early experience with arterial repair of transposition. *Ann Thorac Surg* 1981; 32:8–15.
30. Yacoub MH, Radley-Smith R, Hilton CJ: Anatomical correction of complete transposition of the great arteries and ventricular septal defect in infancy. *Br Med J [Clin Res]* 1976; 1:1112–1114.
31. Yacoub MH, Radley-Smith R, Maclaurin R: Two-stage operation for anatomical correction of transposition of the great arteries with intact interventricular septum. *Lancet* 1977; 1:1275–1278.
32. Yacoub M, Bernhard A, Lange P, et al: Clinical and hemodynamic results of the two-stage anatomic correction of simple transposition of the great arteries. *Circulation* 1980; 62(suppl I):190–196.
33. Fleming WH: Why switch? *J Thorac Cardiovasc Surg* 1979; 78:1–2.
34. Laks H: The arterial switch procedure for the neonate: Coming of age. *Ann Thorac Surg* 1989; 48:3–4.
35. Lincoln CR, Lima R, Rigby ML: Anatomical correction of simple transposition of the great arteries during neonatal transition (letter). *Lancet* 1983; 1:39.
36. Rubay J, de Leval M, Bull C: To switch or not to switch? The Senning alternative. *Circulation* 1988; 78(suppl):1–4.
37. Stark J: Transposition of the great arteries: Which operation (editorial)? *Ann Thorac Surg* 1984; 38:429–431.
38. Yacoub MH: The case for anatomic correction of transposition of the great arteries. *J Thorac Cardiovasc Surg* 1979; 78:3–6.
39. Mustard WT: Successful two-stage correction of transposition of the great vessels. *Surgery* 1964; 55:469–472.
40. Trusler GA, Williams WG, Izukawa T, et al: Current results with the Mustard operation in isolated transposition of the great arteries. *J Thorac Cardiovasc Surg* 1980; 80:381–389.
41. Arensman FW, H-Sievers H, Lange P, et al: Assessment of coronary and aortic anatomoses after anatomic correction of transposition of the great arteries. *J Thorac Cardiovasc Surg* 1985; 90:597–604.
42. Gittenberger-de Groot AC, Sauer U, Quaegebeur J: Aortic intramural coronary artery in three hearts with transposition of the great arteries. *J Thorac Cardiovasc Surg* 1986; 91:566–571.
43. Rossi MB, Ho SY, Anderson RH, et al: Coronary arteries in complete transposition: The significance of the sinus node artery. *Ann Thorac Surg* 1986; 42:573–577.
44. Goor DA, Shem-Tov A, Neufeld HN: Impeded coronary flow in anatomic correction of transposition of the great arteries. *J Thorac Cardiovasc Surg* 1982; 83:747–752.
45. Rowlatt UF: Coronary artery distribution in complete transposition. *JAMA* 1962; 179:109–118.
46. Yacoub MH, Radley-Smith R: Anatomy of the coronary arteries in transposition of the great arteries and methods of transfer in anatomical correction. *Thorax* 1978; 33:418–424.
47. Bergouignan M, Fontan F, Trarieux M, et al: L'enfant au decours d'interventions cardio-chirurgicales sous hypothermie profonde. *Rev Neurol (Paris)* 1961; 105:48–60.
48. Clarkson P, McArthur B, Barrett-Boyes B, et al: Developmental progress after cardiac surgery in infancy utilizing hypothermia and circulatory arrest. *Circulation* 1980; 62:855–861.
49. Ehyai A, Fenichel G, Bender H Jr: Incidence and prognosis of seizures in infants after cardiac surgery with profound hypothermia and circulatory arrest. *JAMA* 1984; 252:3165–3167.

50. Mavroudis C, Greene MA: Cardiopulmonary bypass and hypothermia circulatory arrest in infants, in Jacobs ML (ed): *Current Issues in Pediatric Heart Surgery.* Stoneham, Mass, Butterworth Publishers, in press.
51. Molina J, Einzig S, Mastri A, et al: Brain damage in profound hypothermia. *J Thorac Cardiovasc Surg* 1984; 87:596–604.
52. Treasure T, Naftel D, Conger K, et al: The effect of hypothermic circulatory arrest time on cerebral function, morphology, and biochemistry. *J Thorac Cardiovasc Surg* 1983; 86:761–770.
53. Swain JA, McDonald T, Griffith P, et al: Low flow hypothermic cardiopulmonary bypass protects the brain. Presented at the American Association for Thoracic Surgery meeting, Toronto, May 1990.
54. Greeley WJ, Ungerleider RM, Kern FH, et al: Effect of hypothermic cardiopulmonary bypass and total circulatory arrest on cerebral blood flow and metabolism in neonates and small infants. Presented at the American Association for Thoracic Surgery meeting, Toronto, May 1990.
55. Aoshima M, Yokota M, Shiraishi Y, et al: Prolonged aortic cross-clamping in early infancy and method of myocardial preservation. *J Cardiovasc Surg (Torino) 1988;* 29:591–595.DeLeon SY, Idriss FS, Ilbawi MN, et al: Comparison of single versus multidose blood cardioplegia in arterial switch procedures. *Ann Thorac Surg 1988;* 45:548–553.
56. DeLeon SY, Idriss FS, Ilbawi MN, et al: Comparison of single versus multidose blood cardioplegia in arterial switch procedures. *Ann Thorac Surg* 1988; 45:548–553.
57. Ganzel BL, Katzmark SL, Mavroudis C: Myocardial preservation in the neonate. *J Thorac Cardiovasc Surg* 1988; 96:414–422.
58. Corno AF, Bethencourt DM, Laks H, et al: Myocardial protection in the neonatal heart: A comparison of topical hypothermia and crystalloid and blood cardioplegic solutions. *J Thorac Cardiovasc Surg* 1987; 93:163–172.
59. Yonenaga K, Yasui H, Kado H, et al: Myocardial protection by retrograde cardioplegia in arterial switch operation. *Ann Thorac Surg* 1990; 50:238–242.
60. Lamberti JJ Jr, Cohn LH, Laks H, et al: Local cardiac hypothermia for myocardial protection during correction of congenital heart disease. *Ann Thorac Surg* 1975; 20:446–455.
61. Rheuban KS, Kron IL, Bulatovic A: Internal mammary artery bypass after the arterial switch operation. *Ann Thorac Surg* 1990; 50:125–126.
62. Anderson HL, Attorri RJ, Custer JR, et al: Extracorporeal membrane oxygenation for pediatric cardiopulmonary failure. *J Thorac Cardiovasc Surg* 1990; 99:1011–1021.
63. Wernovsky G, Hougen TJ, Walsh EP, et al: Midterm results after the arterial switch operation for transposition of the great arteries with intact ventricular septum: Clinical, hemodynamic, echocardiographic, and electrophysiologic data. *Circulation* 1988; 77:1333–1344.
64. McGoon DC: Surgery for transposition of the great arteries (editorial). *Circulation* 1972; 45:1147.
65. Bove EL, Beekman RH, Snider AR, et al: Arterial repair for transposition of great arteries and large ventricular septal defect in early infancy. *Circulation* 1988; 78:III26–31.
66. Salerno TA, Chiong MA: The hemodynamic and metabolic effects of cardioplegic rearrest in the pig. *Ann Thorac Surg* 1983; 35:280–287.
67. Wright RN, Levitsky S, Holland C, et al: Beneficial effects of potassium cardioplegia during intermittent aortic cross-clamping and reperfusion. *J Surg Res* 1978; 24:201–209.

68. Yamaguchi M, Hosokawa Y, Imai Y, et al: Early and midterm results of the arterial switch operation for transposition of the great arteries in Japan. *J Thorac Cardiovasc Surg* 1990; 100:261–269.

69. Planche C, Serraf A, Lacour-Gayet F, et al: Arterial switch for transposition of the great arteries and ventricular septal defect, 106 patients. Presented at the American Association for Thoracic Surgery meeting, Toronto, May 1990.

70. Major WK Jr, Matsuda H, Subramanian S: Failure of the Jatene operation in a patient with d-transposition and intact ventricular septum. *Ann Thorac Surg* 1976; 22:386–388.

71. de Leval MR, McKay R, Jones M, et al: Modified Blalock-Taussig shunt: Use of subclavian artery orifice as flow regulator in prosthetic systemic-pulmonary artery shunts. *J Thorac Cardiovasc Surg* 1981; 81:112–119.

72. Nakano H, Ueda K, Saito A, et al: Beneficial preparatory aortopulmonary shunt for anatomic repair of transposition of the great arteries and intact ventricular septum. *Ann Thorac Surg* 1985; 40:512–515.

73. Yasui H, Kado H, Yonenaga K, et al: Arterial switch operation for transposition of the great arteries, with special reference to left ventricular function. *J Thorac Cardiovasc Surg* 1989; 98:601–610.

74. Taussig HB, Bing RJ: Complete transposition of the aorta and a levoposition of the pulmonary artery. *Am Heart J* 1949; 37:551–559.

75. Van Praagh R: What is the Taussig-Bing malformation (editorial)? *Circulation* 1968; 38:445–449.

76. Lev M, Rimoldi HJA, Eckner FAO, et al: The Taussig-Bing heart. Qualitative and quantitative anatomy. *Arch Pathol Lab Med* 1966; 81:24–35.

77. Patrick DL, McGoon DC: An operation for double-outlet right ventricle with transposition of the great arteries. *J Cardiovasc Surg (Torino)* 1968; 9:537–542.

78. Kawashima Y, Fujita T, Miyamoto T, et al: Intraventricular rerouting of blood for the correction of Taussig-Bing malformation. *J Thorac Cardiovasc Surg* 1971; 62:825–829.

79. Snoddy JW, Parr EL, Robertson LW, et al: Successful intracardiac repair of the Taussig-Bing malformation in 2 children. *Ann Thorac Surg* 1978; 25:158–163.

80. Harvey JC, Sondheimer HM, Williams WG, et al: Repair of double-outlet right ventricle. *J Thorac Cardiovasc Surg* 1977; 73:611–615.

81. Kirklin JW, Pacifico AD, Blackstone EH, et al: Current risks and protocols for operations for double outlet right ventricle: Derivation from an 18 year experience. *J Thorac Cardiovasc Surg* 1986; 92:913–930.

82. Yacoub MH, Radley-Smith R: Anatomic correction of the Taussig-Bing anomaly. *J Thorac Cardiovasc Surg* 1984; 88:380–387.

83. Van Praagh: Anatomic correction of the Taussig-Bing anomaly (Comment). *J Thorac Cardiovasc Surg* 1984; 88:387–388.

84. Hightower BM, Barcia A, Bargeron LM Jr, et al: Double-outlet right ventricle with transposed great arteries and subpulmonary ventricular septal defect. The Taussig-Bing malformation. *Circulation* 39&40(suppl I):I207–I213. 1969;

85. Wedemeyer AL, Lucas RV Jr, Castaneda AR: Taussig-Bing malformation, coarctation of the aorta, and reversed patent ductus arteriosus. Operative correction in an infant. *Circulation* 1970; 42:1021–1027.

86. Luber JM, Castaneda AR, Lang P, et al: Repair of double outlet right ventricle. Early and late results. *Circulation* 1983; 68(suppl II):144–147.

87. Ottino G, Kugler JD, McNamara DG, et al: Taussig-Bing anomaly: Total repair with closure of ventricular septal defect through the pulmonary artery. *Ann Thorac Surg* 1980; 29:170–176.
88. Abe T, Komatsu S, Chiba M, et al: Successful modified Senning operation for the repair of Taussig-Bing malformation. *J Cardiovasc Surg (Torino)* 1982; 23:1–5.
89. Muster AJ, Bharati S, Aziz KU, et al: Taussig-Bing anomaly with straddling mitral valve. *J Thorac Cardiovasc Surg* 1979; 77:832–842.
90. Damus PS, Thomson NB Jr, McLoughlin TG: Arterial repair without coronary relocation for complete transposition of the great vessels with ventricular septal defect. *J Thorac Cardiovasc Surg* 1982; 83:316–318.
91. Stansel HC Jr: A new operation for *d*-loop transposition of the great vessels. *Ann Thorac Surg* 1975; 19:565–567.
92. Kaye MP: Anatomic correction of transposition of the great arteries. *Mayo Clin Proc* 1975; 50:638–640.
93. Smith EEJ, Pucci JJ, Walesby RK, et al: A new technique for correction of the Taussig-Bing anomaly. *J Thorac Cardiovasc Surg* 1982; 83:901–904.
94. Binet JP, Lacour-Gayet F, Conso JF, et al: Complete repair of the Taussig-Bing type of double-outlet right ventricle using the arterial switch operation without coronary translocation. Report of one successful case. *J Thorac Cardiovasc Surg* 1983; 85:272–275.
95. Ceithaml EL, Puga FJ, Danielson GK, et al: Results of the Damus-Stansel-Kaye procedure for transposition of the great arteries and for double outlet right ventricle with subpulmonary ventricular septal defect. *Ann Thorac Surg* 1984; 38:433–437.
96. Freedom RM, Culham JAG, Olley PM, et al: Anatomic correction of transposition of the great arteries: Pre- and postoperative cardiac catheterization, with angiocardiography in five patients. *Circulation* 1981; 63:905–914.
97. Parr GVS, Waldausen JA, Bharati S, et al: Coarctation in Taussig-Bing malformation of the heart. Surgical significance. *J Thorac Cardiovasc Surg* 1983; 86:280–287.
98. Quaegebeur JM: The optimal repair for the Taussig-Bing heart (editorial). *J Thorac Cardiovasc Surg* 1983; 85:276–277.
99. Kanter K, Anderson R, Lincoln C, et al: Anatomic correction of double-outlet right ventricle with subpulmonary ventricular septal defect (the "Taussig-Bing" anomaly). *Ann Thorac Surg* 1986; 41:287–292.
100. Ohtake S, Idriss FS, Ilbawi MN, et al: Severe systemic right ventricular dysfunction after Mustard operation for transposition. *Circulation* 1989; 80(suppl II):II–70.
101. Ohtake S, Idriss FS, Backer CL, et al: Fate of tricuspid valve as a systemic atrioventricular valve: A 20 year follow-up of TGA with Mustard repair. *J Am Coll Cardiol* 1990; 15:79A.
102. Mee RBB: Severe right ventricular failure after Mustard or Senning operation. Two-stage repair: Pulmonary artery banding and switch. *J Thorac Cardiovasc Surg* 1986; 92:385–390.
103. Paillole C, Sidi D, Kachaner J, et al: Fate of pulmonary artery after anatomic correction of simple transposition of great arteries in newborn infants. *Circulation* 1988; 78:870–876.
104. Rees A, Solinger R, Elbl F, et al: Conventional Doppler echocardiography and Doppler color flow mapping in the evaluation of the arterial switch operation. *Clin Res* 1989; 37:42.

105. Kanter KR, Anderson RH, Lincoln C, et al: Anatomic correction for complete transposition and double outlet right ventricle. *J Thorac Cardiovasc Surg* 1985; 90:690–699.
106. Martin MM, Snider AR, Bove EL, et al: Two-dimensional and Doppler echocardiographic evaluation after arterial switch repair in infancy for complete transposition of the great arteries. *Am J Cardiol* 1989; 63:332–336.
107. Martin RP, Ettedgui JA, Qureshi SA, et al: A quantitative evaluation of aortic regurgitation after anatomic correction of transposition of the great arteries. *J Am Coll Cardiol* 1988; 12:1281–1284.

Central Nervous System Dysfunction After Cardiac Surgery

Mark Newman, M.D.

Chief of Cardiothoracic Anesthesia, Department of Anesthesiology, Department of the Air Force, Lackland Air Force Base, Texas

Peter Frasco, M.D.

Fellow in Cardiac Anesthesia, Department of Anesthesiology, The Heart Center, Duke University Medical Center, Durham, North Carolina

Frank Kern, M.D.

Assistant Professor, Department of Anesthesiology, Boston Children's Hospital, Boston, Massachusetts

William J. Greeley

Assistant Professor, Department of Anesthesiology; Assistant Professor, Department of Pediatrics, The Heart Center, Duke University Medical Center, Durham, North Carolina

James A. Blumenthal, Ph.D.

Associate Professor, Department of Psychiatry; Assistant Professor, Department of Medicine, The Heart Center, Duke University Medical Center, Durham, North Carolina

J. G. Reves, M.D.

Professor, Department of Anesthesiology, The Heart Center, Duke University Medical Center, Durham, North Carolina

Over time, the incidence of morbidity and mortality following cardiac surgery has declined significantly due to improvements in surgical and anesthetic management.[1] However, despite a decline in neuropsychologic complications, these now represent an important contribution to the overall incidence of postoperative morbidity and mortality. This review summarizes the available information on neuropsychologic morbidity following cardiac surgery and cardiopulmonary bypass (CPB), emphasizing the incidence, etiology, and risk factors thought to be associated with these complications, methods of monitoring neurologic function, and methods of cerebral protection.

Clinical Findings

Clinical reports of neuropsychologic complications following cardiac surgery and CPB were first published in the mid-1950s[2] and were brought to widespread attention in 1965.[3] Neurologic findings vary in their manifestation and severity, and range from transient isolated motor weakness to aphasia, permanent paralysis, cerebrovascular accident, and irreversible coma. Other reports of visual[4] and auditory[5] dysfunction include findings of transient to permanent visual impairment manifested as visual hallucinations, transient ischemic attacks, decreased visual acuity, scotoma, and total permanent blindness as well as unilateral sensorineural hearing loss that is consistent with cochlear lesions. They may be transient or permanent in nature. Postoperative psychologic manifestations.[6, 7] include delayed awakening, confusion and disorientation, anxiety, hallucinations, personality and behavioral changes, depression, delusions, and a syndrome labeled postcardiotomy delirium[8] that occurs after a 2- to 4-day interval of lucidness. Although sensory monotomy or overload and deprivation of sleep in the intensive care environment may contribute to the development of this syndrome, the incidence declines with shorter periods of CPB,[9] suggesting that events during the operative period are important. In addition, more subtle aberrations have been detected by multiple psychometric testing regimens.

Subclinical Findings

In addition to the clinical manifestations just outlined, investigation of various subclinical parameters is yielding information that confirms the widespread extent of the insult to the central nervous system during CPB. Creatine kinase and adenylate kinase, found in the cerebrospinal fluid, are brain-specific biochemical markers of cerebral ischemia. Measurements of these markers confirm the presence of widespread subclinical brain injury and reveal a correlation with the degree of irreversible neuronal damage.[10, 11] Other putative markers of brain ischemia include the brain amines, β-endorphin, and the neurospecific myelin basic protein.[12, 13] More recent work also supports the concept of diffuse impairment of the central nervous system following extracorporeal circulation that is consistent with global brain stunning. Regional cerebral blood flow as determined by single-photon emission computerized tomography both preoperatively and within 10 days postoperatively reveals a uniform decrease in regional CBF despite the absence of motor deficits or focal abnormalities noted on tomograms.[14] Computerized tomography of the brain also has revealed unexpected abnormalities following surgery in patients who have essentially normal results on postoperative neurologic examinations.[15] These findings have been noted for both children and adults and demonstrate that the insult to the central nervous system during CPB is not the exception, but the rule.

Detection and Incidence

Detection

Detection of Neurologic Deficits After Cardiopulmonary Bypass

The detection of neurologic deficits associated with CPB varies with the wide range of severity of injuries seen and the thoroughness of the postoperative assessment. A complete neurologic exam is seldom performed before or after cardiac surgery, and subtle deficits are often missed. Peripheral neuropathies associated with either chest retraction or Favalaro retractor placement often go unnoticed, as do visual field defects.[16-18] The value of an experienced observer in detecting neurologic dysfunction is clear. It has been reported that patients retrospectively analyzed by a non-neurologist had a 6% incidence of postoperative cerebral abnormalities, while patients examined prospectively by neurologists had a 35% incidence of new deficits.[18] Debate on the significance of subclinical neurologic changes or neuropsychologic deficits occurs because the majority of the neuropsychologic deficits tend to be resolved by 6 months. However, a 5-year follow-up study provides disturbing data indicating that these changes are significant, showing transient neuropsychologic deficits to be associated with significant global cerebral dysfunction 5 years postoperatively compared to patients who did not experience these changes.[19] With these neurologic changes ever present, detection of intraoperative changes that could predict poor outcome and allow intervention is the ultimate goal of ongoing research.

Intraoperative Neurologic Monitoring

Attempts to prevent neurologic injury by monitoring the electroencephalogram (EEG) were first employed during CPB in 1957. However, today it is used more frequently to detect brain ischemia during carotid endarterectomy, neurosurgery, and hypotensive anesthesia.[20, 21] The development of computerized EEG monitors to reduce the volume of data and facilitate the recognition of abrupt changes and trends has facilitated interpretation by anesthesiologists and surgeons. The best proven utilization of this technology is for carotid endarterectomies in which abnormalities in the EEG have been correlated with impaired cerebral blood flow and the development of new postoperative neurologic deficits.[20, 21] Unfortunately, CPB is not conducive for EEG monitoring because of the effects of anesthesia, and hypothermia and the likelihood of regional brain injury. Despite this limitation, routine monitoring of the EEG may provide at least potential benefit with virtually no risk. Although there are no large prospective studies demonstrating that routine monitoring of the EEG reduces neurologic sequelae or improves outcome, a recent pilot study has demonstrated that prolonged increases in delta frequencies of processed EEGs during CPB may be predictive of postoperative disorientation. Catastrophic events possibly could be detected and perhaps treated earlier if specific EEG criteria for brain ischemia during CPB are produced.[22]

Evoked potentials also have been advocated by several authors as a means of monitoring cerebral function during CPB.[21, 23-25] Evoked potentials are better preserved than is spontaneous electrical activity (EEG) during hypothermia and deep anesthesia.[26] Unfortunately, intraoperative evoked potential monitoring is technically more difficult to perform and interpret than is processed EEG.[26] These limitations, along with the lack of any prospective trial showing improved outcome, limit the current usefulness of evoked potentials.

Transcranial Doppler assessment of middle cerebral artery flow velocity has been shown to reflect trends in cerebral blood flow and allow continuous measurement.[27] This Doppler ultrasound technology also allows for the detection of middle cerebral artery emboli, (Fig 1), which can be quan-

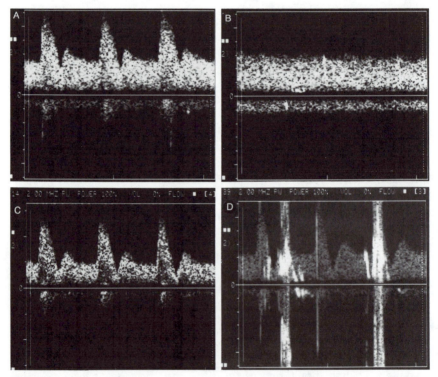

FIG 1.
A and **B,** spectral display of Doppler signal shortly before the institution of cardiopulmonary bypass and during steady-state cardiopulmonary bypass. **C** and **D,** spectral display of Doppler signal at baseline and at release of aortic cross-clamp after aortic valve replacement, demonstrating probable embolic event signified by increased signal intensity.

titated and correlated with surgical events. Recent studies have shown correlation between the number of middle cerebral artery emboli and neuropsychologic outcome.[28] Despite this interesting correlation, a level of embolization requiring intervention or treatment has not been described. Transcranial Doppler must be considered early in its development, and its usefulness requires larger, prospective trials to confirm its value in predicting neurologic or neuropsychologic deficits. Finally, xenon[133] cerebral blood flow measurements have been used for routine monitoring during carotid endarterectomy.[29] Cerebral blood flow measurements are a useful research tool during CPB.[30-32] The amount of equipment necessary for xenon[133] cerebral blood flow monitoring and the fact that continuous on-line measurements are not possible limit the use of this technology in routine clinical practice at this time.

Detection of Psychometric Deficits

Many of the recent studies of neuropsychologic changes focus on identifying those neuropsychologic instruments that are most sensitive to cerebral damage resulting from cardiac surgery and CPB. Among the most commonly reported, those highly sensitive are the Benton Visual Retention Test, the Trail Making Test Part B, the Digit Span and Digit Symbol tests from the Wechsler Adult Intelligence Scale, and the Stroop Test[33-39] (Table 1). These instruments have an advantage over routine clinical observations in that they offer objective and continuous measures of various cognitive functions. Linear regression analysis has been used to construct a test battery that could definitively identify the presence or absence of a neuropsychologic deficit associated with coronary artery bypass grafting.[37] Subsequently, it was suggested that Digit Symbol, the Stroop Test, Word Learning, Trails B, Digit Span (Backwards), and the Benton Visual Retention Test were adequate to detect a deficit. However, this analysis was performed on data from only 20 male subjects and did not include several instruments utilized by other investigators. In general, although no consensus battery of instruments currently exists, speeded tasks that measure attention, concentration, and memory appear to be most sensitive to deficits associated with cardiac surgery. It remains to be proven how important these easily detected deficits are to patients and their families, and to the overall quality of life during initial and late convalescence.

Incidence

Neurologic Injury

The reported incidence of postoperative neuropsychologic morbidity following cardiac surgery varies widely. Many factors are responsible for these discrepancies. Among the most important are the variable definitions of morbidity, the prospective or retrospective nature of the study, the type of surgical procedures performed, the interval after surgery at which findings are reported, and the year in which the study was performed. In 1969,[40] a 53% incidence of transient neurologic dysfunction and a 15% incidence of

TABLE 1.
Common Instruments Used To Assess Cognitive Deficits After Cardiac Surgery*

Instrument	Description	Purpose
Digit Symbol	Requires subjects to reproduce as many coded symbols as possible in a blank box beneath the digit with which it is paired within 90 seconds	Visuomotor coordination, attention, response speed; relatively unaffected by intelligence level, memory, and learning
Benton Visual Retention Test	Requires subjects to draw from memory a series of geometric shapes following a 10-second exposure	Visuomotor coordination, visuo-spatial perception, and intermediate memory
Trail Making (B)	Requires subjects to connect a series of numbers and letters in alternating sequence (e.g., 1-A-2-B-3-C, etc.) that have been randomly distributed on a single piece of paper as quickly as possible	Attention and concentration, visual conceptual, and visuotracking
Digit Span	Requires subjects to repeat a series of digits that have been presented orally forward and, in an independent test, in reverse order	Immediate memory, attention, working memory
The Stroop Test	Requires subjects to name the color of the ink that the words red, blue, or green are printed in; each word is printed in the same or conflicting color	Assesses concentration and the facility with which an individual can shift his/her perceptual set to match changing demands

*From Lezak MD: *Neuropsychological Assessment.* New York, Oxford University Press, 1983. Used by permission.

permanent cerebral deficits at the time of discharge were reported. In 1970, another group[7] found that abnormal neurologic signs developed in 44% of patients at the time of the first examination following surgery. In 1971, one group, in a prospective study,[41] demonstrated neurologic findings in 23% of their patients, and in 1972, using a retrospective[42] analysis, a 19% incidence of neurologic dysfunction was reported. In 1985, a British group[4] noted a 61% incidence of abnormal neurologic findings following extracorporeal circulation and a 1.6% incidence of death or severe disability related to central nervous system injury. The frequency of cerebral infarction after CPB ranges from 0% to 13%.[4, 7, 9, 40, 42–50] The incidence of stroke is higher after intracardiac than extracardiac procedures.[51] Duration or improvement in neurologic status is gradual and dependent on the extent of the initial postoperative deficit.

Cognitive Dysfunction

To provide greater insight into the incidence and particular characterization of postoperative cognitive dysfunction, we selected papers for Tables 2 and 3 that met the following criteria: (1) primarily coronary artery bypass graft patients (rather than valvular or other cardiac surgery); (2) neuropsychologic instruments utilized in the identification of postoperative cognitive deficits; and (3) sample size of at least 20 subjects. Studies that relied solely on clinical neurologic exams were excluded because of potential problems with the lack of objective and quantifiable end points. The incidence and psychometric tests used to detect cognitive dysfunction are listed in the table. It should be noted that the incidence of deficits after CPB is highest in those patients tested earlier and more extensively.[34]

Over the past 30 years, surgical, perfusion, and anesthetic management have improved. Also recently (since the 1970s), the ratio of extracardiac to intracardiac surgical procedures has increased significantly. These facts coincide with the noted decline in the number of neurologic events. The best evidence that cognitive dysfunction has been reduced over time comes from longitudinal studies at a single center. The improvement in neuropsychologic outcome over a 9-year period at one institution has been reported using identical instruments of detection. Reports from 1972 to 1973, 1977, and 1980 noted a decreasing incidence of cerebral complications and associated mortalities of 15% and 3%, 3.5% and 0.5%, and 1.8% and 0.3%, respectively.[52, 69, 70]

Duration

The duration of postoperative neuropsychologic dysfunction after CPB varies between studies. Studies by various groups have shown that 30% to 70% of patients have significant cognitive function deficits on neuropsychologic testing in the first week after CPB.[55, 57, 71] Follow-up testing at 1 to 2 months postoperatively showed a decrease from 7.7% to 12%, and at 6 months 0% to 5%.[55, 57, 71] These studies and others suggest that the majority of cognitive function deficits resolve within the first several months

TABLE 2.
Coronary Artery Bypass Grafting and Cognition*

Author (year)	Subjects†	Design†	Results†
Gilberstadt and Sako (1967)[35]	53 male "open heart" patients (mean age 45 yr) 56 male noncardiac surgery controls (>55 yr)	Pre-post (3 wk)	Cardiac patients showed significant decline on Verbal IQ, Digit Span, and Digit Symbol from WAIS
Lee et al. (1971)[41]	86 cardiac operation patients (mean age 35 yr)	Pre-post (10 days, 3 months)	23% incidence of deficits at 10 days in cardiac group; 0% incidence of deficits at 10 days in noncardiac group; 3 months postoperative mortality was three times greater for cardiac patients with postoperative deficits at 10 days
Frank et al. (1972)[3]	49 patients (>21 yr); 37 valve, 12 miscellaneous "open-heart"	Pre-post (6 mo)	WAIS full IQ, Verbal IQ, information similarities, block, and Benton Visual Retention significantly increased at 6 months
Aberg and Kihlgren (1974)[52]	99 valve; 18 CABG; 27 miscellaneous open-heart (51.6 yr)	Pre-post (8-days); follow-up at 2 mo and 1 yr	16% (age 50–59 yr) died; 30% (age 60–69 yr) died; postoperative deficits on Synonyms Block, Figure rotation, Figure Identification, and Figure classification in cardiac group; at 2 months, 11%–23% of patients demonstrated cognitive deficits; correlates with deficits in perfusion and valvular calcification

Study	Sample	Design	Findings
Willner and Rabiner (1979)[54]	64 CABG and/or valve	Pre-post (10 days); follow-up at 18 mo and 5 yr	No change in WAIS vocabulary; Conceptual Level Analogy Test (CLAT) increase from 10 days to 18 months
Kolkka and Hilberman (1980)[45]	102 CABG alone; 102 CABG and other surgical procedure (56 yr)	Postoperative; pre-post (3–7 days)	17% incidence of neurological dysfunction at discharge; correlates with deficits of advanced age, longer bypass time
Ellis et al. (1980)[55]	30 male CABG (55.4 yr)	Pre-post (7 days); follow-up (4 wk)	75% showed some deficit 1 wk postoperatively; 17% showed some deficit 4 wk postoperatively; ANOVA showed no significant changes over time; memory Quotient declined at 1 wk postoperatively
Savageau et al. (1982)[56]	184 male; 43 female: 172 (76%) CABG; 29 (13%) valve; 26 (11%) both (mean age 54.5 yr)	Pre-post (10 days)	1%–17% showed deficit on at least 1 test; correlates with postoperative deficits of (1) age >60 yr; (2) end-diastolic pressure >30 mm Hg, (3) enlarged heart preoperatively, (4) duration of operation >7 hr, (5) pump time >2 hr, (6) cross-aortic clamp time >2 hr, (7) blood loss >2,000 mL, (8) perioperative hypotension, (9) insertion of intra-aortic balloon, (10) postoperative depression
Savageau et al. (1982)[57]	198 male; 47 female: 185 (75%) CABG; 34 (14%) valve; 26 (11%) both (mean age 54.7 yr)	Pre-post (6 mo)	5% continuing deficit (deficit at 1 wk persisted at 6 mo); 45% of patients with deficits at 1 wk had shown improvement from preoperative scores

(Continued.)

TABLE 2 (cont.).

Author (year)	Subjects[†]	Design[†]	Results[†]
Fish et al. (1982)[37]	20 male coronary artery surgery patients (range 45–70 yr)	4 days preoperative prior to discharge	Digit Span, Stroop, Word Learning, Dig Span (Backwards) and Benton Visual Retention showed significant decrease; linear regression showed Digit Span, Stroop Color/Word, Word Learning, Trails B, Digit Span (Backwards) and Benton Visual Retention adequate to detect deficit; no correlates
Breuer et al. (1983)[50]	361 male; 60 female; all CABG (mean age 57 yr)	Pre-post (4 days); follow-up (6 mo to 1 yr)	11.6% incidence of cerebral damage at day 4; 2% had severe damage; Correlates with postoperative deficits of use of intra-aortic balloon pump and use of pressor drug
Garvey et al. (1983)[58]	2 open-heart patients with arterial filtration with Pall filter; 34 open-heart patients with arterial filtration with Bentley AF-10 filter	Pre-post (7 days)	AF-10 filter group—24% incidence of impairment; Pall filter group—0% incidence; bypass time correlated with deficits in AF-10 filter group

*From Robinson M, Blumenthal JA, Burker EJ, et al: *J Cardiopulmonary Rehabil* 1990; 10:180–189. Used by permission.
†CABG = coronary artery bypass grafting; pre-post = preoperative-postoperative testing; WAIS = Wechsler Adult Intelligence Scale; ANOVA = analysis of variance.

TABLE 3.
Coronary Artery Bypass Grafting and Cognition*

Author (year)	Subjects†	Design†	Results†
Coffey et al. (1983)[59]	1,669 CABG	Retrospective analysis of cerebral complications	3.8% incidence of cerebral complications, 29% mortality at 1 yr postoperatively; no correlation between year of operation and incidence of cerebral damage
Aberg et al. (1984)[15]	94 CABG and/or valve patients	Pre-post (7 days, SD-2.3)	No decline in group performance postoperatively; deficits not correlated to type of oxygenator, degrees of valvular calcification, or length of perfusion; correlates with deficits of amount of adenylate kinase in cerebrospinal fluid postoperatively
Pears et al. (1984)[38]	54 CABG or valve patients	1 week preoperatively, 2 weeks postoperatively; follow-up (3 mo)	Group decline on Benton Visual Retention, Weschler Memory Scale, and Digit Symbol. Deficits persisted at 3 mo on Benton Visual Retention
Raymond et al. (1984)[36]	Cardiac group—31 CABG, 28 male, 3 female, (mean age 56 yr); Surgical control group—16 non-ECC surgery patients, 10 male, 6 female, (mean age 60 yr)	Pre-post (1–2 wk); follow-up (6–8 wk)	CABG—significant decline on WAIS performance IQ, Symbol Digit, Buschke Word List; control—significant increase on WAIS Verbal IQ and Full Scale IQ
Elsass (1984)[60]	19 open-heart (mean age 48 yr); 17 open-chest, noncardiac (mean age 57 yr)	Pre-post (1, 2, 6, days)	RT significantly slower in cardiac group on day 1 and day 2 (than control); no difference at day 6; correlates with deficits of mean perfusion pressure during ECC, duration of ECC, duration of MABP <50 mm

(Continued.)

TABLE 3 (cont.).

Author (year)	Subjects†	Design†	Results†
Walsh et al. (1986)[61]	30 CABG; 15 oxygenated with bubble oxygenator; 15 oxygenated with membrane oxygenator	Pre-post (7–10 days); follow-up (6 wk)	Membrane did significantly better on Digit Span at 6 wk; bubble did significantly better on verbal learning at 1 wk and 6 wk
Nussmeier et al. (1986)[33]	182 CABG	Pre-post (5 days)	34% incidence of postoperative deficits on Trails A, Trails B, or both
Smith et al. (1986)[62]	CABG, 51 male, 4 female (mean age 54.7 yr); surgical control (mean age 58 yr)	Pre-post (8 days); follow-up (8 wk)	CABG at 8 days—35% severe deficits, 30% moderate deficits. At 8 wk—0% severe deficits, 40% moderate deficits; Control at 8 days—15% severe deficits, 44% moderate deficits. At 8 wk—15% severe deficits, 30% moderate deficits
Shaw et al. (1986)[34]	298 CABG, 276 male, 36 female (mean age 53.4 yr, SD = 7.4); 20 nonsurgery control, 15 male, 5 female	Pre-post (mean 7.4 days)	24% moderate impairment; 48% mild impairment; significant group deficits on Trails B, Orientation, Mental Control, Logical Memory, Digit Span, Associative Learning, Vocabulary
Shaw et al. (1987)[63]	259 CABG, 234 male, 25 female (mean age 53.5 yr range = 33–70 yr)	Pre-post (6 mo)	5% incidence of impairment
Nevin et al. (1987)[64]	65 CABG	Pre-post (3 and 7 days)	Patients whose cerebral blood volume was carefully regulated—3 days, 40% incidence (20 or more tests), 7 days, 13% incidence of impairment; patients whose cerebral blood volumes was regulated normally—3 days, 71%, 7 days, 26%.

Study	Sample	Testing	Results
Fish et al. (1987)[39]	100 male CABG (mean age 58.1 yr, SD = 6.2)	Pre-post (1 wk and 2 mo)	Significant decline on Stroop, Symbol Digit, Benton Visual Retention, Trails B, Buschke Word; significant increase on Benton Visual Retention, Trails B, Trails B at 2 mo.
Folks et al. (1988)[65]	83 CABG; 34 male; 49 female	Pre-post (4 days)	Correlates with deficits in postoperative depression, lower educational level, and lower socioeconomic status.
Hammeke (1988)[66]	46 male CABG (mean age 60.3 yr, SD = 7.3); 14 male noncardiac surgery controls (mean age 60.8 yr, SD = 8.2); 26 male nonsurgery controls (mean age 59.0 yr, SD = 5.2)	Pre-post (2–3 wk and 6 mo)	CABG group had 24% incidence of deficits postoperatively; CABG deficits primarily on attention, concentration, and psychomotor speed; follow-up showed little or no incidence of continuing deficits
Newman et al. (1989)[67]	62 CABG; 57 male (mean age 55.2 yr); 5 female (mean age 54.5 yr)	Pre-post (13 mo)	Subjects self-reported deficits were correlated to depression and anxiety levels, not to actual deficits on tests
Townes et al. (1989)[68]	90 surgical patients; CABG 65; valvular 25; controls 47 (nonsurgery)	Pre-post (7 mo)	Surgical patients showed acute (early) impairment that resolved over time (late); no difference between valve and CABG; only predictor of negative outcome was advanced age; No effect of blood pressure or time on bypass

*From Robinson M, Blumaenthal JA, Burker EJ, et al: *J Cardiopulmonary Rehabil* 1990; 10:180–189. Used by permission.
†CABG = coronary artery bypass grafting; WAIS = Wechsler Adult Intelligence Scale; Pre-post = preoperative-postoperative testing.

after CPB. Whether there is true improvement in function or whether the improvement represents a practice effect on the examinations is sometimes debated.[52, 53, 72] A decline in the incidence of cognitive deficits over time suggests that a majority of them are transient and that most patients return to preoperative levels within 6 months of surgery. However, the possibility of selective attrition (most impaired patients die or fail to return for follow-up) also should be considered. This information places greater significance on the prevention of "transient" neuropsychologic deficits, and questions how "transient" they truly are.[19]

Risk Factors

Risk factors for postoperative neuropsychologic dysfunction are listed in Table 4. The presence of valvular heart disease poses risk, since patients undergoing surgery for the replacement of a valve sustain damage to the central nervous system severalfold more frequently than do those undergoing intracardiac surgery for other conditions.[3, 40, 42, 51, 69, 73, 79–83] The duration of CPB[7] and concurrent cerebrovascular disease[42, 79] (especially significant bilateral carotid stenoses) also represent incremental risk factors for an adverse neurologic outcome.

Advanced age has been implicated as a risk factor [3, 40, 42, 45, 55, 70, 73, 80–89] for neuropsychologic injury after CPB. Explanations for the susceptibility of elderly patients include unknown previous cerebrovascular disease, impaired cerebral autoregulation, and possibly altered drug metabolism. Concerns over altered cerebral autoregulation as a cause for this injury in the geriatric patient remain unresolved. In a pilot study, we found that cerebral blood flow is independent of perfusion pressure over a range of mean arterial pressures of 20 to 90 mm Hg, in 11 patients over the age of 65 years (mean age of 72 years) when alpha-stat blood gas regulation was used. Compared to nine patients under the age of 50 years (mean age of 42 years), no discernible difference can be made in the relationship of cerebral blood flow and mean arterial pressures[90] (Fig 2). These data suggest that cerebral blood flow autoregulation remains intact in the geriatric population. However, as the surgical management of coronary artery disease becomes more aggresive in patients of advanced age, we find ourselves caring for an ever-increasing percentage of septuagenarian and octogenarians. In this age range, alterations in autonomic function may affect cerebral autoregulation. The normal increase in systemic vascular resistance needed to distribute a greater amount of cardiac output to the cerebral circulation during periods of reduced pump flow may be impaired in the elderly, who have decreased baroreflex responsiveness and vasoconstrictor response to cold stress.[91] Cerebral blood flow is reduced by approximately 20% by the age of 60 to 70 years and by as much as 40% by the age of 90 years compared to young, healthy adults. These reductions in blood flow parallel age-related changes in neuronal loss.[92] Clearly, more research into the mechanism of central nervous system injury in elderly patients is urgently needed.

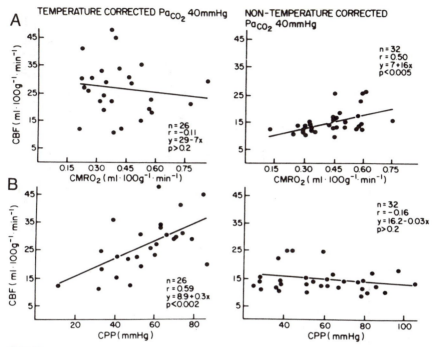

FIG 2.
Linear regression of cerebral pressure *(CPP)* or cerebral oxygen consumption *(CMRO₂)* vs. cerebral blood flow *(CBF)* for temperature-corrected and non–temperature-corrected. **A,** in the temperature-corrected group, there was no significant correlation between CBF and $CMRO_2$. **B,** in the temperature-corrected group, CBF was significantly correlated with CPP. In the non–temperature-corrected group, CBF was independent of CPP. (From Murkin JM, Farrar JK, Tweed WA, et al: *Anesth Analg* 1987; 66:825–832. Used by permission.)

Initial investigations into the question of adequate cerebral perfusion pressure demonstrated that postoperative neuropsychologic dysfunction was related to periods of intraoperative hypotension. Later studies, however, demonstrate that hypotension during CPB is not, in itself, a risk factor (Tables 5 and 6). It is unclear why initial studies differ in result from more current investigations. Surely, changes in bypass and anesthesia techniques, the use of arterial in-line filters, and increased awareness have played some role. However, one must consider the gradual change over the last decade in the intraoperative management of acid-base status. Early in the history of CPB (when hypotension was a demonstrated risk factor for neuropsychologic dysfunction), blood gas values for pH, PaO_2, and $PaCO_2$ were corrected for the decrease in temperature by the addition of CO_2 to the bypass circuit, i.e., pH-stat management. The resultant hypercarbia has been shown to alter the coupling of cerebral blood flow and cerebral metabolic rate for oxygen[30] and to alter pressure flow

TABLE 4.
Risk Factors for Postoperative Neuropsychologic Dysfunction*

Study	Number of Patients	Perspective	Operation	Observation	Risk Factors Identified
Lee et al. (1971)[41]	71	P	I	C&Ps	Symptom duration, valve replacement, bypass duration
Stockard et al. (1973)[73]	25	P	I&E	C	Age, hypotension
Aberg and Kihlgren (1974)[52]	197	P	I&E	C&Ps	Age, bypass duration, valve calcification
Branthwaite (1975)[74]	528	R	I&E	C	Age, preoperative neurologic abnormality, sanguineous prime, duration of bypass
Aberg and Kihlgren (1977)[69]	223	P	I&E	C&Ps	Duration of bypass
Kolkka and Hilberman (1980)[45]	204	P	I&E	C&Ps	Intracardiac procedures, age, bypass
Savageau et al. (1982)[56]	227	P	I&E	Ps	Age, left ventricular end-diastolic pressure >30, cardiomegaly on chest x-ray, duration of bypass/surgery, blood loss >2,000 mL, hypotension, need for intra-aortic balloon pump, postoperative electrolyte abnormalities

Study	N				Risk factors
Slogoff et al. (1982)[51]	204	P	I&E	C&Ps	Age, intracardiac procedures
Lederman et al. (1982)[75]	421	R	E	C	Male gender, use of hypothermia
Gardner et al. (1985)[76]	3,279	R	E	C	Age, cerebrovascular disease, atherosclerosis of ascending aorta, duration of bypass, hypotension
Nussmeier et al. (1986)[33]	187	P	I	C&Ps	Age, aortic valve replacement, duration of bypass, calcification of replaced valve
Newman et al. (1987)[77]					Age, duration of bypass
Venn et al. (1987)[78]	66	P	E	Ps	Age, duration of bypass/operation
Townes et al. (1989)[68]	90	P	I&E	Ps	Age

*P = prospective; R = retrospective; I = intracardiac; E = extracardiac; C = clinical; Ps = psychometric.

TABLE 5.
Hypotension is Not a Risk Factor for Perioperative
Neuropsychologic Dysfunction*

Study	Number of Patients	Perspective	Operation	Observation
Kolkka and Hilberman (1980)[15]	204	P	I&E	C&Ps
Ellis et al. (1980)[55]	30	P	E	C&Ps
Sotaniemi et al. (1981) [71]	49	P	I	C&Ps
Slogoff et al. (1982)[51]	204	P	I&E	C&Ps
Govier et al. (1984)[32]	17	P	E	C&Ps
Nussmeier et al. (1986) [33]	187	P	I	C&Ps
Townes et al. (1989)[68]	90	P	I&E	Ps

*P = prospective; I = intracardiac; E = extracardiac; C = clinical; Ps = psychometric.

autoregulation[30-32] (Fig 3). This subsequently may lead to pressure-passive cerebral hemodynamics such that cerebral blood flow becomes dependent upon mean arterial pressure. The alpha-stat management strategy suggests that the decrease in $Paco_2$ and increase in pH that occurs with decreasing temperature is the appropriate response to hypothermia. Temperature correction is not necessary and CO_2 is not added to

TABLE 6.
Hypotension is a Risk Factor for Perioperative Neuropsychologic
Dysfunction*

Study	Number of Patients	Perspective	Operation	Observation
Gilman (1965)[93]	35	P	I	C&Ps
Javid et al. (1969)[40]	100	P	I	C
Tufo et al. (1970)[7]	85	P	I	C&Ps
Lee et al. (1971)[41]	71	P	I	C&Ps
Stockard et al. (1973)[73]	25	P	I&E	Ps
Branthwaite (1975)[94]	528	R	I&E	C
Savageau et al. (1982) [56]	227	P	I&E	Ps

*P = prospective; R = retrospective; I-intracardiac; E = extracardiac; C = clinical; Ps = psychometric.

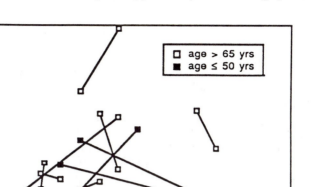

FIG 3.
Shown is a plot of data from patients with observations of cerebral blood flow at two different mean arterial pressures, demonstrating that changes in pressure have no uniform effect on cerebral blood flow. (From Brusino FG, Reves JG, Smith LR, et al: *J Thorac Cardiovasc Surg* 1989; 97:541–547. Used by permission.)

the bypass circuit. Autoregulation and flow metabolism coupling is maintained during alpha-stat management. We speculate that the change in acid-base strategy distinguishes the early studies from later ones in which hypotension did not correlate with neuropsychologic dysfunction (see Table 4).

To summarize, there is a wide range in the reported incidence of neuropsychologic dysfunction after cardiac surgery, dependent on the sensitivity of the methods used for detection. However, two trends have become apparent. First, the incidence of neuropsychologic morbidity and mortality has declined over the past 30 years, presumably due to improvements in surgical and anesthetic management as well as CPB techniques. Unfortunately, the increasingly elderly patient population undergoing cardiac surgery is counterbalancing this trend. Second, intracardiac procedures are associated with a greater incidence of morbidity and mortality than is extracardiac surgery.

Causes of Injury

Embolization

Emboli are postulated to be the major cause of neuropsychologic and neurologic deficits after CPB. Embolization can be divided into microembolization and macroembolization according to differences in etiology, incidence, and significance.

Microemboli can be detected in the arterial-line blood of all patients undergoing CPB.[95-98] Their transmission to the cerebral circulation has been documented by middle cerebral artery transcranial Doppler and retinal angiography showing emboli during CPB.[17, 99] Despite the introduction of arterial line filters and membrane oxygenators, microemboli continue to occur.[97] Evaluation of microemboli has identified multiple sources including platelet aggregates, air, particulate matter, lipid droplets, calcium fragments, leukocytes, antifoam particles, and protein particles. Light, scanning, and transmission electron microscopy along with chemical identification have been used to document these emboli in multiple tissue beds.

CPB exposes platelets to nonendothelial surfaces, causing platelet activation and aggregation. Heparin is used during bypass to potentiate the inhibitory effect of antithrombin III or thrombin. The use of heparin, however, does not prevent platelet activation with the possibility of aggregation and embolization. The oxygenator tubing, traumatized by the nonocclusive roller pump, also can be a source of microemboli.[98] Particulate matter, particularly within the oxygenator, is another source of microemboli. These very small particulates are reduced significantly by circulation through a 5-μm filter for 15 to 30 minutes.[100] During CPB, gaseous emboli are a major concern with both open and closed cardiac surgery. Air microemboli can arise from gases used to oxygenate the blood, rewarming of liquid within the CPB circuit, venting of the left ventricle, and other sources. Gaseous microemboli are detected in the middle cerebral artery by transcranial Doppler throughout CPB, with the number decreased by the use of membrane rather than bubble oxygenators.

Microembolization from the surgical field is frequently identified as a common cause of cerebral dysfunction.[15, 33, 49-51, 69, 83, 93, 101-105] This is confirmed by the higher incidence of neurologic deficits after open cardiac procedures (i.e., valve replacement, repair of septal defect, etc.) compared with coronary artery bypass grafting (7.5% vs. <2%). Debris from the surgical field and air emboli from air trapped in the heart at closing are more common during open cardiac procedures and account for the higher incidence of permanent defects in these procedures.

Macroembolization does occur during coronary artery bypass grafting, most likely from application of the aortic cross-clamping in an area of calcified atherosclerosis and from air introduced by venting of the left atrium or ventricle. Studies indicating a higher incidence of deficits with severely calcified aortic valves support this conclusion.[33, 69, 83] Even with the multiple advances made in filtering and oxygenation, prevention of macroembolization from the aorta and intracardiac chambers depends primarily upon meticulous surgical technique.[33, 106, 107] Increased surgical awareness of the consequences has documented to produce improvement in neuropsychologic outcome at two institutions.[33, 57] Hand-held echocardiographic probes to characterize ascending aortic atherosclerotic plaques,[108] have proven useful in predicting the type of aortic plaque and a safe cannulation site.[108, 109] The evacuation of intracardiac air following open cardiac procedures is also helpful. Transesophageal two-dimensional echocardiography is a very sensitive monitor for intracardiac air, but quantification is difficult.[110] Typically, aggressive lung inflations push air from the pulmonary veins. The patient is placed in steep Trendelenburg prior to aortic cross-clamp removal and allowed to remain in this position for 10 minutes or more to allow any residual air to be directed away from the carotid arteries and cerebral circulations.[111] The use of transesophageal two-dimensional echocardiography to assist the surgeon in the evacuation of air may contribute to the recently reported[112] similar incidence of cognitive dysfunction in valvular and coronary artery bypass graft patients.

Abnormalities in Flow/Metabolism

Under normal circumstances, cerebral blood flow is regulated to the metabolic needs of regional areas of the brain. This has been termed "cerebral flow/metabolism coupling" and is an important feature of cerebral homeostasis[113-116] (Fig 4). In the healthy awake human, a mean cerebral metabolic rate for oxygen of 3.0 to 4.0 mL/100 g/min is coupled to a cerebral blood flow of 45 to 60 mL/100 g/min, for a cerebral blood flow/cerebral metabolic rate for oxygen ratio of 13 to 20.[115] This ratio is main-

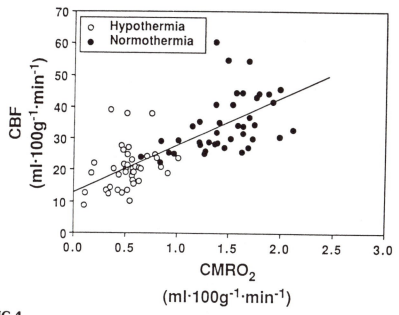

FIG 4.
The direct effect of temperature condition on cerebral oxygen consumption *(CMRO$_2$)* and cerebral blood flow *(CBF)* is evident when measured in 41 patients during hypothermia and normothermia.

tained unless marked physiologic alterations in mean arterial pressure, $Paco_2$, Pao_2 or glucose regulation occur. Mean arterial pressure or, more precisely, cerebral perfusion pressure, may vary widely, yet cerebral blood flow is maintained at a constant level.[117, 118] In general, in awake patients, cerebral blood flow is independent of cerebral perfusion pressure between a range of 50 to 130 mm Hg. This is referred to as "pressure flow autoregulation." During CPB with hypothermia and alpha-state blood gas management, the range of autoregulation is extended down to a mean arterial pressure of 30 mm Hg in adults[32] (Fig 5) and 20 mm Hg in children.[119] Besides marked elevations in blood pressure or significant hypotension, other abnormal physiologic states that result in hypercarbia or severe hypoxemia will cause significant cerebral vasodilation, which overrides this normal pressure flow autoregulation. Certain illnesses such as insulin-dependent diabetes, seizure disorders, and severe pulmonary disease also can alter flow-metabolism coupling. Age alters cerebral metabolic coupling in addition. In neonates (0 to 2 months of age), the cerebral blood flow/cerebral metabolic rate for oxygen ratio is generally higher than in adults.[120] This is believed to be due to increased metabolic demand for neuronal growth, myelinization, etc. In the elderly, however, there is a blunting of

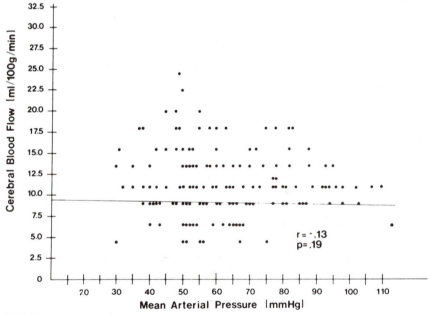

FIG 5.
Mean arterial pressure vs. cerebral blood flow during cardiopulmonary bypass. Note that there is poor correlation between cerebral blood flow and mean arterial pressure. Autoregulation appears to be constant to a mean arterial pressure of 30 mm Hg. (From Govier AV, Reves JG, McKay RD, et al: *Ann Thorac Surg* 1984; 38:592–600. Used by permission.)

the cerebrovascular response to hypercarbia and hyperoxia and an overall reduction in cerebral blood flow that parallels the loss of neuronal tissue.[92] In general, the brain is very efficient at maintaining an adequate cerebral blood flow-to-metabolism ratio except in the presence of marked physiologic alterations, as listed previously. Considering that CPB produces marked physiologic alterations in overall body blood flow and metabolism, these could be a possible mechanism for brain injury. Some of the specific alterations during CPB relevant to adequate cerebral perfusion and central nervous system dysfunction are discussed in the following sections.

Pump Flow Rates

Customary (routine) pump flow rates during CPB have been suggested for adults and children based on body surface area and the maintenance of efficient organ perfusion as determined by arterial blood gases, acid-base balance, and whole body oxygen consumption during hypothermic CPB.[32, 121, 122] In practice, however, pump flow rates may be reduced drastically below these customary rates to facilitate cardiac repair when organ protection is provided with hypothermia. Clinical experience suggests that brief periods of low-flow bypass are well tolerated at moderate hypothermia and that periods of no flow are tolerated for up to 60 to 80 minutes with profound hypothermia at 18° C.[123–125] These periods of circulatory arrest may result in abnormalities in cerebral blood flow and metabolism during reperfusion. On the other hand, customary pump flow rates resulted in normal to increased cerebral blood flow and cerebral metabolic rate for oxygen during reperfusion after CPB when circulatory arrest was not utilized.[119, 125]

In terms of flow requirements, one can quantitate the degree of cerebral metabolic reduction as it relates to brain temperature and, based on this, predict a minimally safe pump flow rate. There are some recent laboratory studies pertinent to this issue. Data in mature cynomolgus monkeys in which flow was reduced to 25% of calculated at 20° C revealed no change in the cerebral metabolic rate for oxygen,[122] attesting to the adequacy of this decrease in flow at profound hypothermia. A recent report has shown that flow rates of 10 mL/kg/min at 15° C for periods of up to 2 hours in sheep maintain normal levels of adenosine triphosphate and phosphocreatine, and a normal brain pH.[126] When flow is reduced to 5 mL/kg/min at 15° C, organic phosphates become depleted and brain pH begins to fall after only 15 minutes. The effect of 5-mL/kg/min flow rates on cerebral metabolic factors is indistinguishable from a similar undergoing circulatory arrest at 15° C in a similar group of sheep.[126] In a canine study performed at 20° C and a flow rate of 2.5 mL/kg/min, there was a reduction in brain pH and Po_2, and an elevation of brain Pco_2 after rewarming from CPB. This would suggest that flow was inadequate to meet metabolic demand.[127] Using a predicted cerebral metabolic rate for oxygen reduction based on temperature of the patient, adequate pump flow can be predicted (see later).

There are mechanisms by which the brain compensates for reduction of flow. Animal studies show that the brain tolerates reductions in pump flow during profound CPB by redistributing perfusate from the body to the brain and increasing cerebral oxygen extraction.[122] Despite these compensatory mechanisms, there most certainly is a critical flow level below which ischemic injury occurs. This critical level, which is dependent on temperature and probably other factors, remains to be determined in man.

Nonpulsatile Perfusion

The degree to which nonpulsatile perfusion causes central nervous system injury is not known. It has been found that nonpulsatile flow plays a minor role in brain metabolic reduction. Nine percent of the reduction in cerebral metabolic rate for oxygen cannot be accounted for by temperature reduction alone during CPB and therefore can be attributed to the overall effect of nonpulsatile CPB perfusion.[125] Nonpulsatile flow most likely alters the distribution of flow throughout the cerebral microcirculation. This flow alteration could be deleterious. Laboratory evidence exists for improved cerebral perfusion with the addition of pulsatile flow at a pump flow rate of 25 mL/kg/min in a dog model. This is reflected in improved brain pH, Pco_2, and Po_2 with the addition of pulsatile flow over nonpulsatile flow at this marginal perfusion rate.[127]

Cerebral Perfusion Pressure

With moderate hypothermia ($\geq 26°$ C) and intact autoregulation, concerns have been raised about cerebral injury due to inadequate cerebral perfusion pressures. Several studies have shown that the brain alters cerebral vascular resistance to maintain cerebral blood flow in response to metabolic need during variations in pump flow rate and perfusion pressure.[32, 122] Preservation of autoregulation during CPB explains the fact that seemingly low (≤ 50 min Hg) perfusion pressures are well tolerated.[32] Cerebral injury due to inadequate cerebral perfusion pressure during CPB has been theorized, but not documented in recent studies. Adding to this information, preliminary data from our institution in 19 patients found no neuropsychologic dysfunction with a perfusion pressure of less than 50 mm Hg for an average of 32 ± 17 minutes.[128] With intact autoregulation in patients managed with alpha-stat blood gas, a perfusion pressure of 30 mm Hg or more should be well tolerated. Patients with hypertension, diabetes, and/or cerebrovascular disease and those managed with pH-stat blood gas may require a perfusion pressure higher than 30 mm Hg.

Abnormalities of Autoregulation During Hypothermic Cardiopulmonary Bypass

The previous discussion of flow rates assumes that normal autoregulatory mechanisms are intact. We know, however, that under certain conditions cerebral blood flow autoregulation is lost. Profound hypothermia (temperatures $<22°$ C), elevated CO_2 levels, diabetes, and hypertension all disrupt normal flow/metabolism coupling. Cerebral blood flow becomes dependent on pump flow rate and perfusion pressure with the loss of autoregulation and the brain could be harmed by the loss of pressure or oxygen-carrying capacity of the blood (anemia).

Carbon Dioxide and Temperature Correction of Blood Gases.—Elevation in $Paco_2$ results in increased cerebral blood flow in excess of metabolic demand. This may be beneficial in terms of improved oxygen delivery to cerebral tissue. Alternatively, it may be deleterious due to the theoretical risk of increased delivery of air particulate emboli with an unregulated increase in cerebral blood flow. In addition, the cerebral cellular acidosis that occurs with increased $Paco_2$ may interfere with normal neuronal and glial function and result in the inefficient use of cellular oxygen. Several studies have addressed these issues. The use of the pH-stat blood gas management strategy involving the addition of CO_2 to the pump) results in a significantly lower brain pH than does the use of alpha-stat regulation during the rewarming phase of CPB after circulatory arrest in a canine model.[127] This information is important, since it suggests that patients managed with the pH-stat blood gas strategy during CPB may have an acidotic brain pH. This would interfere with normal metabolic function and create a metabolic debt for the patient during rewarming. If one added marginal perfusion or, more to the point, decreased oxygen delivery after separation from CPB, a greater potential for cerebral injury may exist.

The issue of temperature correction of blood gases has not been addressed fully. To date, there has been only one study evaluating neuropsychologic outcome in patients using alpha-stat or pH-stat management, and it found no difference among 86 patients undergoing CPB.[68, 129] Although differences were not found, the average age of the patient population was relatively young (60 ± 10 years), the pH and Pco_2 differences were relatively small (7.38 ± 0.03 vs. 7.32 ± 0.04 and 40.2 ± 1.3 vs. 47.3 ± 3.4, respectively), and the mean arterial pressure was maintained between 60 and 80 mm Hg. Advanced age and mean arterial pressure may be important adjunct factors in determining the risk of pH-stat management. If CO_2 is added to raise Pco_2 in temperature-corrected management, the result is relative hypercarbia and, with that, the loss of normal autoregulatory processes. It has become increasingly popular not to correct blood gas for temperature in order to preserve normal cerebral autoregulatory mechanisms during CPB, and we concur with this practice.

Diabetes and Hypertension.—We have demonstrated altered autoregulation in patients with diabetes undergoing CPB (Figs 6 and 7).[130] In these patients, cerebral blood flow is independent of cerebral metabolic rate for oxygen and falls with decreasing cerebral perfusion pressure. As a result, the brain must rely on increasing O_2 extraction to meet its metabolic needs, a fact that has been documented by measuring arteriovenous saturation differences across the brain.[131] This implies that the principal mechanism for cerebral protection during CPB, i.e., flow/metabolism coupling, is impaired in diabetic patients, and under these circumstances higher perfusion pressures and less anemia may be warranted to prevent cerebral injury. The mechanism by which diabetes alters cerebral autoregulation is unknown, but one may speculate that it is part of the general autonomic neuropathy associated with this disease.[131]

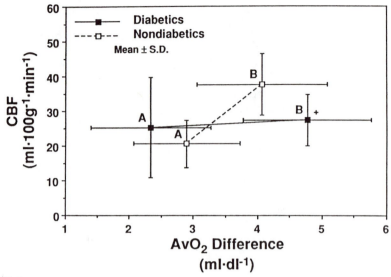

FIG 6.
The effect of a change in temperature (from 26.6 ± 2.4° C to 36.9 ± 0.6° C in diabetic patients and from 28.4 ± 2.8° C to 36.5 ± 0.5° C in nondiabetics) on cerebral blood flow *(CBF)* and arteriovenous oxygen *(AVD₂)* difference is known. The change in AvO_2 difference is significantly (P = .01) greater in diabetic patients (as indicated by the plus sign). (From Croughwell N, Lyth M, Quill TJ, et al: *Circulation* 1990; 82(5 Suppl): IV 407–412.)

Uncontrolled hypertension has been shown to alter pressure/flow autoregulation in the awake individual. Autoregulation is not lost, but rather is shifted to the right, so that the lower limit of acceptable cerebral perfusion pressure may be 70 mm Hg rather than 50 mm Hg. The implications of this are that uncontrolled hypertensive patients may require a higher perfusion pressure on pump to assure adequate cerebral perfusion.[132] Since autoregulation will return toward normal after several weeks in treated hypertensive patients with effective blood pressure control,[115] perfusion pressure is less likely to be important in well-controlled hypertensive patients.

Profound Hypothermia.—During profound hypothermia, cerebral blood flow exceeds metabolic demand with the ratio of cerebral blood flow to cerebral metabolic rate for oxygen over 75:1. This compares to 20:1 for normothermic temperatures and to about 25:1 for moderate hypothermic conditions.[125] Despite this loss of cerebral blood flow metabolism coupling, when cerebral blood flow becomes perfusion-pressure–and CPB-flow–dependent, there still is a degree of luxuriant perfusion and the risk of injury seems quite remote. The mechanism of profound hypothermic disruption of autoregulation is unknown and we speculate a cold-induced vasoparesis.

Unexplained Causes.—We recently have found that a significant proportion of patients experience significant jugular bulb desaturation (a jugu-

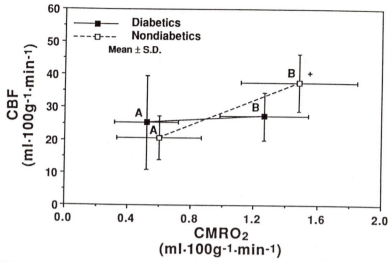

FIG 7.
The effect of a change in temperature on cerebral blood flow *(CBF)* and cerebral oxygen consumption *(CMRO$_2$)* is shown in diabetic and nondiabetic patients. With increased temperature from 26.6 ± 2.4° C to 36.9 ± 0.06° C (diabetic) and from 28.4 ± 2.8° C to 36.5 ± 0.5° C (nondiabetic), the change in CBF is significantly (*P* = .001) greater in nondiabetics, as indicated by the *plus sign*. This demonstrates impairment of cerebral metabolic autoregulation in diabetic patients. (From Croughwell N, Lyth M, Quill TJ, et al: *Circulation* 1990; 82(5 Suppl): IV 407–412.)

lar vein O$_2$ of less than 70%) during rewarming while on CPB. In 22% of these patients, jugular venous desaturations were extreme (≤40%). The desaturation reflects an increase in extraction and appears to be compensation for an increased cerebral metabolic rate of oxygen without a compensatory increase in cerebral blood flow.[133] These alpha-stat–managed patients did not have preexisting cerebral vascular disease, diabetes, or uncontrolled hypertension to explain this uncoupling of flow and metabolism, but they did experience a relatively high cerebral metabolic rate of oxygen during rewarming. Why these patients did not autoregulate remains a mystery. We could not appreciate an increased incidence of neuropsychologic impairment in them. However, these patients would seem to be at increased risk if further impairment of cerebral perfusion due to low cardiac output after separation from CPB ensued.

Miscellaneous Causes of Injury

In both animal and human studies, hyperglycemia has been shown to increase greatly the severity of ischemic brain damage.[134-137] In retrospective and prospective studies, diabetics and nondiabetics who were hyperglycemic had poorer neurologic outcome after stroke.[136] Retrospective analysis of a small group of pediatric patients who underwent profound hypothermic cardiac arrest revealed that those who had markedly elevated glucose levels had a much higher rate of neurologic deficits than did those who were normoglycemic.[138] Although large, prospective studies are lacking, it seems prudent to follow the recommendation of withholding glucose or giving it in moderation to keep the level below 200 mg/dL whenever brain ischemia may occur intraoperatively.[139]

Cerebral Protection

At present, and until the cause(s) of brain injury are fully determined and eliminated, research must be directed toward the development of better methods of cerebral protection from ischemic injury. This research should lead to clinical methods of cerebral protection, of which currently there are several.

Hypothermia

The cerebral metabolic rate for oxygen is related directly to brain temperature[140, 141] (Figs 8 and 9). Reducing the brain cerebral metabolic rate for oxygen should minimize injury in conditions of oxygen deprivation and/or reduced supply. A convenient expression of the effect of temperature on this rate is to calculate the ratio of metabolism at a temperature gradient of

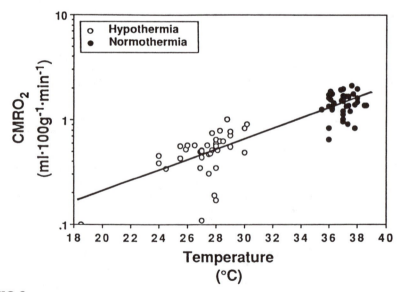

FIG 8.
Cerebral metabolism (CMRO$_2$) measurements expressed logarithmically at stable hypothermia (27 $\pm$ 2.0° C) and normothermia (37 $\pm$ 0.7° C). There is a significant difference ($P <$ .0001) in CMRO$_2$ between the two temperatures.

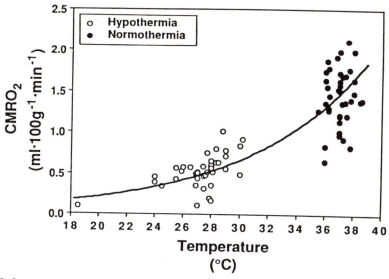

FIG 9.
Cerebral metabolism *(CMRO₂)* is expressed in relation to temperature based on the equation log $(CMRO_2)$ = $9+b*T$, where log (°) is the natural logarithm function, T is the temperature, ° C is the intercept, and b is the slope.

10° C, called the Q10.[142] Cerebral oxygen consumption in a dog model using closed-circuit spirometry revealed a Q10 of 2.2.[140] In 41 adult patients, we calculated a median Q10 in humans on CPB of 2.8. This means a reduction in cerebral oxygen consumption of 68%.[141]

Metabolic reduction is exponentially related to temperature, so an equation can be derived to predict the degree of metabolic reduction for each degree Centigrade of reduction in temperature during CPB. The equation, cerebral metabolic rate for oxygen = $.021e^{,1147T}$ best describes this data in adults and allows one to predict a the rate at different temperatures. Thus, at 37° C, the cerebral metabolic rate for oxygen is 1.46; at 32° C, it is 0.82 (44% reduction); at 27° C, it is 0.44 (68% reduction); at 20° C, it is 0.21 (85% reduction); and at 15° C, it is 0.12 (92% reduction).[141] Both human and animal data suggest that these figures are reasonable approximations of oxygen requirements. The requisite flow to meet these requirements can be calculated from this equation as long as oxygen carrying capacity is unchanged.

Although hypothermia alone affords cerebral protection, it is worth noting that in examining the effect of temperature on metabolism, all of the animal and human investigations have the confounding effects of general anesthesia and temperature. It appears that temperature and general anesthesia, even though they both reduce the cerebral metabolic rate for oxygen in a dose-dependent manner, do not act by the same mechanism. It has been postulated,[143] and experimentally confirmed in animals[144] and humans,[145] that general anesthesia and temperature affect brain oxidative metabolism differently. Cerebral metabolism supports (1) cellular function (electrical activity of neuronal transmission of impulses) and (2) cellular integrity (maintenance of cellular homeostasis). The functional component of cerebral metabolism accounts for 60% of metabolism, while cellular integrity accounts for the remainder.[143] The functional component is affected primarily by general anesthetics, whereas both function and integrity are affected by temperature. In clinical studies, there always will be a combined effect of general anesthesia and hypothermia, but, as shown in dogs, it is temperature that provides the most significant cerebral protection from anoxia.[143] This was proven in animals by reducing temperature to 30° C and giving thiopental (46 mg/kg) at normothermia. Each condition reduced the cerebral metabolic rate for oxygen by the same amount from control, but temperature produced significantly greater cerebral protection as measured by adenosine triphosphate loss and lactate production 4 minutes after decapitation.

Others have examined the cerebral protective effect of profound hypothermia to a temperature of 20° C on cerebral metabolism by measuring high-energy phosphate compounds with [31]phosphate nuclear magnetic resonance.[146–148] One author reported that while adenosine triphosphate fell to 34% of preischemic values at a temperature of 37° C, it remained unchanged from control if the temperature was lowered to 20° C during ischemia (Fig 10). More pertinent to adult cardiac surgery are studies examining the effect of slight hypothermia (32° C) on cerebral metabolism. With ischemic injury (induced by four-vessel occlusion), there is an increase in the release of glutamate and dopamine that may play a major role in mediating cellular injury (as measured by histopathologic examination of the hippocampal neurons of the killed rat models).[149] When the temperature is lowered from 36° C to 33° C, the expected rise in glutamate release does not occur and dopamine levels actually fall. Studies in the cat model[148] exposed to 16 minutes of bilateral carotid occlusion followed by 1 to 2 hours of recirculation demonstrated that hypothermia (between 27° C and 35° C) significantly reduced cerebral intracellular acidosis and resulted in a more rapid return of high-energy phosphate compounds compared to normothermic controls. Interestingly, this study also demonstrated that animals protected with slight hypothermia at 34° C and moderate hypothermia at 27° C behave similarly in response to ischemia and recirculation. There was no significant difference between pH and adenylate phosphate concentration at slight hypothermia (34° C) compared to moderate hypothermia (27° C). This protective effect of slight hypothermia is supported by other studies.[150–152] Slight hypothermia (34° C) prevented the ischemic neuronal injury in the CA-1 layer of the hippocampus as compared to normothermic controls. Moderate hypothermia was no more protective than was this slight level of hypothermia. These data may demonstrate that hypothermia does not affect the extent of ischemic injury through a reduction in cerebral blood flow or high-energy phosphate metabolism. Preventing the release of excessive amounts of neurotransmitters may mediate the protective effects of hypothermia.

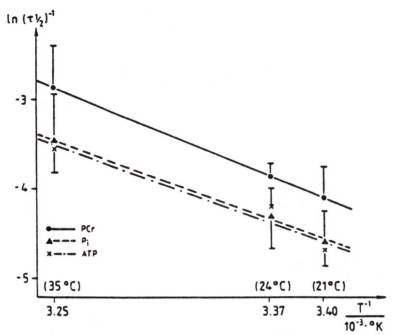

FIG 10.
Logarithm plot of average reaction rates $[\ln(t_{1/2}^{-1})]$ phosphocreatine *(PCr)*, adenosine triphosphate *(ATP)*, and inorganic phosphate *(Pi)* vs. the inverse absolute temperature, showing an increase in the decay half-time $(t_{1/2})$ in ATP, PCr, and Pi. (From Stocker F, Herschkowitz N, Bossi E, et al: *Pediatr Res* 1986; 20:867–871. Used by permission.)

Other investigators have studied the effect of hypothermia on various metabolic parameters: cellular release of creatine phosphokinase,[153] calcium release,[154] local tissue pH,[127, 155] cerebral blood flow,[32, 156, 157] and glucose and lactate metabolism.[143] Each study has demonstrated that hypothermia "protects" the metabolic variable studied. Despite the widespread use of hypothermia in clinical cardiac surgery, no study to date has examined the effects of differing levels of hypothermia on neurologic outcome, metabolic parameters, and cerebral blood flow rates. Do the predicted decreases in the cerebral metabolic rate for oxygen of moderate hypothermia provide greater protection to the brain than does slight hypothermia? Many questions remain regarding the use and efficacy of hypothermia as it relates to cerebral protection. Whether there is an optimal perfusate temperature for brain protection during CPB is not known.

Other Measures

Although hypothermia, as described previously, is an important mechanism of cerebral protection, unfortunately, it is not always available at those periods of highest risk for embolization during CPB (aortic cannulation, aortic cross-clamping, cross-clamp release, and placement of the aortic side-biting clamp). Thus, other mechanisms of protection have been sought. These are primarily pharmacologic and include barbiturates, inhaled anesthetics, calcium channel blockers, and free radical scavengers.

The clinical use of barbiturates, particularly thiopental for cerebral protection, was brought to the forefront in 1986 in patients undergoing intracardiac surgery. In this study, those patients in whom an isoelectric EEG was induced with large doses of thiopental during CPB showed a statistically significant decrease in persistent neurologic complications compared to controls.[33] The early dysfunction postoperatively was similar, indicating that thiopental may have decreased the clinical expression of focal ischemic insults, but not the frequency of symptomatic embolization.[33] Unfortunately, the study was performed without the use of hypothermia or arterial line filters, confusing the clinical significance of the results. A larger study using hypothermia and arterial line filters in coronary artery bypass graft patients showed no improvement in neurologic outcome with thiopental given in doses to produce burst suppression on EEG during CPB.[158] Therefore, early work may have validated barbiturates as cerebral protectants, but further studies with hypothermia and arterial line filters are necessary to reveal the appropriateness of this therapy in current clinical practice.

Isoflurane, like thiopental, causes significant decreases in the cerebral metabolic rate and will induce an isoelectric EEG at 1.5 to 2.0 minimum alveolar concentration.[159, 160] In several animal models, isoflurane provided a degree of cerebral protection similar to that of thiopental.[159, 160] In normothermic humans during carotid endarterectomy, the critical cerebral blood flow (i.e., that below which ischemia occurs as measured by EEG change) is reduced significantly to 8 to 10 mL/100 g/min during isoflurane anesthesia compared with that seen during enflurane or halothane anesthesia (18 to 20 mL/100 g/min).[29] This has led to the consideration that isoflurane could cause intracerebral steal. A recent study of incomplete focal ischemia in the primate model seems to confirm this, since isoflurane-anesthetized animals had significantly worse outcome with respect to frequency and size of infarct than did thiopental-treated primates.[161] The confounding variable between the study group and the controls was a 20–mm Hg difference in mean arterial pressure in the isoflurane group (vs. the thiopental group), which may make the significance of these results questionable. More recent studies without significant pressure differences between control and study subjects showed similar neurologic outcomes with isoflurane and thiopental.[162, 163] Clinical studies with isoflurane during CPB are needed to determine its effectiveness in reducing neurologic and neuropsychologic deficits. Other anesthetic drugs such as etomidate, midazolam, phenytoin, and lidocaine have been postulated as cerebral protectants with evidence in animal models and ongoing investigations that they could reduce the severity of focal ischemia.[164–167] The efficacy of these drugs for cerebral protection during CPB is untested

A group of drugs showing great promise in cerebral protection is the calcium entry blockers. Nimodipine reduced the deleterious effects of vasospasm in patients suffering from subarachnoid hemorrhage.[168] In global cerebral ischemia, a reactive hyperemia is followed in 20 to 30 minutes by a delayed postischemic hypoperfusion state.[169] In animal studies, nimodipine given either before or after the ischemic episode attenuated this hypoperfusion state and improved neurologic outcome.[170–173] Flunarizine, another calcium entry blocker, also has been shown to reduce significantly the area of infarction in focal ischemia.[174] Recent prospective data indicated that those patients receiving chronic calcium channel blockers prior to their open cardiac procedures had a significant reduction in the incidence of postoperative neurologic dysfunction.[175] These data strongly support the effectiveness of calcium entry blockers in preventing postoperative neurologic sequelae and warrant further study.

Despite theoretical evidence that other agents such as free radical scavengers, deferoxamine, catalase, or superoxide dismutase would minimize free radical damage and improve neurologic outcome, these have failed to improve neurologic outcome in higher animal models.[176, 177] Antagonists of excitatory amino acid inhibitors also have been postulated as possible cerebral protective agents. Several investigators have found protection with these agents against focal or global ischemia in animals, while others showed no prevention of ischemic neuronal damage in cats.[178–180] The efficacy of these drugs in humans or against CPB-associated injury has not been tested.

References

1. Pryor DB, Harrell FE, Rankin JS, et al: The changing survival benefits of coronary revascularization over time. *Circulation* 1987; 76:V13–V21.
2. Clowes GHA, Neville WE, Hopkins A, et al: Factors contributing to success or failure in the use of a pump oxygenator for complete bypass of the heart and lung; experimental and clinical. *Surgery* 1954; 36:557–579.
3. Kornfield DS, Zimberg S, Malm JR: Psychiatric complications of open-heart surgery. *N Engl J Med* 1965; 273:287–292.
4. Shaw PJ, Bates D, Cartlidge NEF, et al: Early neurological complications of coronary artery bypass surgery. *Br Med J [Clin Res]* 1985; 291:1384–1387.
5. Plasse HM, Mittleman M, Frost JO: Unilateral sudden hearing loss after open heart surgery: A detailed study of seven cases. *Laryngoscope* 1981; 91:101–109.
6. Kimball CP: The experience of open heart surgery. 3. Toward a definition and understanding of post cardiotomy delirium. *Arch Gen Psychiatry* 1972; 27:57–63.
7. Tufo HM, Ostfeld AM, Shekelle R: Central nervous system dysfunction following open heart surgery. *JAMA* 1970; 212:1333–1340.
8. Blachy PH, Starr A: Post-cardiotomy delirium. *Am J Psychiatry* 1964; 121:271–275.
9. Heller SS, Frank KA, Malm JR, et al: Psychiatric complications of open-heart surgery. A re-examination. *N Engl J Med* 1970; 283:1015–1020.
10. Taylor KM, Devlin BJ, Mittra SM, et al: Assessment of cerebral damage dur-

ing open-heart surgery. A new experimental model. *Scand J Thorac Cardiovasc Surg* 1980; 14:197–203.

11. Aberg T, Ronquist G, Tyden H, et al: Release of adenylate kinase into cerebrospinal fluid during open-heart surgery and its relation to postoperative intellectual function. *Lancet* 1982; 1:1139–1142.

12. Alling C, Karlsson B, Vallfors B: Increase in myelin basic protein in CSF after brain surgery. *J Neurol* 1980; 223:225–230.

13. Thomas DGT, Palfreyman JW, Ratcliffe JG: Serum myelin basic protein assay in diagnosis and prognosis of patients with head injury. *Lancet* 1978; 1:113–116.

14. Henriksen L: Evidence suggestive of diffuse brain damage following cardiac operations. *Lancet* 1984; 1:816–820.

15. Aberg T, Ronquist G, Tyden H, et al: Adverse effects on the brain in cardiac operations as assessed by biochemical, psychometric, and radiologic methods. *J Thorac Cardiovasc Surg* 1984; 87:99–105.

16. Hanson MR, Breuer AC, Furlan AJ, et al: Mechanism and frequency of brachial plexus injury in open heart surgery: A prospective analysis. *Ann Thorac Surg* 1983; 36:675–679.

17. Blauth CI, Arnold JV, Schulenberg WE, et al: Cerebral microembolism during cardiopulmonary bypass. *J Thorac Cardiovasc Surg* 1988; 95:668–676.

18. Sotaniemi KA: Cerebral outcome after extracorporeal circulation: Comparison between prospective and retrospective evaluations. *Arch Neurol* 1983; 40:75–77.

19. Sotaniemi KA, Mononer H, Hokkanen TE: Long-term cerebral outcome after open-heart surgery. *Stroke* 1986; 17:410–416.

20. Theye RA, Patrick RT, Kirklin JW: The electroencephalograph in patients undergoing intracardiac operations with the aid of extracorporeal circulation. *J Thorac Cardiovasc Surg* 1957; 34:706–716.

21. Pronk RAF, Simons AJR: Processing the electroencephalogram in cardiac surgery. *Comput Programs Biomed* 1984; 18:181–190.

22. Edmonds HL Jr, Griffiths LK, Shields CB: Online statistical analysis of the EEG predicts postoperative neurologic dysfunction during cardiopulmonary bypass (CPB) surgery Presented at the 12th Annual Meeting of the Society of Cardiovascular Anesthesiologists, Orlando, Florida, May, 1990.

23. Plum F, Posner JB: *The Diagnosis of Stupor and Coma.* Philadelphia, FA Davis, 1980.

24. Levy WJ, Grundy BL, Smith NT: Monitoring the electroencephalogram and evoked potentials during anesthesia, in Saidman LJ, Smith NT (eds): *Monitoring in Anesthesia,* ed 2. Boston, Butterworths, 1984, pp 227–267.

25. Mohr JP: Neurological complications of cardiac valvular disease and cardiac surgery including systemic hypotension, in Vinken PJ, Bruyn GW, Klawans HL (eds): *Handbook of Clinical Neurology, vol 38, Neurological Manifestations of Systemic Diseases, Part I.* New York, North-Holland, 1979, pp 143–171.

26. Grundy BL: Intraoperative monitoring of sensory-evoked potentials. *Anesthesiology* 1983; 58:72–87.

27. Lundar T, Lindegaard KF, Froysaker T, et al: Cerebral perfusion during non-pulsatile cardiopulmonary bypass. *Ann Thorac Surg* 1985; 40:144–148.

28. Newman S: The incidence and nature of neuropsychological morbidity following cardiac surgery. *Perfusion* 1989; 4:93–100.

29. Casement B, Messick J, Milde L, et al: "Critical" CBF during isoflurane anesthesia in man. *Anesthesiology* 1985; 63:A406.

30. Murkin JM, Farrar JK, Tweed AW, et al: Cerebral autoregulation and flow/ metabolism coupling during cardiopulmonary bypass. *Anesth Analg* 1987; 66:825–832.
31. Prough DS, Stump DA, Roy RC, et al: Response of cerebral blood flow to changes in carbon dioxide tension during hypothermic cardiopulmonary bypass. *Anesthesiology* 1986; 64:576–581.
32. Govier AV, Reves JG, McKay RD, et al: Factors and their influence on regional cerebral blood flow during nonpulsatile cardiopulmonary bypass. *Ann Thorac Surg* 1984; 38:592–600.
33. Nussmeier NA, Arlund C, Slogoff S: Neuropsychiatric complications after cardiopulmonary bypass: Cerebral protection by a barbiturate. *Anesthesiology* 1986; 64:165–170.
34. Shaw PJ, Bates D, Cartledge NEF, et al: Early intellectual dysfunction following coronary bypass surgery. *Q J Med* 1986; 225:59–68.
35. Gilberstadt H, Sako Y: Intellectual and personality changes following open-heart surgery. *Arch Gen Psychiatry* 1967; 16:210–214.
36. Raymond M, Conklin C, Schaeffer J, et al: Coping with transient intellectual dysfunction after coronary bypass surgery. *Heart Lung* 1984; 13:531–539.
37. Fish KJ, Helms K, Sarnquist FH, et al: Neuropsychological dysfunction after coronary artery surgery. *Anesthesiology* 1982; 57:A55.
38. Pears E, Bowman R, Kincey J, et al: Does prostacyclin prevent cognitive deficits after open heart surgery? *Psychol Med* 1984; 14:213–214.
39. Fish KJ, Helms KN, Sarnquist FH, et al: A prospective, randomized study of the effects of prostacyclin on neuropsychologic dysfunction after coronary artery operation. *J Thorac Cardiovasc Surg* 1987; 93:609–615.
40. Javid H, Tufo HM, Najafi H, et al: Neurologic abnormalities following open-heart surgery. *J Thorac Cardiovasc Surg* 1969; 58:502–509.
41. Lee WH Jr, Brady MP, Rowe JM, et al: Effects of extracorporeal circulation upon behavior, personality, and brain function. II. Hemodynamic, metabolic, and psychometric correlations. *Ann Surg* 1971; 173:1013–1023.
42. Branthwaite MA: Neurological damage related to open-heart surgery. A clinical survey. *Thorax* 1972; 27:738–753.
43. Hutchinson JE, Green GE, Mekhjian HA, et al: Coronary bypass grafting of 376 consecutive patients, with three operative deaths. *J Thorac Cardiovasc Surg* 1974; 67:7–16.
44. Loop LD, Cosgrove DM, Lytle BW, et al: An 11 year evolution of coronary arterial surgery (1967–1978). *Ann Surg* 1979; 190:444–445.
45. Kolkka R, Hilberman M: Neurologic dysfunction following cardiac operation with low-flow, low-pressure cardiopulmonary bypass. *J Thorac Cardiovasc Surg* 1980; 79:432–437.
46. Turnipseed WD, Berkoff HA, Belzer FO: Postoperative stroke in cardiac and peripheral vascular disease. *Ann Surg* 1980; 192:365–368.
47. Cannon DS, Miller DC, Shumway NE, et al: The long term followup of patients undergoing saphenous vein bypass surgery. *Circulation* 1974; 49:77–85.
48. Hodgman JR, Cosgrove DM: Post-hospital course and complications following coronary bypass surgery. *Cleve Clin Q* 1976; 43:125–129.
49. Gonzalez-Scarano F, Hurtig HL: Neurologic complications of coronary artery bypass grafting: Case-control study. *Neurology* 1981; 31:1032–1035.
50. Breuer AC, Furlan AJ, Hanson MR, et al: Central nervous system complications of coronary artery bypass graft surgery: Prospective analysis of 421 patients. *Stroke* 1983; 14:682–687.

51. Slogoff S, Girgis KZ, Keats AS: Etiologic factors in neuropsychiatric complications associated with cardiopulmonary bypass. *Anesth Analg* 1982; 61:903–911.
52. Aberg T, Kihlgren M: Effects of open heart surgery on intellectual function. *Scand J Thorac Cardiovasc Surg* 1974; 15:1–63.
53. Frank KA, Heller SS, Kornfeld DS, et al: Long-term effects of open heart surgery on intellectual functioning. *J Thorac Cardiovasc Surg* 1972; 64:811–815.
54. Willner AE, Rabiner CJ: Psychopathology and cognitive dysfunction five years after open heart surgery. *Compr Psychiatry* 1979; 20:409–418.
55. Ellis RJ, Wigniewski A, Potts R, et al: Reduction of flow rate and arterial pressure at moderate hypothermia does not result in cerebral dysfunction. *J Thorac Cardiovasc Surg* 1980; 79:173–180.;
56. Savageau JA, Stanton BA, Jenkins CD, et al: Neuropsychological dysfunction following elective cardiac operation—early assessment. *J Thorac Cardiovasc Surg* 1982; 84:585–594.
57. Savageau JA, Stanton BA, Jenkins CD, et al: Neuropsychological dysfunction following elective cardiac operation: A six month reassessment. *J Thorac Cardiovasc Surg* 1982; 84:595–600.
58. Garvey JW, Willner A, Wolpowitz A, et al: The effect of arterial filtration during open heart surgery on cerebral function. *Circulation* 1983; 68:125–128.
59. Coffey CE, Massey EW, Roberts DB: Natural history of cerebral complications of coronary artery bypass graft surgery. *Neurology* 1983; 33:1416–1421.
60. Elsass P: Acute cerebral dysfunction after open heart surgery. A reaction-time study. *Scand J Thorac Cardiovasc Surg* 1984; 18:161–165.
61. Walsh GW, Hearn S, O'Reilly W: A comparison of psychological test results in patients post cardiopulmonary bypass using membrane and bubble oxygenators. *Proceedings of the American Academy of Cardiovascular Perfusion* 1983; 7:35–38.
62. Smith PLC, Newman SP, Ell PJ, et al: Cerebral consequences of cardiopulmonary bypass. *Lancet* 1986; 1:823–826.
63. Shaw PJ, Bates D, Cartlidge NEF, et al: Long-term intellectual dysfunction following coronary artery bypass graft surgery: A six month follow-up study. *Q J Med* 1987; 239:259–268.
64. Nevin M, Colchester ACF, Adams S, et al: Evidence for involvement of hypocapnia and hypoperfusion in aetiology of neurological deficit after cardiopulmonary bypass. *Lancet* 1987; 2:1493–1495.
65. Folks DG, Freeman AM, Sokol RS, et al: Cognitive dysfunction after coronary artery bypass surgery: A case-controlled study. *South Med J* 1988; 81:202–206.
66. Hammeke TA: Neuropsychologic alterations after cardiac operation. *J Thorac Cardiovasc Surg* 1988; 96:326–331.
67. Newman S, Klinger L, Venn G, et al: Subjective reports of cognition in relation to assessed cognitive performance following coronary artery bypass surgery. *J Psychosom Res* 1989; 33:227–233.
68. Townes BD, Bashein G, Hornbein TF, et al: Neurobehavioral outcome in cardiac operations. A prospective controlled study. *J Thorac Cardiovasc Surg* 1989; 98:774–782.
69. Aberg T, Kihlgren M: Cerebral protection during open heart surgery. *Thorax* 1977; 32:525–533.

70. Aberg T, Kihlgren M, Johnsson I, et al: Improved cerebral protection during open heart surgery, in Becker R, Katz J, Polonius M–J (eds) *Psychopathological and Neurological Dysfunctions Following Open-Heart Surgery.* Heidelberg, Springer, 1982, pp 343–351.
71. Sotaniemi KA, Juolasmaa AN, Hokkanen ET: Neuropsychologic outcome after open heart surgery. *Arch Neurol* 1981; 38:2–8.
72. Juolasmaa A, Outakoski J, Hirvenoja R, et al: Effect of open heart surgery on intellectual performance. *J Clin Neurol* 1981; 3:181–197.
73. Stockard JJ, Bickford RG, Schauble JF: Pressure-dependent cerebral ischemia during cardiopulmonary bypass. *Neurology* 1973; 23:521–529.
74. Branthwaite MA: Prevention of neurological damage during open heart surgery. *Thorax* 1975; 30:258–261.
75. Lederman RJ, Breuer AC, Hanson MR, et al: Peripheral nervous system complications of coronary artery bypass graft surgery. *Ann Neurol* 1982; 12:297–301.
76. Gardner TJ, Horneffer PJ, Manolio TA, et al: Stroke following coronary artery bypass grafting: A ten year study. *Ann Thorac Surg* 1985; 40:574.
77. Newman S, Smith P, Treasure T, et al: Acute neuropsychological consequences of coronary artery bypass surgery. *Curr Psych Res Rev* 1987; 6:115.
78. Venn GE, Klinger L, Newman S, et al: The neuropsychologic sequelae of bypass 12 months following coronary artery surgery. *Br Heart J* 1987; 57:565.
79. Hertzer NR, Loop FC, Taylor PC, et al: Staged and combined surgical approach to simultaneous carotid and coronary vascular disease. *Surgery* 1978; 84:803–811.
80. Diethrich EB, Reiling M, Ibrahim F, et al; Stroke screening prior to coronary artery bypass. *Cardiovasc Dis/Bull Texas Heart Inst* 1977; 4:262.
81. Silverstein A, Jacobson E, Krell I, et al: Effects on the brain of extracorporeal circulation in open-heart surgery: A neurologic, electroencephalographic, psychometric and neuropathologic study. *Neurology* 1960; 10:987–992.
82. Reul GJ, Morris GC, Howell JR, et al: Current concepts in coronary artery surgery: A critical analysis of 1,287 patients. *Ann Thorac Surg* 1972; 14:243–257.
83. Sotaniemi KA: Brain damage and neurological outcome after open-heart surgery. *J Neurol Neurosurg Psychiatry* 1980; 43:127–135.
84. Ashor GW, Meyer BW, Lindesmith GG: Coronary artery disease: Surgery in 100 patients 65 years of age and older. *Arch Surg* 1973; 107:30–33.
85. Branthwaite MA: Detection of neurological damage during open heart surgery. *JAMA* 1970; 212:1333–1336.
86. Hochberg MS, Morrow AG, Michaelis LL, et al: Aortic valve replacement in the elderly. *Arch Surg* 1977; 112:1475–1480.
87. Stephenson LW, MacVaugh H, Edmunds LH: Surgery using cardiopulmonary bypass in the elderly. *Circulation* 1978; 58:250–254.
88. Higginbothom M, Hunt D, White A, et al: Surgical treatment of angina pectoris in the elderly. *Med J Aust* 1981; 2:664–666.
89. Bergdahl L, Bkork VO, Jonasson R: Aortic valve replacement in patients over 70 years. *Scand J Thorac Cardiovasc Surg* 1981; 15:123–128.
90. Brusino FG, Reves JG, Smith LR, et al: The effect of age on cerebral blood flow during hypothermic cardiopulmonary bypass. *J Thorac Cardiovasc Surg* 1989; 97:541–547.
91. Collins KJ, Exton-Smith AN, James MH, et al: Functional changes in autonomic nervous system responses with aging. *Age Ageing* 1980; 9:17.

92. Rogers RL, Meyer JS, Mortel KF, et al: Age-related reductions in cerebral vasomotor reactivity and the law of initial value: A 4-year prospective longitudinal study. *J Cereb Blood Flow Metab* 1985; 5:79.
93. Gilman S: Cerebral disorders after open-heart operations. *N Engl J Med* 1965; 272:489–498.
94. Robinson M, Blumaenthal JA, Burker EJ, et al: Coronary artery bypass grafting and cognitive function: A review. *J Cardiopulmonary Rehabil* 1990; 10:180–189.
95. Clark RE, Dietz DR, Miller JG: Continuous detection of microemboli during CPB in animals and man. *Circulation* 1976; 54:74–78.
96. Guidoin RG, Kenedi RM: Thrombus formation and microaggregate removal during extracorporeal membrane oxygenation. *J Biomed Mater Res* 1979; 13:317–335.
97. Pederson T, Hatteland K, Semb BK: Bubble extraction by various arterial-filters measured in vitro with doppler ultrasound techniques. *Ultrasound Med Biol* 1982; 8:77–81.
98. Orenstein JM, Sato N, Aaron B, et al: Microemboli observed in deaths following cardiac surgery. *Hum Pathol* 1982; 13:1082–1090.
99. Deverall PB, Padayachee TS, Parsons S, et al: Ultrasound detection of micro-emboli in the middle cerebral artery during cardiopulmonary bypass surgery. *Eur J Cardiothorac Surg* 1988; 2:256–260.
100. Reed CC, Romagnoli A, Taylor DE, et al: Particulate matter in the bubble oxygenators. *J Thorac Cardiovasc Surg* 1974; 68:971–974.
101. Martin WRW, Hashimoto SA: Stroke in coronary bypass surgery. *Can J Neurol Sci* 1982; 9:21–26.
102. Oka Y, Moriwaki KM, Hong Y, et al: Detection of air emboli in the left heart by M-mode transesophageal echocardiography following cardiopulmonary bypass. *Anesthesiology* 1985; 63:109–113.
103. Ghatak NR, Sinnenberg RJ, Deblois GG: Cerebral fat embolism following cardiac surgery. *Stroke* 1983; 14:619–621.
104. McKibbin DW, Bulkley BH, Green WR, et al: Fatal cerebral atheromatous embolization after cardiopulmonary bypass. *J Thorac Cardiovasc Surg* 1976; 71:741–745.
105. Briely JB: Brain damage complicating open-heart surgery: A neuropathological study of 46 patients. *Proc R Soc Med* 1967; 60:858–859.
106. Lawrence GH, McKay HA, Sherensky RT: Effective measures in the prevention of intraoperative aeroembolus. *J Thorac Cardiovasc Surg* 1971; 62:731–735.
107. Mills NL, Ochsner JL: Massive air embolism during cardiopulmonary bypass: Causes, prevention and management. *J Thorac Cardiovasc Surg* 1980; 80:708–717.
108. Barzilai B, Saffitz JE, Miller JG, et al: Quantitative ultrasonic characterization of the nature of atherosclerotic plaques in human aorta. *Circ Res* 1987; 60:459–463.
109. Barzilai B, Marshall WG Jr, Saffitz JE, et al: Avoidance of embolic complications by ultrasonic characterization of the ascending aorta. *Circulation* 1989; 80:I275–I279.
110. Topol EJ, Humphrey LS, Borkon AM, et al: Value of intraoperative left ventricular microbubbles detected by transesophageal 2-dimensional echocardiography in predicting neurologic outcome after cardiac operations. *Am J Cardiol* 1985; 56:773–775.
111. Gomes OM, Pereira SN, Catagna RC, et al: The importance of the different

sites of air injection in the tolerance of arterial air embolism. *J Thorac Cardiovasc Surg* 1973; 65:563–568.

112. Blumenthal JA, Burker EJ, Schneibolk S, et al: The effects of cardiac surgery on neuropsychological functioning. Presented at the 12th Annual Meeting of the Society of Cardiovascular Anesthesiologists, Orlando, Florida, May, 1990.

113. Kety SS, Schmidt CF: The determination of cerebral blood flow in man by the use of nitrous oxide in low concentrations. *Am J Physiol* 1945; 143:53–60.

114. Scheinberg P, Stead EA: The cerebral blood flow in male subjects as measured by the nitrous technique: Normal values for blood flow, oxygen utilization, glucose utilization, and peripheral resistance with observations on the effect of lilting and anxiety. *J Clin Invest* 1949; 28:1163–1168.

115. Michenfelder JD: *Anesthesia and the Brain*. New York, Churchill Livingstone, Inc, 1988.

116. Stullken EH Jr, Milde JH, Michenfelder JD, et al: The non-linear responses of cerebral metabolism to low concentrations of halothane, enflurane, isoflurane and thiopental. *Anesthesiology* 1977; 46:28.

117. Lassen NA: Autoregulation of cerebral blood flow. *Circ Res* 1964; 15:I201–I204.

118. Lassen NA, Christenson MS: Physiology of cerebral blood flow. *Br J Anaesth* 1976; 48:719–734.

119. Greeley WJ, Ungerleider RM, Kern FH, et al: Effects of cardiopulmonary bypass on cerebral blood flow in neonates, infants and children. *Circulation* 1989; 80:I205–I209.

120. Rosenberg AA, Jones MD Jr, Traystman RJ, et al: Response of cerebral blood flow to changes in pCO_2 in fetal, neonatal and adult sheep. *Am J Physiol* 1982; 242:H863–H866.

121. Fox LS, Blackstone EH, Kirklin JW, et al: Relationship of whole body oxygen consumption to perfusion flow rate during hypothermic cardiopulmonary bypass. *J Thorac Cardiovasc Surg* 1982; 83:239–248.

122. Fox LS, Blackstone EH, Kirklin JW, et al: Relationship of brain blood flow and oxygen consumption to perfusion flow rate during profound hypothermic cardiopulmonary bypass. *J Thorac Cardiovasc Surg* 1984; 87:658–664.

123. Messmer BJ, Schallberger U, Gattiker R, et al: Psychomotor and intellectual development after deep hypothermic circulatory arrest in early infancy. *J Thorac Cardiovasc Surg* 1976; 72:494–502.

124. Mohri H, Barnes RW, Winterscheid LC, et al: Challenge of prolonged suspended animation: A method of surface-induced hypothermia. *Ann Surg* 1968; 168:779–787.

125. Greeley WJ, Kern F, Ungerleider RM, et al: The effect of hypothermic cardiopulmonary bypass and total circulatory arrest on cerebral metabolism in neonates, infants and children. *J Thorac Cardiovasc Surg*, in press.

126. Swain JA, Griffith PK, Balabal RS, et al: Low flow hypothermic cardiopulmonry bypass protects the brain. *J Thorac Cardiovasc Surg*, in press.

127. Watanabe T, Orita H, Kobayashi M, et al: Brain tissue pH, oxygen tension and carbon dioxide tension in profoundly hypothermic cardiopulmonary bypass. *J Thorac Cardiovasc Surg* 1989; 97:369–401.

128. Stanley TE III, Smith LR, White WD, et al: Effect of cerebral perfusion pressure during cardiopulmonary bypass on neuropsychiatric outcome following coronary artery bypass grafting. Presented at the 12th Annual Meeting of the Society of Cardiovascular Anesthesiologists, Orlando, Florida, May, 1990.

129. Bashein G, Townes BD, Nessly ML, et al: A randomized study of carbon dioxide management during hypothermic cardiopulmonary bypass. *Anesthesiology* 1990; 72:7–15.
130. Croughwell N, Lyth M, Quill TJ, et al: Diabetic patients have abnormal cerebral autoregulation during cardiopulmonary bypass. *Circulation,* 1990; 82(5 Suppl): IV 407–412.
131. Ewing DJ, Campbell IW, Clarke BF: Assessment of cardiovascular effects in diabetic autonomic neuropathy and prognostic implications. *Ann Intern Med* 1980; 92:308–311.
132. Jones JV, Fitch W, MacKenzie ET, et al: Lower limit of cerebral blood flow autoregulation in experimental renal vascular hypertension in the baboon. *Circ Res* 1976; 39:555–561.
133. Croughwell N, Newman M, Quill T, et al: Warming during cardiopulmonary bypass is associated with jugular bulb desaturation. *Anesth Analg* 1990; 70:S72.
134. Ginsberg MD, Welsh FA, Budd WW: Deleterious effect of glucose pretreatment on recovery from diffuse cerebral ischemia in the cat. *Stroke* 1980; 11:347–354.
135. Pulsinelli WA, Levy DE, Duffy TE: Regional cerebral blood flow and glucose metabolism following transient forebrain ischemia. *Ann Neurol* 1982; 11:499–509.
136. Pulsinelli WA, Levy DE, Sigsbee B, et al: Increased damage after ischemic stroke in patients with hyperglycemia with or without established diabetes mellitus. *Am J Med* 1983; 74:540–544.
137. Berger L, Hakim AM: The association of hyperglycemia with cerebral edema in stroke. *Stroke* 1986; 17:865–897.
138. Steward DJ, DaSilva CA, Fiegel T: Elevated blood glucose may increase the danger of neurologic deficit following profoundly hypothermic/cardiac arrest. *Anesthesiology* 1988; 68:653.
139. Sieber FE, Smith DS, Traystman RJ, et al: A reevaluation of its intraoperative use. *Anesthesiology* 1987; 67:72–81.
140. Michenfelder JD, Theye RA: Hypothermia: Effect on canine brain and whole-body metabolism. *Anesthesiology* 1968; 29:1107–1112.
141. Croughwell N, Smith LR, Quill T, et al: The effect of temperature on cerebral metabolism and blood flow in adults during cardiopulmonary bypass. *J Thorac Cardiovasc Surg,* in press.
142. Croughwell, Quill T, Newman M, et al: The Q10 for cerebral oxidative metabolism during CPB in man. Presented at the 12th Annual Meeting of the Society of Cardiovascular Anesthesiologists, Orlando, Florida, May, 1990.
143. Michenfelder JD, Theye RA: The effects of anesthesia and hypothermia on canine cerebral ATP and lactate during anoxia produced by decapitation. *Anesthesiology* 1970; 33:430–439.
144. Steen PA, Newberg L, Milde JH, et al: Hypothermia and barbiturates: Individual and combined effects on canine cerebral oxygen consumption. *Anesthesiology* 1983; 58:527–532.
145. Woodcock TE, Murkin JM, Farrar JK, et al: Pharmacologic EEG suppression during cardiopulmonary bypass: Cerebral hemodynamic and metabolic effects of thiopental or isoflurane during hypothermia and normothermia. *Anesthesiology* 1987; 67:218–224.
146. Stocker F, Herschowitz N, Bossi E, et al: Cerebral metabolic studies in situ by [31]phosphorus nuclear magnetic resonance after hypothermic circulatory arrest. *Pediatr Res* 1986; 20:867–871.

147. Norwood WI, Norwood CR, Ingwall JS, et al: Hypothermic circulatory arrest: ^{31}Phosphorus nuclear magnetic resonance of isolated perfused neonatal rat brain. *J Thorac Cardiovasc Surg* 1979; 78:823–830.
148. Chopp M, Knight R, Tidwell CD, et al: The metabolic effects of mild hypothermia on global cerebral ischemia and recirculation in the cat: Comparison to monothermia and hypothermia. *J Cereb Blood Flow Metab* 1989; 9:141.
149. Globus MY-T, Busto R, Dietrich WD, et al: Intra-ischemic extracellular release of dopamine and glutamate is associated with striatal vulnerability to ischemia. *Neurosci Lett* 1988; 91:36.
150. Berntman L, Welsh FA, Harp JR: Cerebral protective effect of low grade hypothermia. *Anesthesiology* 1981; 55:495.
151. Keykhah MM, Welsh FA, Hagerdal M, et al: Reduction of the cerebral protective effect of hypothermia by oligemic hypotension during hypoxia in the rat. *Stroke* 1982; 13:171.
152. Busto R, Dietrich WD, Globus MY-T, et al: Small differences in the intra-ischemic brain temperature critically determine the extent of ischemic neuronal injury. *J Cereb Blood Flow Metab* 1987; 7:729.
153. Ekroth R, Thompson RJ, Lincoln C, et al: Elective deep hypothermia with total circulatory arrest: Changes in plasma creatine kinase BB, blood glucose, and clinical variables. *J Thorac Cardiovasc Surg* 1984; 97:30–35.
154. Blackman CF, Benane SG, Elder JA, et al: Induction of calcium ion efflux from brain tissue by radio frequency radiation: A set of sample number and modulation frequency on the power density window. *Bioelectromagnetics* 1980; 1:35–43.
155. Sako K, Kobatuke K, Yamamoto YL, et al: Correlation of local cerebral blood flow, glucose utilization and tissue pH following a middle cerebral artery occlusion in the rat. *Stroke* 1985; 16:828.
156. Venn GE, Sherry K, Klinger L, et al: Cerebral blood flow determinants and their derived implications during cardiopulmonary bypass. *Perfusion* 1988; 3:271–280.
157. Wollman H, Stephen GW, Clement AJ, et al: Cerebral blood flow in man during extracorporeal circulation. *J Thorac Cardiovasc Surg* 1966; 52:558–564.
158. Zaidan JR, Martin W, Klochang A: Preservation of CNS function with thiopental after coronary artery surgery. *Anesthesiology* 1989; 71:A283.
159. Newberg LA, Milde JH, Michenfelder JD: The cerebral metabolic effects of isoflurane at and above concentrations that suppress cortical electrical activity. *Anesthesiology* 1983; 59:23–28.
160. Newberg LA, Michenfelder JD: Cerebral protection by isoflurane during hypoxemia or ischemia. *Anesthesiology* 1983; 59:29–35.
161. Nehls DG, Todd MM, Spetzler RF, et al: A comparison of the protective effects of isoflurane and thiopental in a primate model of temporary focal cerebral ischemia. *Anesthesiology* 1987; 66:453.
162. Baughman VL, Hoffman WE, Thomas C, et al: The interaction of nitrous oxide and isoflurane with incomplete cerebral ischemia in the rat. *Anesthesiology* 1989; 70:767–774.
163. Michenfelder JD: Does isoflurane aggravate regional cerebral ischemia. *Anesthesiology* 1987; 66:451–452.
164. Nugent M, Artu AA, Michenfelder JD: Cerebral metabolic, vascular, and protective effects of midazolam maleate. *Anesthesiology* 1982; 56:172–176.
165. Ashton D, Van Reempts J, Wanquier A: Behavioural electroencephalographic and histological study of the protective effect of etomidate against his-

totoxic dysoxia produced by cyanide. *Arch Int Pharmacodyn* 1981; 254:196–210.

166. Astrup J, Skovsted P, Gjerris F, et al: Increase in extracellular potassium in the brain during circulatory arrest: Effects of hypothermia, lidocaine, and thiopental. *Anesthesiology* 1981; 55:256–262.

167. Artru AA, Michenfelder JD: Anoxic cerebral potassium accumulation reduced phenytoin: Mechanism of cerebral protection? *Anesth Analg* 1981; 60:41–45.

168. Allen GS, Ahn HS, Spetzler RF, et al: Cerebral arterial spasm—a controlled trial of nimodipine in patients with subarachnoid hemorrhage. *N Engl J Med* 1983; 308:619–624.

169. Steen PA, Milde JH, Michenfelder JD: Cerebral metabolic and vascular effects of barbiturate therapy following complete global ischemia. *J Neurochem* 1978; 31:1317–1324.

170. Steen PA, Newberg LA, Milde JH, et al: Nimodipine improves cerebral blood flow and neurologic recovery after complete cerebral ischemia in the dog. *J Cereb Blood Flow Metab* 1983; 3:38–43.

171. Steen PA, Newberg LA, Milde JH, et al: Cerebral blood flow and neurologic outcome when nimodipine is given after complete cerebral ischemia in the dog. *J Cereb Blood Flow Metab* 1984; 4:82–87.

172. Steen PA, Gisvold SE, Milde JH, et al: Nimodipine improves outcome when given after complete cerebral ischemia in primates. *Anesthesiology* 1985; 62:406–414.

173. Rolfsen ML, Davis WR: Cerebral function and preservation during cardiac arrest. *Crit Care Med* 1989; 17:283–292.

174. Wauquier A, Ashton D, Clincke G, et al: Calcium entry blockers as cerebral protecting agents: Comparative activity in tests of hypoxia and hyperoxicitability. *Jpn J Pharmacol* 1985; 38:1–7.

175. Tuman KJ, McCarthy RJ, Spiess BD, et al: Do calcium channel blockers decrease neurologic deficits after intracardiac operations. *Anesth Analg* 1990; 70:S413.

176. Fleischer JE, Lanier WL, Milde JH, et al: Failure of deferoxamine, an iron chelator, to improve neurologic outcome following complete cerebral ischemia in dogs. *Stroke* 1987; 18:124–127.

177. Forsman M, Fleischer J, Milde JH, et al: Superoxide dismutase and catalase failed to affect neurologic outcome following complete cerebral ischemia in dogs. *Stroke* 1987; 18:124.

178. Duverger D, Benavides J, Cudennec A, et al: A glutamate antagonist reduces infarction size following focal cerebral ischemia independently of vascular and metabolic changes. *J Cereb Blood Flow Metab* 1987; 7:S144.

179. Oyzurt E, Graham DI, McCulloch J, et al: The NMDA receptor antagonist MK-801 reduces focal ischemic brain damage in the cat. *J Cereb Blood Flow Metab* 1987; 7:S146.

180. Block GA, Pulsinelli WA: Excitatory amino acid receptor antagonists: Failure to prevent ischemic neuronal damage. *J Cereb Blood Flow Metab* 1987; 7:S149.

Epicardial Echocardiography During Repair of Congenital Heart Defects

Ross M. Ungerleider, M.D.

Assistant Professor, General and Thoracic Surgery; Chief, Pediatric Cardiac Surgery, Department of Surgery, Duke University Medical Center, Durham, North Carolina

The surgical correction of congenital heart defects has evolved to its own subspecialty within the field of cardiac surgery. Surgeons who concentrate on this aspect of the profession are creating more imaginative and aggressive methods to repair or reconstruct complex cardiac defects, even in tiny infants. Many of these approaches are made possible by advances in technology that enable the safe application of cardiopulmonary bypass to the very young.[1] Furthermore, understanding of the impact of profound hypothermia with periods of total circulatory arrest on cerebral metabolism[2] has led surgeons to use this technical option more readily (and safely) to extend their capabilities further during complicated intracardiac procedures. It is becoming increasingly clear that achieving survival, except in certain high-risk lesions, is not the only standard by which to evaluate successful surgical results. Indeed, the quality of the repair may relate importantly to the expected long-term outcome after surgical correction. Routine intraoperative assessment of the quality of surgical repair in patients with congenital heart disease must be able to examine accurately residual shunts, gradients, valve function, flow through and around baffles, and the function of both the right and left ventricles. Methods available have been limited in the past to techniques such as oximetry or green dye curves. These methods can be cumbersome and time-consuming, and, because they are "indirect" techniques, may lack accuracy. New techniques, such as echocardiography with Doppler color flow imaging (echo-DCFI) have been evaluated recently as alternative approaches to the older modalities.[3–7] Echo-DCFI is uniquely suited for this purpose, as it provides readily available images of complex spatial anatomic arrangements as well as information about blood flow that can lead to clear delineation of abnormal flow patterns (such as those seen with residual shunts or stenoses) and precise localization of these problems with respect to intracardiac structures.

Because of the anticipated advantages of learning to apply echo-DCFI in the operating room environment during the repair of congenital heart defects, we began investigating (in a prospective fashion) the merits of routine intraoperative echo-DCFI applied both before and after cardiopulmonary bypass for infants, children, and adults undergoing repair of congenital heart defects.

Techniques

Echocardiography can be performed by either the transesophageal or the direct epicardial approach. Although transesophageal echocardiography, which has become so popular in adult patients,[8] is possible in infants and small children, especially with some of the more recently introduced transducers, we feel that epicardial application of the transducer provides greater flexibility and possibly more information in patients with potentially complex intracardiac defects that require unique image production and do not always lend themselves well to "standard views." Although epicardial scanning requires active involvement of the surgeon with temporary "interruption" of the process of operating, the surgeon is also the individual who is most affected by the information generated and who best understands the spatial relationships of the surgical reconstruction to the underlying defect. All echocardiographic exams at the Duke Heart Center are performed using a Hewlett-Packard HP77020CF color flow imaging device equipped with multiple transducers. Most examinations are best accomplished using the 5.0-MHz short focus transducer, but in certain cases (e.g., for larger patients) the 5.0-MHz medium focus or 2.5-MHz transducer are helpful. On some occasions, a nonimaging 1.9-MHz continuous wave Doppler probe is useful to provide spectral information regarding flow gradients or direction. Prior to imaging, the transducer and cable are cleaned with a commercially available glutaraldehyde solution and left wrapped in a glutaraldehyde-soaked towel for at least 10 minutes. Particular care is taken to keep the liquid from entering the electrical contacts on the transducer assembly. The transducer is then wiped with sterile saline and taken to the patient's head, where it can be introduced by the surgeon into a sterile sheath containing 20 mL of sterile ultrasound gel. The sheath is then secured to the surgical side of the ether screen (Fig 1).

All images should be analyzed "on-line" in real time and decisions made in each case on the basis of echo-DCFI as well as any other relevant clinical observations that are available. At our center, all echo-DCFI data are evaluated mutually and by consensus of the attending surgeon, anesthesiologist, and cardiologist present during the procedure. New findings from the intraoperative echo-DCFI study are judged in comparison to the preoperative echo-DCFI and any available catheterization data. Data from each study are then entered into a data bank for later retrieval and analysis. Comparisons of echo-DCFI findings, as they relate to both operative planning and postoperative course, are performed by the standard chi-squared test using a Bonferroni correction factor to allow for multiple vari-

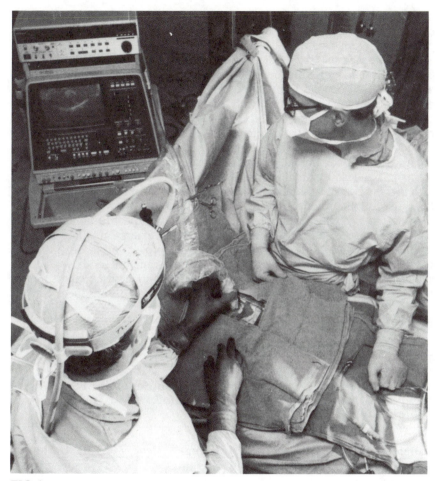

FIG 1.
Placement of the ultrasound transducer into a sterile sheath makes it readily accessible to the surgeon at any time during the operation. Here the prebypass evaluation of a patient with an atrioventricular canal defect is being performed. It is notable how little space this technology occupies in the operating room compared to the enormous amount of information that it provides. (From Ungerleider RM: *Echocardiography* 1990; 7:289–304. Used by permission.)

ables. A P value of $<.01$ is significant. Some of our data are presented below.

Although we have acquired experience with intraoperative echo-DCFI only during the repair of intracardiac lesions through a median sternotomy, application of the probe through a thoracotomy incision certainly would be feasible and, with experience, useful view orientations probably could be obtained. This might be especially helpful for tricuspid or mitral valve repair or replacement, or for atrial septal defect closure through a right thoracotomy. The use of transesophageal methods for these patients might be particularly attractive.

Initial practice with epicardial echo-DCFI during the operative repair of congenital heart defects should be acquired in an environment as rich in experience as possible. For this reason, a cardiologist who is familiar with echocardiography as well as with congenital heart disease should be present in the operating room to assist and educate the surgeon for each examination. Review of our experience (Table 1) demonstrates that the first few prebypass ("initial") examinations performed by a team just learning how to produce helpful images can last as long as 12 minutes and that postbypass ("last") examination can take up to 23 minutes. Nevertheless, with increasing expertise and familiarity with this technique, the lengthy interrogations that are encountered when first learning these methods can be expected to decrease drastically; overall, we now expect to obtain a complete prebypass or postbypass examination in less than 4 minutes, and often in less than 1 minute for some of the less complex and more "routine" defects (e.g., secundum atrial septal defect or perimembranous ventricular septal defect). It is also very helpful to elicit full-time systematic support from a trained echocardiology technician. Because the transducer is ster-

TABLE 1.
Duke University Medical Center
Intraoperative Echocardiography With Doppler Color Flow Imaging for Congenital Heart Repair: Number and Times of Examinations in 414 Patients*

Variable	Minimum	Maximum	Mean = 2.73	Standard Deviation
Number of examinations	1	7		1.10
Duration of examinations (in minutes)				
Initial examination	0.18	12.78	3.93	1.91
Last examination	0.17	23.83	3.41	2.34
Total time/case	2.02	35.83	9.35	4.78
Average time/exam/case	0.61	17.91	3.55	1.65

*Patients had between one and seven intraoperative epicardial examinations done per case, although most frequently only the prebypass and postbypass examinations were required. "Initial examination" refers to the prebypass examination, with the minimum and maximum times demonstrating the range for prebypass exams. "Last examination" refers to the final examination after repair with minimum and maximum times again representing the range.

TABLE 2.
Duke University Medical Center
Intraoperative Echocardiography With Doppler Color Flow
Imaging for Congenital Heart Repair in 414 Patients

Complications	Number of Patients (%)
None	368 (89%)
Mild ectopy	37 (9%)
Moderate ectopy	7 (2%)
Severe ectopy (stop study)	1 (<1%)
Infections (mediastinal)	1 (<1%)

ilely ensheathed on the surgical field, it conveniently can be left in place during the entire procedure while the machine is moved, as necessary, to other operating rooms (or sites where it might be needed in the hospital). The machine then is returned when the surgeon is ready to obtain further studies.

It is important for the team to record, in some prospective and retrievable fashion, the information generated by these studies. Only in this manner can they begin to use the experience obtained to help guide procedures in the future. Recognition of which defects (by echocardiography) correlate with good long-term outcome and which echocardiographic patterns give cause for concern probably will be individualized for each team, but once patterns become predictable, intraoperative decisions can be made on the basis of echo findings. Table 2 demonstrates that complications are minimal.

Transducer Orientation

Placement of the transducer on the epicardial surface provides the opportunity to obtain some unique and high-resolution images. With a little practice, the various orientations that are most helpful for highlighting different congenital heart defects will become established views in the operating room and quite simple to reproduce. Nevertheless, certain complex forms of cardiac anatomy will require more individualized transducer position. The more commonly useful views in our experience are described below.

Long Axis.—For this image, the transducer is placed on the epicardial surface (usually near the anterior atrioventricular groove). The echo plane should extend from the apex to the base of the heart (Fig 2). This view is especially helpful for evaluating the mitral valve, aortic valve, interventricular septum, and ventricular function. By angling the transducer to include

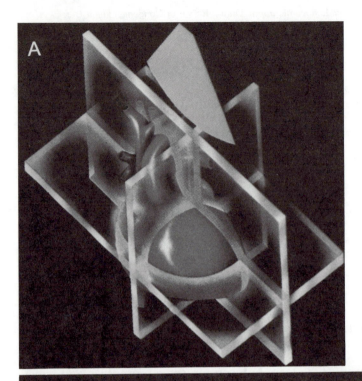

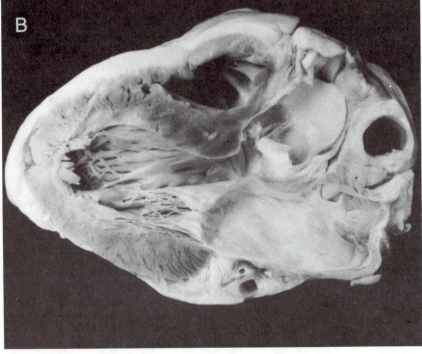

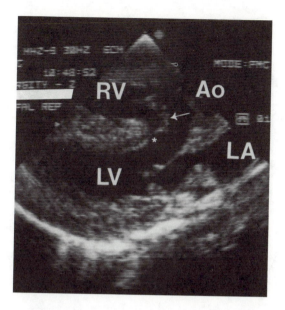

FIG 3.
This long-axis image obtained from a 9-month-old with tetralogy of Fallot demonstrates attachment of the chordal apparatus *(arrow)* of the tricuspid valve to the crest of the interventricular septum *(asterisk)*. Although initial inspection of this ventricular septal defect at the time of cardiotomy produced concern that the defect was not repairable due to straddling chords, the echocardiogram image encouraged it to be closed with confidence. The patient had an uneventful recovery. AO = aorta, LA = left atrium, LV = left ventricle; RV = right ventricle. (From Ungerleider RM, Greeley WJ, Sheikh KH: *J Thorac Cardiovasc Surg* 1990; 100:297–309. (Used by permission.)

the atrium, it is also possible to interrogate the atrial septum and tricuspid valve (Figs 3 to 7).

Short Axis.—The transducer is placed perpendicular to the long axis plane and then can be angled toward the base or apex of the heart to obtain the desired image. This orientation can allow the evaluation of ventricular function when the image is obtained from the mid-papillary muscle

---

FIG 2.
When the transducer is oriented so that the image plane bisects the heart from base to apex **(A),** a long-axis view of the heart is obtained **(B)**. This image enables ready evaluation of the left atrium, left ventricle, interventricular septum, and aortic and mitral valves. Flow also can be appreciated easily in the pulmonary artery (below the aorta) and the size of the coronary sinus (below the left atrium) can be seen; this will be enlarged when there is a persistent left superior vena cava. (From Leech G, Kisslo J: *Principles and Practice of Echocardiography.* London, MediCine Ltd, 1981.)

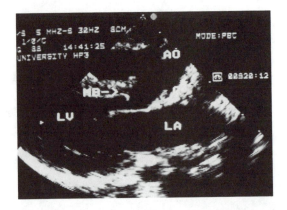

FIG 4.
In this patient with double outlet right ventricle, prebypass epicardial scanning reveals a ridge of obstructing tissue *(MB)* in the subaortic area of the left ventricular outflow tract. Recognition of this anatomic feature (previously unappreciated) enabled adequate resection of this potential source of left ventricular outflow tract obstruction after intracardiac repair of this defect. *AO* = aorta; *LA* = left atrium; *LV* = left ventricle.

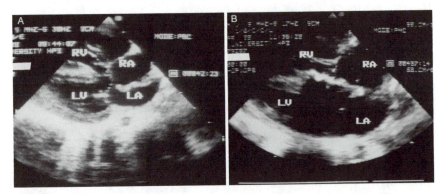

FIG 5.
A, image obtained from a patient with a complete atrioventricular canal defect. The common atrioventricular valve bridges the intraventricular septum with attachments to the septal crest. **B,** epicardial image produced after repair of this defect demonstrates the patch now septating the left and right sides of the heart with valve tissue suspended from this patch. Color flow mapping revealed an excellent result with no residual shunting or mitral insufficiency. *LA* = left atrium; *LV* = left ventricle; *RA* = right atrium; *RV* = right ventricle. (Part B from Ungerleider RM, Kisslo JA, Greeley WJ, et al: *J Thorac Cardiovasc Surg* 1989; 98:90–100. Used by permission.)

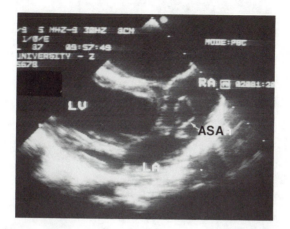

FIG 6.
An intra-atrial septal aneurysm is nicely displayed from this epicardial image. This view is a variation of the long-axis orientation with the transducer angled toward the atria to display the intra-atrial septum. *ASA* = atrial septal aneurysm; *RA* = right atrium; *LA* = left atrium; *LV* = left ventricle. (From Ungerleider RM, Greeley WJ, Sheikh KH: *J Thorac Cardiovasc Surg* 1990; 100:297–309. Used by permission.)

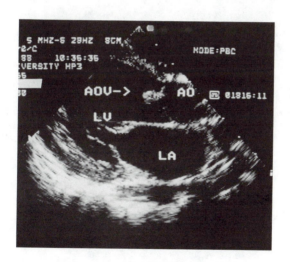

FIG 7.
AOV indicates an avulsed aortic valve leaflet after failed balloon angioplasty. Color flow mapping demonstrated severe aortic insufficiency. This image obtained prior to aortic valve repair demonstrated the nature of the valvular defect and helped to guide the intraoperative repair. Postbypass images, revealed an excellent result of valve repair in this instance. *AO* = aorta; *LA* = left atrium; *LV* = left ventricle. (From Ungerleider RM, Greeley WJ, Sheikh KH, et al: *Ann Surg* 1989; 210:526–534. Used by permission.)

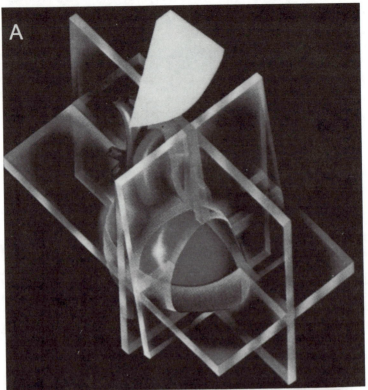

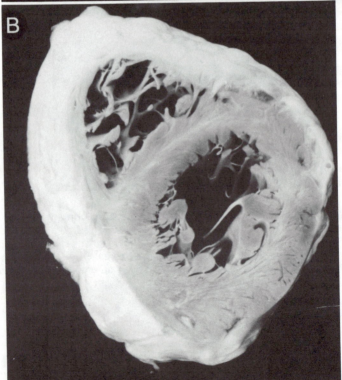

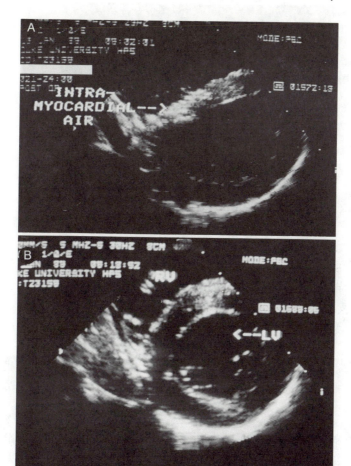

FIG 9.
A, a mid-myocardial short-axis view of a patient whose hemodynamic problems after being weaned from cardiopulmonary bypass can be seen clearly to be due to air within the ventricular septum in the distribution of the right coronary artery. **B,** after treatment with an alpha agent, the patient's myocardial air has disappeared and ventricular function has returned to normal, obviating the need for an inotropic agent. *LV* = left ventricle; *RV* = right ventricle.

FIG 8.
A, angling the short-axis image orientation toward the ventricular apex provides an excellent view **(B)** of the left ventricular and right ventricular muscle mass. This view is usually obtained at the level of the papillary muscles and is superb for evaluating ventricular function and chamber size. (From Leech G, Kisslo J: *Principles and Practice of Echocardiography.* London, Medi-Cine Ltd, 1981. Used by permission.)

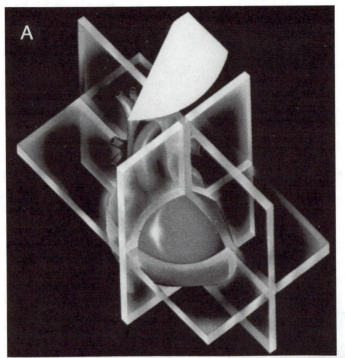

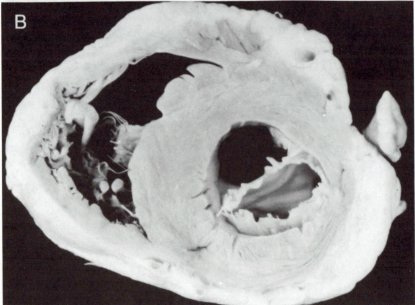

FIG 10.
A, the short-axis view at the mid-myocardial level enables evaluation of **(B)** the mitral valve, the left ventricular outflow tract, and the intraventricular septum. (From Leech G, Kisslo J: *Principles and Practice of Echocardiography.* London, Medi-Cine Ltd, 1981. Used by permission.)

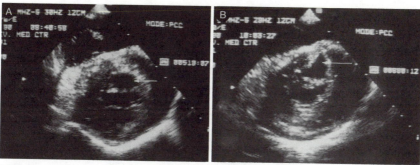

FIG 11.
A, a mid-myocardial view obtained from a patient with idiopathic hypertrophic subaortic stenosis. The left ventricular outflow tract *(arrow)* can be seen before and **(B)** after septal myectomy. Enlargement of the left ventricular outflow tract is evident and demonstrates a generous excision of muscle, indicating a good surgical result.

level (Figs 8 and 9), or of the mitral valve and left ventricular outflow tract if anatomy is viewed from the mid-myocardial level (Figs 10 to 12). If the transducer is aimed toward the base of the heart (Fig 13), a very instructive and informative image is created which demonstrates the interatrial septum, tricuspid valve, right ventricular outflow tract, pulmonary valve, and aortic valve. This image orientation is especially helpful for identifying the location of a ventricular septal defect, since the perimembranous type is visible near the tricuspid valve while the supracristal type is found below the pulmonary valve (Fig 14). Variations of this view can display the pulmonary artery bifurcation (a view useful for demonstrating a patent ductus

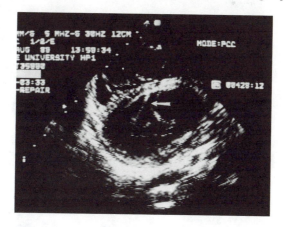

FIG 12.
A mid-myocardial image from a patient with an ostium primum atrial septal defect (partial atrioventricular canal defect). The cleft in the mitral valve is easily visualized, looking like an inverted "V" attached to the interventricular septum *(arrow)*. A cleft in the mitral valve always can be identified by this image orientation.

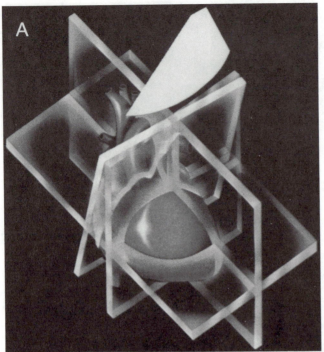

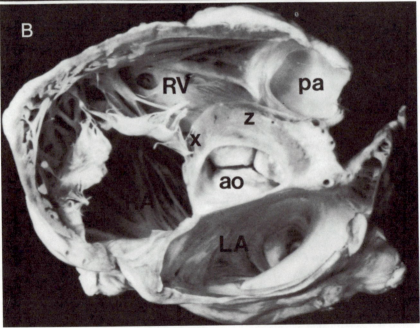

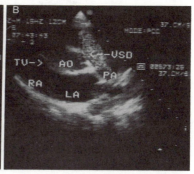

FIG 14.
A, this patient has a perimembraneous ventricular septal defect that can be appreciated clearly in the short-axis view by its proximity to the tricuspid valve *(TV)*. **B,** in this patient, the ventricular septal defect is supracristal (or subpulmonary) and is clearly quite far removed from the tricuspid valve. The approach to this ventricular septal defect should be transventricular or transpulmonary more often than transatrial. *AO* = aorta; *LA* = left atrium; *PA* = pulmonary artery; *RA* = right atrium; *RV* = right ventricle; *VSD* = ventricular septal defect. (From Ungerleider RM, Greeley WJ, Sheikh KH: *J Thorac Cardiovasc Surg* 1990; 100:297–309. Used by permission.)

arteriosus; Fig 15) or the sinus venosus portion of the atrial septum (Fig 16).

Other Views.—An advantage of epicardial echo-DCFI is that the images can be obtained from several unique and creative approaches to demonstrate various anatomic features (Figs 17 and 18). The transducer can be placed on a great vessel as well as on the epicardial surface. Unusual views are frequently necessary in patients with complex forms of congenital heart disease, such as those with heterotaxy syndromes and abnormal cardiac position. Although color flow mapping is extremely helpful in elucidating flow patterns within the cardiac structures, occasionally it is necessary to use microcavitation techniques to delineate pathologic flow clearly. An example of this is given in Figure 19, in which a large sinus venous defect and hypoplastic superior vena cava resulted in the produc-

---

FIG 13.
A, by angling the short-axis orientation toward the base of the heart, an image can be obtained that **(B)** depicts the left atrium *(LA)*, right atrium *(RA)*, right ventricle *(RV)*, and pulmonary and aortic valves. The interventricular septum is also identified and this view is particularly helpful in demonstrating the location of a perimembranous ventricular septal defect *(X)* and distinguishing it from a supracristal ventricular septal defect *(Z)*. *AO* = aorta; *PA* = pulmonary artery. (From Leech G, Kisslo J: *Principles and Practice of Echocardiography*. London, Medi-Cine Ltd, 1981. Used by permission.)

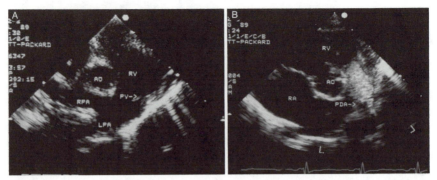

FIG 15.
A, variation of a short-axis view demonstrates the pulmonary outflow tract and the bifurcation into the right and left pulmonary artery. **B,** when color flow imaging is applied, the presence of a patent ductus arteriosus *(PDA)* can be appreciated. *AO* = aorta; *RA* = right atrium; *RV* = right ventricle.

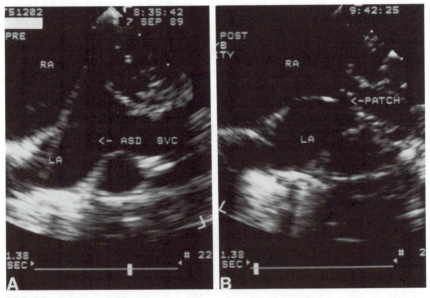

FIG 16.
A, a sinus venosus atrial septal defect *(ASD)* is visible and it can be seen that this defect is really absence of the common wall between the superior vena cava *(SVC)* and left atrium *(LA)*. **B,** the defect is shown postrepair and the pericardial patch used to separate the left atrium from the SVC and right atrium *(RA)* can be seen nicely.

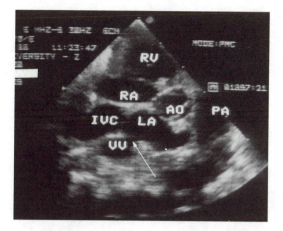

FIG 17.
A postrepair image obtained after successful correction of total anomalous pulmonary venous drainage (type III-infradiaphragmatic). Note the large anastomosis *(arrow)* between the vertical vein *(VV)* and left atrium *(LA)*. Spectral analysis across this region showed no significant Doppler shift, confirming unobstructed communication. The patient is now doing well 3 years postoperatively. *IVC* = inferior vena cava; *RA* = right atrium; *RV* = right ventricle; *AO* = aorta; *PA* = pulmonary artery. (From Ungerleider RM, et al: *Echocardiography* 1990; 7:289. Used by permission.)

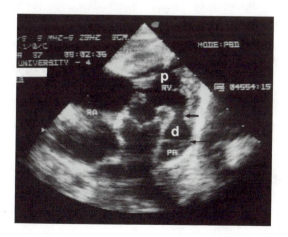

FIG 18.
Using echocardiography, the anatomy of a double chamber right ventricle can be depicted so that the defect is clearly understood. The proximal chamber *(P)* of the right ventricle *(RV)* is separated from the distal chamber *(D)* by hypertrophy in the infundibulum *(thick arrow)*. The distal (low pressure) chamber is still clearly below the pulmonary valve *(thin arrow)*. *PA* = pulmonary artery; *RA* = right atrium. (From Ungerleider RM, Sabiston DC: Tetralogy of Fallot, in Sabiston DC Jr, Spencer FC (eds): *Surgery of the Chest.* Philadelphia, WB Saunders Co, 1990, pp 1332–1358. Used by permission.)

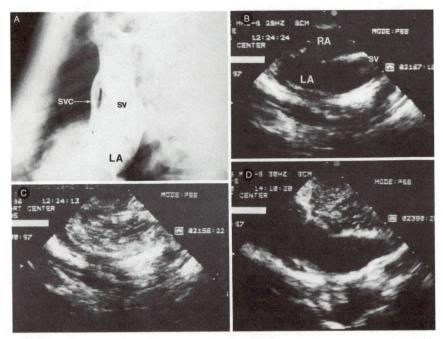

FIG 19.
A, an angiogram obtained from a patient with a large sinus venosus atrial septal defect *(SV)* and an extremely hypoplastic superior vena cava *(SVC)* that the angiography catheter traverses. This patient appeared to have communication between the SVC and left atrium *(LA)* and presented with marked cyanosis. **B,** intraoperative echocardiographic image reveals the right atrium *(RA)* and left atrium, but the SV defect, which was high in the SVC, could not be seen clearly by this image. **C,** the injection of microbubbles into a right internal jugular intravenous line showed the appearance of microcavitations quickly within the left atrium, confirming the defect demonstrated by angiography. **D,** after repair of this defect, a similar injection of microbubbles now demonstrates that the systemic venous return has been diverted to the right atrium and no longer produces a right-to-left shunt.

tion of a significant right-to-left shunt, causing cyanosis. The physiology of this flow was delineated clearly by microcavitation, but due to the nature of the defect, it could not be appreciated by color flow techniques. Furthermore, the success of the cardiac repair also could be demonstrated clearly using microcavitation techniques.

Results

Four hundred and fourteen patients undergoing repair of a variety of congenital heart defects (Table 3) through a median sternotomy at the Duke Heart Center between March, 1987 and March, 1990 provide information relating to the usefulness of these techniques. These patients ranged in age

TABLE 3.
Duke University Medical Center
Intraoperative Echocardiography With Doppler Color Flow
Imaging for Congenital Heart Repair in 414 Patients*

Principal Diagnoses	Number of Patients
Tetralogy of Fallot	50
Ventricular septal defect	56
Atrial septal defect (primum and sinus venosus)	68
Atrioventricular septal defect	37
Valvular regurgitation	40
Congenital valvular aortic stenosis	20
Transposition of the great vessels	19
Univentricular heart (includes HLHS)†	19
Pulmonary atresia	16
Tricuspid atresia/stenosis	18
Subvalvular aortic stenosis	12
Double outlet right ventricle	13
Aortic arch anomaly	11
Total anomalous pulmonary venous return	8
Coronary anomaly	5
Corrected transposition of the great vessels	4
Truncus arteriosus	3
Others	15

*Patients are coded with respect to principal diagnosis. Many patients had several diagnoses and, as is typical for congenital cardiac lesions, it is sometimes difficult to determine which category the patient best falls within. Nevertheless, each patient is counted only once with respect to what was felt to be a major congenital defect.
†HLHS = hypoplastic left heart syndrome.

from 1 day to 59 years (mean = 6.3 years), with the majority of them being less than 3 years old and more than one third less than 1 year old. The smallest patient was 1.8 kg and underwent closure of a ventricular septal defect.

It is difficult to quantitate the usefulness of intraoperative echocardiography performed prior to bypass, since the findings often have equivocal impact on the case. Nevertheless, in as objective a fashion as possible, we attempted to record the instances in which we felt the intraoperative study provided information that was not clearly appreciated prior to the examination and called these "anatomic details" (Table 4). In many cases, these were "trivial" and would either have been discovered easily when the heart was opened or had little if any impact on the operative plan. Furthermore, review of the preoperative transthoracic echocardiogram and cardiac catheterization (when performed) often revealed that the presence of these "details" had just gone "unrecognized" until the intraoperative ex-

TABLE 4.
Duke University Medical Center
Intraoperative Echocardiography With Color Flow Imaging for
Congenital Heart Repair: 80 Anatomic Details in 72 Patients
(17%)

Anomaly	Number of Patients
Atrial septal defect (none suspected)	13
Interatrial septal aneurysm	5
Multiple ventricular septal defects	6
Multiple atrial septal defects	6
Ventricular septal defect (none suspected)	4
Atrioventricular septal defect (complete)	1
Ventricular inlet/outlet	
Valvular anatomic or functional anomaly	9
Left or right ventricular outflow anomaly	3
Atrioventricular valve leaflet chordal anomaly	2
Functional flow anomaly (Tet spell)	2
Ventricular morphologic abnormality	2
Mitral systolic anterior motion	1
Subaortic membrane	2
Venous drainage	
Aberrant left superior vena cava	6
Anomalous pulmonary veins	1
Others	
Found normal anatomic structures thought absent	8
Patent ductus arteriosus	4
Residual shunt (Blalock-Taussig)	1
Located anomalous coronary different than at catheterization	4

amination. Nevertheless, the ability to appreciate the anatomy and physiology of a defect with exquisite clarity at the time of operative repair does provide the surgeon with a lucid mental image of all pertinent information that he or she needs to focus on in order to provide an optimal result. Occasionally, the intraoperative echocardiogram provided information of compelling importance (such as previously unappreciated multiple ventricular septal defects or persistent left superior vena cavae) that had significant impact on the operative plan (Table 5). With experience, the impact that intraoperative echo-DCFI has on the conduct of an operation is modified by several factors. Not insignificant among these is the tendency for surgeons continually to change their approach to certain problems and to evolve improved methods for dealing with congenital heart disease. Echocardiography probably plays a role in helping surgeons acquire the experience that leads to better recognition of the patterns of congenital heart disease and improved methods of reconstructing some of these complex conditions.

TABLE 5.
Duke University Medical Center
Intraoperative Echocardiography With Doppler Color Flow
Imaging for Congenital Heart Repair: Impact on Case Planning*

Impact	Number of Patients
Influence operative plan prior to cardiopulmonary bypass	
Change diagnosis	4
Change operation	20
Repair unsuspected lesion	20
Influence approach to lesion	32
Alter cardiopulmonary bypass plan	16
Total	92
Guide the intraoperative approach	
Clarify valve and/or chordal commitments	28
Indicate best manner for valve repair	19
Identify precise location of defect	18
Specify how to repair	56
Total	121
Alter Anesthesia Conduct Before Cardiopulmonary Bypass	10

*Echocardiography with Doppler color flow imaging impacted planning 223 times in 175 patients (42%).

Perhaps the most significant role for intraoperative echocardiography is demonstrating the adequacy of the repair. In 44 of our patients (11%), the repair was revised prior to removing them from the operating room (Table 6), and in 24 instances, this revision was based on echocardiographic findings alone. Of particular interest, when the revision was performed in patients who had no clinically evident problems, the likelihood of achieving an acceptable result (by echocardiographic standards) was quite high (21 of 24). However, when echocardiography confirmed the presence of a problem suspected in a patient who was not clinically stable, the chance of an acceptable outcome was much lower (11 of 20). These patients most often had problems that transcended the capabilities of surgical repair, as opposed to those in the first group, whose defects were usually residual (or previously unappreciated, e.g., a second ventricular septal defect or suboptimal valve repair (Fig 20) and were more easily corrected. Echocardiography is also extremely helpful in delineating the precise location of a residual defect so that it can be identified quickly and successfully upon re-exploration, resulting in a more satisfactory result. Of special interest is the tremendous learning aid that echocardiography provides the surgeon by producing an immediate appraisal of the surgical result, quickly rein-

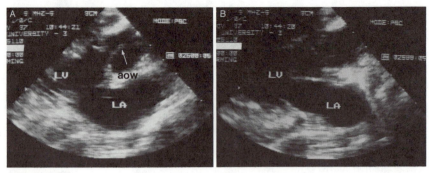

FIG 20.
A, in this patient, who weaned from cardiopulmonary bypass without difficulty after placement of an aortic valve homograft for congenital aortic stenosis, the noncoronary sinus of the homograft *(arrow)* can be seen to have disrupted from the
aortic wall *(AOW).* This was recognized easily by epicardial echocardiography and
B, repaired so that the aortic homograft replacement could produce a more optimal result. *LA* = left atrium; *LV* = left ventricle.

TABLE 6.
Duke University Medical Center
Intraoperative Echocardiography with Doppler Color Flow
Imaging for Congenital Heart Repair: Reason for Revision in 44
(11%) Patients*

Indication for Revision	Number of Repairs Redone	Number With Acceptable Echocardiographic Result After Revision
Clinical problem (echocardiography with Doppler color flow imaging confirms)	20	11
Echocardiography with Doppler color flow imaging alone	24	21
Total	44	32

*Forty-four patients underwent revision of their repair prior to leaving the operating room. In
24 instances, the indication for repair was provided by echocardiographic data alone,
whereas in 20 instances, the patient exhibited clinical signs of a suboptimal repair. Prior to
leaving the operating room, the acceptability of the patient's final echocardiographic result
was recorded.

forcing successful methods and allowing those techniques that should be improved to be recognized.

With experience, the postbypass echocardiogram can provide excellent prognostic information regarding the sufficiency of the repair. We have learned to grade the postoperative result as (1) echocardiogram perfect—no demonstrable problems; (2) acceptable residual—a small defect demonstrated by echocardiogram felt not to need further treatment; or (3) unacceptable residual—a more significant residual problem easily recognizable by epicardial echocardiogram. Table 7 correlates the final postbypass echocardiogram impression in our patients with their "long-term" outcome with respect to objective parameters of a failed operation (death or the need for reoperation). Thanks to the diligence of our cardiologists, follow-up has been 100%. Patients with echocardiographically perfect repairs as well as those with acceptable residual defects (by echocardiogram) clearly have had a better outcome, and it appears that patients who leave the operating room with an unacceptable residual defect have only an 18% chance for a good long-term result. Increased appreciation for how to interpret the echocardiographic images should lead to even better correlation of acceptable residual defects with a good outcome; our more recent experience reflects this enhanced learning of what truly constitutes an acceptable residual defect such that we no longer have any difference in outcome between echocardiographically perfect results and those with small (acceptable) residual defects. This constitutes the "learning curve" for intraoperative echocardiography. By carefully comparing results to echocardiographic images, each surgeon will be able to ascertain for himself or herself which echocardiographic findings require revision prior to leaving the operating room in order to produce the optimal likelihood of a good result. Using this method of evaluation, we were able to demonstrate a substantial difference amongst our patients who had revision of their residual problem prior to leaving the operating room vs. those whose residual problem was left untouched (Table 8).

One echocardiographic parameter that seems to correlate closely with outcome is ventricular function after bypass (Table 9). Dysfunction of either the right or left ventricle was associated with an increased mortality compared to no ventricular dysfunction. Biventricular dysfunction was a particularly ominous sign and was reflected in a 74% risk of death. Echocardiography was always able to establish whether or not ventricular dysfunction (as opposed to a technical or anatomic problem) played a role in any hemodynamic instability that the patient manifested after repair and directed treatment toward the proper mechanism. Occasionally, the echocardiogram demonstrated an easily reversible form of ventricular dysfunction (such as myocardial air) that would be treated more appropriately in a manner other than by the institution of inotropic therapy (see Fig 9).

Overall, the ability of intraoperative epicardial echocardiography to predict outcome, after experience is acquired with its use, can be useful for determining the quality of an operative result. Patients who leave the operating room without any echocardiographic indication for concern (such

TABLE 7.
Duke University Medical Center
Intraoperative Echocardiography With Doppler Color Flow Imaging for Congenital Heart Repair: Outcome Relating to Final Echocardiographic Results in 414 Patients*

Residual Defect (echocardiographically)	Number of Patients	Acceptable Outcome	Reoperated	Surgical Death	Later Death
Echocardiographically "perfect"	262 (63%)†	228 (87%)	2 (1%)	30 (11%)	2 (1%)
Acceptable residual	115 (28%)†	91 (79%)	9 (8%)‡	10 (9%)	5 (4%)
Unacceptable residual	34 (8%)†	6 (18%)‡	12 (35%)‡	13 (38%)‡	3 (9%)
No impression	3 (1%)†	2 (67%)	0	1 (33%)	0

*Outcome with respect to reoperation or surgical death was recorded for all patients and correlated with the echocardiographic result at the time they left the operating room. The data base is current and records all reoperations or deaths. Late deaths were recorded after hospital discharge regardless of cause.
†Percent of entire series.
‡P < .001 by chi-square (compared to echocardiographically "perfect").

TABLE 8.
Duke University Medical Center
Intraoperative Echocardiography With Doppler Color Flow
Imaging for Congenital Heart Repair: Impact of Residual Defect
by Echocardiogram*

Time of Repair	Number of Patients	Number of Patients Reoperated
Repair before leaving operating room	33	1
No repair before leaving operating room	27	12†

*Residual defects observed by the final postrepair echocardiogram in the operating room are correlated with the incidence of late reoperation depending upon whether or not these defects were revised prior to the patient leaving the operating room.
†$P < .001$ by chi-square (compared to repair before leaving operating room).

TABLE 9.
Duke University Medical Center
Intraoperative Echocardiography With Doppler Color Flow
Imaging for Congenital Heart Repair: Outcome Relating to Final
Echocardiographic Results in 414 Patients*

Ventricular Function by Echocardiogram	Number of Patients (%)	Surgical Deaths (%)
No right or left ventricular problem	320 (78)†	10 (3%)
Only right ventricular problem	22 (5%)†	10 (45%)‡
Only left ventricular problem	49 (12%)†	17 (35%)‡
Both right and left ventricular problems	23 (5%)†	17 (74%)‡

*Patients with ventricular dysfunction of either the right or left ventricle or of both ventricles were identified and mortality for these patient groups is tabulated.
†Percent of entire series.
‡$P < .001$ by chi-square (compared to no right or left ventricular problems).

TABLE 10.
Duke University Medical Center
Intraoperative Echocardiography With Doppler Color Flow Imaging for Congenital Heart Repair: Outcome Relating to Final Echocardiographic Results in 414 Patients*

Echocardiographic Outcome	Number of Patients (%)[†]	Acceptable Outcome	Reoperated	Surgical Death	Later Death
No problems of concern	295 (71%)[†]	273 (92%)	8 (3%)	9 (3%)	5 (2%)
Problems of concern	119 (29%)[†]	54 (45%)[‡]	15 (13%)[‡]	45 (38%)[‡]	5 (4%)

*Patients who left the operating room with any residual problem of concern by echocardiogram (residual defect, ventricular dysfunction, technical or anatomic imperfection, etc.) were compared to those whose final postrepair echocardiogram posed no problems of concern and are related to long-term outcome with respect to indices of "operation failure" such as death or the need for a reoperation.
[†]Percent of entire series.
[‡]$P < .001$ by chi-square (compound to no problems of concern).

as a residual defect, ventricular dysfunction, or technical or anatomic inadequacy) were found to have a 92% likelihood of a good outcome (Table 10). As we have become more experienced in interpreting echocardiographic images, our more recent data allow us to predict that these patients will have a 97% chance of a good outcome. In contrast, patients who leave the operating room with a problem for concern have less chance for a good result.

Conclusions

Echocardiography is a tool that helps the surgeon to appreciate clearly the anatomy of a cardiac lesion at the time of repair and to evaluate the quality of the reconstruction after it is complete, but while the patient is still in an environment where revisions can be performed easily. Just as successful surgical repair of congenital heart disease requires skill and experience, constructive application of intraoperative echo-DFCI demands patience and learning. Use of this technology is not essential for producing excellent results in pediatric cardiac surgery and actually may serve only to demonstrate to surgeons the imperfections of techniques that were felt to be "flawless." For younger, less experienced surgeons, intraoperative echocardiography provides a superb mechanism for shortening the "learning curve" by supplying immediate reinforcement of good techniques. Epicardial scanning requires participation by the surgeon and enhances interaction between the cardiology, anesthesiology, and surgery personnel, thereby intensifying teamwork in the operating room. The techniques, once learned, are simple, safe, and quick. The information, once understood, can be extraordinarily helpful, refining appreciation for congenital heart disease and its surgical solutions.

References

1. Ungerleider RM, Greeley WJ, Philips J, et al: Routine intraoperative color flow imaging prevents surgically unacceptable results in repair of congenital heart lesions, in *Perspectives in Pediatric Cardiology*, vol 2, *Pediatric Cardiac Surgery*, part 3. Mount Kisco, NY, Futura Publishing Co, 1990.
2. Greeley WJ, Kern FH, Ungerleider RM, et al: The effect of hypothermic cardiopulmonary bypass and total circulatory arrest on cerebral metabolism in neonates, infants, and children. *J Thorac Cardiovas Surg* 1991; 101:783–794.
3. Hagler DJ, Tajik AJ, Seward JB, et al: Intraoperative two-dimensional Doppler echocardiography. *J Thorac Cardiovasc Surg* 1988; 95:516–522.
4. Ungerleider RM, Kisslo JA, Greeley WJ, et al: Intraoperative prebypass and postbypass epicardial color flow imaging in the repair of atrioventricular canal defects. *J Thorac Cardiovasc Surg* 1989; 98:90–100.
5. Ungerleider RM, Greeley WJ, Sheikh KH, et al: The use of intraoperative echo with Doppler color flow imaging to predict outcome following repair of congenital cardiac defects. *Ann Surg* 1989; 210:526–534.

6. Canter CE, Sekarski DC, Martin TC, et al: Intraoperative evaluation of atrio-ventricular septal defect repair by color flow mapping echocardiography. *Ann Thorac Surg* 1989; 48:544–550.
7. Ungerleider RM, Greeley WJ, Sheikh KH, et al: Routine use of intraoperative epicardial echocardiography and Doppler color flow imaging to guide and evaluate repair of congenital heart lesions. A prospective study. *J Thorac Cardiovasc Surg* 1990; 100:297–309.
8. de Bruijn NP, Clements FM: *Transesophageal Echocardiography.* Boston, Martinus Nijhoff Publishing Co, 1987.

Renal Failure in the Perioperative Patient

Saleh Salehmoghaddam, M.D.

Assistant Clinical Professor, Medicine/Nephrology, University of California, Los Angeles School of Medicine, Los Angeles, California

Edwin J. Jacobson, M.D.

Associate Clinical Professor, Medicine/Nephrology, University of California, Los Angeles School of Medicine, Los Angeles, California

Acute renal failure (ARF) in the setting of cardiac surgery and cardiac transplantation remains one of the most difficult management problems for the surgical team as well as one of the most serious complications for the patient. For patients without significant preexisting renal disease, the incidence of mild to moderate postoperative renal insufficiency may be as high as 20% to 30%.[1] More profound degrees of renal insufficiency (creatinine >5.0 mg/dL) are seen in 2% to 5% of patients undergoing cardiac surgery and are accompanied by a postoperative mortality rate approaching 80% to 90%.[2] Also, postoperative days in intensive care units, total hospital days, and multi-organ complications are significantly increased in patients with ARF. Therefore, it is necessary to identify those patients at increased risk for the development of postoperative ARF, and to modify or correct attendant risk factors as possible. Patients with preexisting renal disease may undergo cardiac surgery with acceptable risk, provided there is careful preparation and perioperative management, and appropriate dialytic therapy available.

Pathophysiology

The pathophysiology of ARF associated with heart surgery is not entirely clear. Renal injury from exposure to nephrotoxic agents as well as that caused by endotoxins such as myoglobin and hemoglobin may occur during the preoperative and intraoperative periods. Prerenal causes such as decreased intravascular volume or decreased renal perfusion (as seen in congestive heart failure) also may lead to a decline in renal function, as can postrenal obstruction of an anatomic or functional nature. The vast majority of ARF associated with heart surgery, however, is the result of inadequate perfusion of the kidneys during surgery and resultant ischemic injury.

Several theories have developed as to the physiologic changes that occur during the "initiation" phase of ARF (Fig 1). Acute and profound constriction of the afferent arteriole is a consistent finding in experimental models.[3] This intense vasoconstriction, which appears to be hormonally regulated, causes a marked decrease in glomerular filtration rate (GFR). Portions of the renin-angiotensin system, as well as certain prostaglandins, have been implicated as responsible mediators, but definitive proof is lacking at present.[4] Ischemic ARF also may result from changes in the glomerulus itself. Loss of structural integrity of the glomerular capillary may result in decreases in permeability and/or loss of glomerular surface area with accompanying reduction of GFR. Finally, tubular mechanisms such as direct necrosis of tubular cells with loss of function, plugging of the tubule with cellular debris, and possible back leak of tubular filtrate into the vascular compartment may contribute to renal failure. An interesting recent experimental observation has been the finding of increased oxygen radicals in the tubular wall associated with an influx of calcium into the tubular cells. A decrease in intracellular adenosine triphosphate levels may result. An understanding of the chemical interactions occurring at the subcellular level may lead to future development of therapeutic interventions.[5]

It is only during the initiation phase of ARF that its course may be altered by intervention. Once the process is established, and the ARF enters

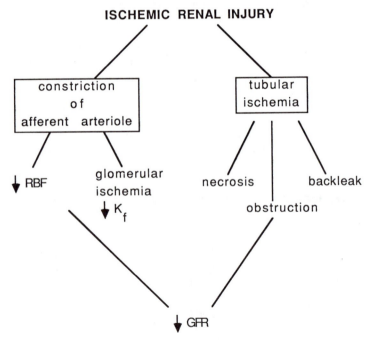

FIG 1.
Physiologic changes occurring during "initiation" phase of ARF.

the "maintenance and recovery phase," little can be done but to support the patient.

Postoperative Acute Renal Failure—Risk Factors

Risk factors associated with the development of renal failure after major surgery are well documented (Table 1). Many patients undergoing heart surgery have been exposed to various nephrotoxins, most commonly contrast dye in the preoperative period. Allowing renal function to return to normal, or at least to baseline level, prior to surgery will decrease significantly the risk of worsening renal failure postoperatively. Avoiding expo-

TABLE 1.
Postoperative Acute Renal Failure

I. Preoperative risk factors.
  A. Preexisting renal disease.
  B. Volume depletion.
    1. Diuretics.
    2. Osmotic agents.
      a. Glucose.
      b. Urea.
      c. Contrast material.
      d. Mannitol.
    3. Fasting.
    4. Nasogastric suction.
    5. Bowel preparation.
  C. Decreased effective arterial volume.
    1. Congestive heart failure.
    2. Low cardiac output states.
    3. Cirrhosis with ascites.
    4. Nephrotic syndrome.
  D. Nephrotoxic agents.
    1. Endogenous.
      a. Pigments.
      b. Bacterial endotoxins and
        exotoxins.
    2. Exogenous.
      a. Drugs.
      b. Contrast material.
II. Intraoperative risk facotrs.
  A. Anesthetics.
  B. Hemodynamic changes
    (hypotension).
  C. Cardiopulmonary bypass.

sure to other nephrotoxins, such as aminogylcoside antibiotics, is advisable.

A recent clinical study by Corwin et al.[1] found three preoperative variables that predicted 72% of the cases of ARF that occurred following heart surgery. Specifically, these were an elevated preoperative serum creatinine level (1.6 ± 0.2 mg/dL vs. 1.3 + 0.3 mg/dL), advanced age (69 ± 8 years vs. 63 ± 12 years), and concurrent valve and bypass operations vs. bypass alone. The latter variable may reflect indirectly time on bypass, longer operations, and higher doses of intraoperative vasopressors. In addition, preoperative congestive heart failure was a significant risk factor for those patients developing ARF, but did not function as a predictive variable. Advanced age or extreme youth also may predispose the patient to postoperative ARF. Obviously, optimization of intravascular volume status and hemodynamics is mandatory in any patient at increased risk of developing postoperative ARF.

Intraoperative events common to all surgical patients, such as exposure to potentially nephrotoxic anesthesia (e.g., methoxyflurane),[6] antibiotics (particularly aminoglycosides), and endotoxins, (e.g., free hemoglobin and myoglobin), likewise occur in patients undergoing heart surgery. However, there are several intraoperative events unique to heart surgery that may profoundly affect postoperative renal function. These events involve the use of cardiopulmonary bypass and the renal structural and hemodynamic abnormalities that consequently occur.

Cardiopulmonary Bypass and Acute Renal Failure

GFR and renal blood flow decrease approximately 30% during cardiopulmonary bypass, resulting in an increase in renal vascular resistance.[7] Because the majority of ARF associated with heart surgery is felt to be ischemic in origin, the length of time on bypass may be of critical importance, as may be the need for extensive use of pressors intraoperatively.[8, 9] The various methods of cardiopulmonary bypass used and the effectiveness of their proposed renoprotective benefits is more controversial. Some investigators have shown that nonpulsatile, low-flow, low-pressure cardiopulmonary bypass (flow rates in the range of 1.61 L/min/m^2 and a sustained mean arterial pressure of 30 mm Hg) may actually serve to decrease the incidence of postoperative renal dysfunction.[8, 9] Others, however, have shown that this type of bypass reduces postoperative renal function due to arterial vasoconstriction and a persistent, low cardiac output state.[10, 11] Yeboah et al.[12] have demonstrated that the maintenance of a mean perfusion pressure of >80 mm Hg while on cardiopulmonary bypass significantly reduces the incidence of ARF, but that when mean perfusion pressure falls below 60 mm Hg, there is a high likelihood of the development of severe ARF. Maintenance of an intraoperative cardiac index above 2.5 L/min/m^2 further reduces the incidence of postoperative renal failure.[9] If poor cardiac output extends into the second postoperative day, an even greater incidence of ARF is noted.[13] The extended use of postoperative, intermittent positive-pressure breathing, without a compensatory increase in cardiac output to offset decreased venous return caused by this modality, is also associated with an increased incidence of ARF following cardiopulmonary bypass.[14]

Evaluation and Treatment

ARF will occur in 1% to 2% of adults undergoing cardiopulmonary bypass, even in the absence of preexisting risk factors. When ARF develops in a patient after heart surgery, it should be evaluated rapidly, in much the same manner as are other forms of ARF. An algorithm for this evaluation is shown in Figure 2. The extent of the evaluation will depend upon the clinical setting and the degree of suspicion for causes other than ischemic ARF. Appropriate action should be taken within the first few hours after the "initiation" of ARF, to allow for the correction of any reversible components.

During the immediate postoperative period, oliguria is generally not related to cardiopulmonary bypass unless there has been prolonged severe intraoperative hypotension. During this period, the most likely causes of renal failure are contrast-induced nephropathy (if angiography was done on the day prior to surgery), bleeding, cardiac tamponade, or severely compromised myocardial function. Fluid administration may be the first therapeutic measure taken in the postoperative patient, but care should be exercised to avoid fluid overload by repeated fluid boluses. If contrast-induced ARF is suspected, optimization of hemodynamics and the administration of large doses of loop diuretics, low-dose dopamine, and, at times, mannitol, can restore urine output while the renal failure resolves spontaneously.

Cardiac tamponade is difficult to establish even by echocardiography in the immediate postoperative period. However, cardiac surgeons are highly attuned to this problem and have little hesitation in reexploring the chest. Correction of this problem usually results in correction of the oliguria within a very short time, provided there has been no severe, prolonged hemodynamic compromise. Severe myocardial dysfunction is easily diagnosed by echocardiography, and when appropriate measures are taken to improve cardiac output in such situations, renal function usually improves.

If the ARF does prove to be ischemic in origin, two patterns seem to emerge. The first form is that of ARF which develops 12 to 18 hours postoperatively. The patient is usually oliguric or may be anuric and displays marked resistance to renal pressors or diuretics. Such patients may become rapidly volume overloaded. Creatinine and blood urea nitrogen tend to increase slowly, but potassium may rise precipitously due to hemolysis and the use of stored blood during the procedure. This "rapid-onset" ARF has been thought to be more directly related to the cardiopulmonary bypass procedure itself, with activation of a portion of the complement path-

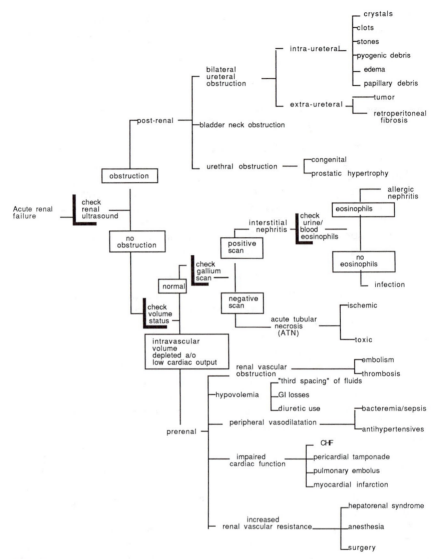

FIG 2.
Algorithm for the evaluation of ARF after the patient has undergone heart surgery.

way leading to intense vasoconstriction in the renal arterioles. Early dialysis may be necessary due to intractable volume overload or life-threatening hyperkalemia.

A second, more common, form of ARF develops 3 to 4 days postoperatively. It is usually nonoliguric, but tends to have a more rapidly rising creatinine and blood urea nitrogen. Dialysis may be necessary if the ARF lasts more than 5 to 7 days, or symptoms of uremia intervene. The etiology of this form of ARF is thought to resemble more closely that of the traditional form of ischemic ARF.

In general, if a patient is oliguric and not volume-contracted, the administration of a low dose of dopamine (1 to 3 µg/kg/min) and large doses of loop-acting diuretics may increase urine output enough to avoid dialysis while the cause of renal failure is being sought. Establishing urine output by this means, however, should not preclude an exhaustive search for the cause of the oliguria.[15] ARF thought to be secondary to intraoperative factors such as cardiopulmonary bypass can be treated by optimizing hemodynamic parameters and administering dopamine, diuretics, and mannitol. Mannitol is given as an intravenous bolus in dosages of 6 to 12 g, and should be used with caution in oliguric patients who may be fluid-overloaded. Renal failure after cardiopulmonary bypass usually resolves over the ensuing few days if it is not severe.

Renal failure with onset beyond 48 hours postoperatively usually occurs in patients as a sequela of preexisting renal disease or for a variety of other reasons, including sepsis and exposure to nephrotoxic agents. If conservative management of this form of renal failure is unsuccessful, dialysis should be instituted. Although attempts should be made to avoid dialysis if possible, it should be kept in mind that dialysis is a life-saving procedure when used in a timely and appropriate manner. Indications for dialysis in postcardiac surgical renal failure are the same as those for other conditions. The temptation to "avoid dialysis at all costs" should be ignored, since the correction of fluid overload and other metabolic disorders may hasten a patient's recovery and allow appropriate nutritional support.

Preexistent Renal Insufficiency—Specific Concerns

Patients with preexisting renal insufficiency who undergo heart surgery may present potentially difficult intraoperative and postoperative problems. Until recently, the end-stage renal failure patient on dialysis was felt to pose an unacceptable risk for cardiac surgery, especially coronary artery bypass. However, two recent studies have shown that with careful perioperative management and the proper use of dialysis, mortality and morbidity is only slightly higher in these patients than in those without end-stage renal failure.[16-19]

For patients with moderate renal insufficiency, few abnormalities are detectable as long as the creatinine clearance remains above 25 mL/min. However, these patients do exhibit a higher incidence of postoperative renal failure. The moderately impaired kidney is more susceptible to nephrotoxic agents; therefore, dosages must be adjusted carefully. These patients may have impaired ability to excrete large potassium, magnesium, or phosphate loads, as well as impaired free water excretion and an increased incidence of hyponatremia.

Patients with severe renal insufficiency (creatinine clearance 10 to 24 mL/min) who are not yet on dialysis require that particular attention be paid to their fluid and electrolyte management, acid-base status, possibility of bleeding diathesis, and risk of infection. Impaired ability to excrete both sodium and free water can lead rapidly to volume overload and hyponatremia. A serum sodium level of 125 to 135 mEq/L is common, but it may drop to the range of 110 to 120 mEq/L after the infusion of hypotonic solutions. Life-threatening hyperkalemia can occur following even small increases in endogenous or exogenous potassium loads (Table 2). Phosphorus and magnesium should be carefully monitored also and intake of these ions limited so as to keep levels within normal range. Most patients with this degree of renal insufficiency will have an underlying hyperchloremic metabolic acidosis. A superimposed anion gap acidosis or hypoventilation may cause profound decreases in arterial pH.

A severe coagulopathy may accompany renal insufficiency and is related directly to the degree of uremia. The etiology is multifactorial and not completely understood, but a disturbance of platelet function is the most common abnormality. This platelet function abnormality can be measured by the template bleeding time. A bleeding time greater than 9 minutes may be associated with increased postsurgical bleeding. The platelet function abnormality may be caused by direct interference with platelet factor III by guanidinosuccinic acid, some portion of the prostacyclin/prostaglandin cycle, or some as yet unknown toxic molecule. Deficiencies in factor VIII also may contribute. The platelet deficiency is correctable with aggressive dialysis to remove potential toxins, and the administration of cryoprecipitate or desmopressin (1-desamino-8-D-arginine vasopression;d DAVP). The des-

---

TABLE 2.
Hyperkalemia in Renal Insufficiency

I. Exogenous sources of potassium.
   A. Intravenous or oral potassium supplements.
   B. Potassium-containing drugs (K salts of many antibiotics).
   C. Administration of stored blood.
   D. Salt substitutes.

II. Endogenous sources of potassium.
   A. Hemolysis.
   B. Tissue trauma or necrosis.
   C. Rhabdomyolysis.
   D. Depolarizing drugs such as succinylcholine.

---

mopressin is thought to act by increasing von Willebrand antigen concentration and factor VIII coagulant activity. Because the risks of administering large quantities of blood products may not be acceptable, desmopressin and/or dialysis are the methods of choice for correcting the bleeding abnormality of uremia. Dialysis, if felt appropriate, should be performed in the 24 hours prior to surgery. Desmopressin in a dosage of 0.3 µg/kg is given in 50 cc of normal saline over 30 minutes at the time of the first incision and may be administered again 24 to 48 hours later. Desmopressin loses its effectiveness rapidly, and may be useful for only 1 to 2 days postoperatively. After this point, dialysis may be needed to continue to correct the bleeding abnormalities. Of interest are two recent studies that demonstrated a decrease in postoperative bleeding after heart surgery with the use of desmopressin, even in patients with normal renal function.[20, 21]

Immune function is impaired in all patients with renal insufficiency due to reduction in total white cells, bone marrow response, chemotaxis, phagocytosis, and mixed leukocyte culture reactivity. The lungs and urinary tract are the most frequent sites of infection, but multiple indwelling lines and catheters are also frequent sources of serious infection.

The use of muscle relaxants during anesthesia in patients with advanced renal insufficiency creates special problems. Many of these agents are excreted by mechanisms that include the kidney, and adjustments in dosages are required. Pseudocholinesterase levels are diminished in patients following dialysis, and this may result in prolonged paralysis when depolarizing agents are used.[22] Succinylcholine causes a rapid transient rise in serum potassium during the initial dose. In the face of preexistent hyperkalemia, as may occur with renal failure, life-threatening potassium levels can result.[23]

A significant problem with the use of curare-like drugs is the phenomenon of recurarization.[23] This event occurs several hours after termination of the surgical procedure. Recurrence of paralysis results in impaired respiratory effort and prolonged need for intubation. Recurarization occurs as a result of a combination of events. Metabolic acidosis and electrolyte imbalance both affect the action of nondepolarizing agents. Patients may be hypothermic during the surgical procedure, and rewarming also may result in renewed activity of the drug with restored paralysis. In addition, plasma pancuronium levels decline much more slowly in patients with renal failure. These effects may be responsible for underestimation of the degree of residual muscle relaxation postoperatively. Curariform agents, therefore, should be used with caution in patients with advanced renal failure.

Management of the Patient With End-Stage Renal Disease and Established Need for Dialysis

For patients with end-stage renal disease on dialysis, the institution of aggressive preoperative and postoperative dialysis has made surgery possible in many who previously were felt to pose unacceptable risks. Dialysis may be performed on a daily basis for several days prior to surgery in order to optimize hemodynamics and volume status, correct electrolyte and acid-base abnormalities and any existing coagulopathy. If possible, dialysis should be avoided for a period of 12 to 16 hours immediately prior to surgery so as to allow for reversal of heparin effects and reequilibration of intracellular and extracellular fluid and electrolytes.

Some patients may be managed more easily by intraoperative hemodialysis. This technique better controls intravascular volume and allows compensation for large infusions or shifts of electrolytes, especially potassium. Intraoperative dialysis also may aid in management of the patient's acid-base status, allowing for optimization of the effects of drugs and pressors which may be partially pH-dependent. Concurrent hemodialysis and cardiopulmonary bypass have been described previously.[25] A modification of the technique has been adopted in our institution and is shown in Figure 3. Scrupulous attention to the dialysis access during the surgery is fundamental.

Postoperatively, the patient with end-stage renal disease again should be managed with aggressive dialysis. Several options are available. Traditional hemodialysis offers rapid, high-efficiency dialysis, but poses potential prob-

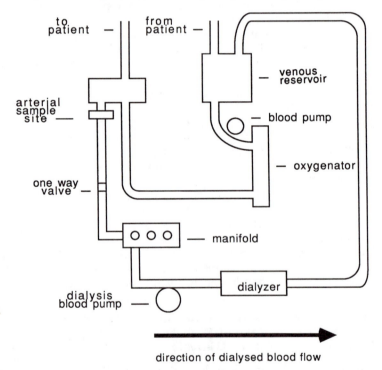

FIG 3.
A modification of the concurrent hemodialysis and cardiopulmonary bypass techniques. Attention to the dialysis access during the surgery is fundamental.

lems with heparinization and hemodynamic instability, Peritoneal dialysis has been proposed as an alternative, but respiratory compromise from fluid in the peritoneum may occur, giving rise to an increased incidence of postoperative atelectasis and difficulty with extubation. More recently, continuous arteriovenous hemodialysis (CAVHD) has been proposed as an alternative to traditional hemodialysis. This technique, however, while theoretically less prone to problems of hemodynamic instability, is extremely nurse-intensive and has limited practical usage. Using these techniques, mortality rates of patients with end-stage renal disease undergoing cardiac surgery have been reported to be as low as 6.2%.[16] The patients' chances of long-term survival and meaningful rehabilitation are excellent and appear to be not significantly different from those of end-stage renal disease patients as a whole.

Cardiac Transplantation and Acute Renal Failure

The same factors that result in ARF following heart surgery in general also apply to the cardiac transplant patient. In addition, there are other important considerations that bear upon renal function. These include the severity of pretransplant heart failure, the administration of cyclosporine, and the adequacy of the transplanted heart to support circulation.

Pretransplant evaluation of renal function includes the taking of a thorough history and, when appropriate, the performance of renal ultrasound, urinalysis, and a 24-hour urine collection for total protein and creatinine clearance. The University of California, Los Angeles heart transplant program generally excludes patients with proteinuria greater than 500 to 600 mg/24 hr because of the possibility of the presence of intrinsic renal disease, in addition to any renal dysfunction resulting from cardiac failure. If the ultrasound is normal and the total protein is less than 500 mg/24 hr, it is assumed that any renal dysfunction present is secondary to heart failure. The lower the GFR pretransplant, the greater the risk of postoperative renal failure. Patients have been transplanted, however, with creatinine clearances as low as 30 mL/min without requiring posttransplant dialysis.

Renal failure after cardiac transplantation currently can be divided into three phases, the first of which encompasses renal failure arising in the first 16 to 24 hours immediately after transplantation. During this period, the most common causes of renal failure are undue bleeding with volume depletion, and right ventricular dysfunction. Right ventricular dysfunction is a common occurrence in patients who have undergone cardiac transplantation. It may be caused by high pulmonary vascular resistance, poor preservation of the donor heart, severe tricuspid insufficiency, or fluid overload.

Right ventricular dysfunction is characterized by a rising right atrial pressure, a decrease in systemic mean arterial pressure, usually low to normal left atrial or precapillary wedge pressure, and a decrease in cardiac output.

This situation may result in various degrees of oliguria depending on the severity of the right ventricular dysfunction.

Renal failure secondary to right ventricular dysfunction is best treated by the use of inotropic agents in conjunction with measures to decrease pulmonary vascular resistance. Isoproterenol is a potent inotrope with pulmonary vasodilatory properties. The usefulness of this agent is limited, however, by its propensity to cause arrhythmias and tachycardia. Prostaglandin E_1 is a potent pulmonary vasodilator and, when used in conjunction with isoproterenol or other inotropic agents, it can serve to decrease pulmonary vascular resistance and increase cardiac output. This approach, in our hands, almost always has been effective in reversing the oliguria associated with right ventricular dysfunction. The maximum dose of isoproterenol is 0.01 mg/kg/min by intravenous infusion. Prostaglandin E_1 is started at a dose of 0.005 to 0.01 μg/kg/min and titrated up in increments of 0.005 up to 0.1 μg/kg/min or until the desired effect on hemodynamics and urine output is achieved. Generally, the agent is well tolerated and blood pressure increases despite a concomitant decrease in the peripheral vascular resistance. Once the hemodynamic status of the patient is stabilized, diuretics are administered in sufficient doses to produce a diuresis. An attempt is made to lower right atrial pressures to 6 to 8 mm Hg, provided systemic blood pressure remains stable. Volume overload during the first 24 hours after transplantation can worsen right ventricular dysfunction significantly with its attendant complications. It should be avoided by minimization of fluid administration during this period.

The second phase of renal failure after transplantation begins 24 hours postoperatively when the effects of cardiopulmonary bypass and intraoperative hemodynamic insult to the kidney become apparent. This period is heralded by a decrease in urine output, which up to that point may have been adequate. During this period, response to diuretics is poor and, at our institution, the administration of prostaglandin E_1 has met with variable success in reversing the oliguria. The renal dysfunction usually lasts 12 to 72 hours, depending on the severity of the perioperative insult to the kidney, as well as the severity of preoperative renal dysfunction. Furthermore, cyclosporine administration impacts maximally on renal function during this post-transplant phase. If volume overload is present during this period, the patient's chances of requiring dialysis are relatively high. A valuable strategy is to attempt diuresis in the first 24 hours following surgery in order to be able to wait out the subsequent period of oliguria. If the patient can be managed conservatively for 12 to 48 hours, he usually will not require dialysis. Conservative management includes meticulous attention to fluid and electrolyte abnormalities and hemodynamic parameters. During this period, there is a rise in blood urea nitrogen and creatinine, but unless patients become severely uremic, encephalopathic, or hyperkalemic, dialysis is not instituted. Dialytic therapy, when initiated electively, is almost always hemodialysis via temporary subclavian venous access. When dialysis is instituted emergently, the femoral vein route is utilized. Patients who require dialysis in the first 72 hours after cardiac transplantation usually experience a prolonged course of renal failure lasting 1 to 4 weeks, and generally require dialysis on an ongoing basis during this time. Infectious complications remain the most serious during this period.

The contribution of cyclosporine to renal failure after transplantation is substantial. The major impact of cyclosporine toxicity is most apparent during the first 48 hours after transplantation, when the kidney is most susceptible to ischemic insults. Cyclosporine is usually administered intravenously or via nasogastric tube in the immediate post-transplant period. Intravenous cyclosporine may be more nephrotoxic than the oral form because of its vehicle cremaphor, which has been demonstrated to increase vascular resistance in the kidney. Cyclosporine toxicity is thought to be secondary to afferent arteriolar vasoconstricture resulting from an imbalance in renal prostaglandins[26] as well as the contribution of the sympathetic system to renal vasoconstriction.[27] Various strategies have been used to minimize the contribution of cyclosporine to renal failure after transplantation. Some groups avoid the use of cyclosporine in the immediate post-transplant period until renal function is established. Others start with small doses, which are increased to tolerance according to renal function measurement.

In addition to oliguria and rising levels of blood urea nitrogen and creatinine, cyclosporine toxicity can result in hyperkalemia and a mild metabolic acidosis,[28] as well as hypomagnesemia.[29] These disturbances should be sought systematically and addressed with appropriate measures. Cyclosproine therapy is monitored using blood and serum levels. Cyclosporine monitoring is not a foolproof means of avoiding either nephrotoxicity or rejection, but it is a useful adjunct when combined with other clinical data.[30, 31]

The third phase of renal failure occurs beyond 48 to 72 hours after transplantation and usually is caused by transplant rejection, cardiac tamponade, infection, or cyclosporine toxicity. If the cause of renal failure during this period is determined carefully and corrected, the duration of the renal failure may be shortened, even if patients require dialysis.

Some complications of hemodialysis are unique to patients who have undergone cardiac transplantation. Hypotension is the major complication of hemodialysis. Normally, the major defense against dialysis-induced hypotension is reflex tachycardia. Cardiac transplant patients cannot mount such a defense due to cardiac denervation. Thus, pressor support should be used liberally to avoid major hypotensive episodes during hemodialysis. Hemodialysis is especially hazardous in the first 24 hours after transplantation, when patients have right ventricular dysfunction and are dependent on high filling pressures. In this situation, continuous arteriovenous hemofiltration (CAVH), with its ability to control intravascular volume more closely, may be preferable, so as to minimize hemodynamic instability.

In summary, ARF is a serious potential complication of all forms of cardiac surgery. Renal failure may be prevented or at least modified in the majority of patients if it is recognized early. This chapter has outlined the causes and treatment of renal failure following cardiac surgery and transplantation. The early recognition of this disorder and prompt institution of corrective measures cannot be overemphasized.

References

1. Corwin HL, Sprague S, DeLaria GA, et al: Acute renal failure associated with cardiac operations. *Thorac Cardiovasc Surg* 1989; 98:1107–1112.
2. Leurs PB, Mulder AW, Fiers HA, et al: Acute renal failure after cardiovascular surgery. Current concepts in pathophysiology, prevention and treatment. *Eur Heart J* 1989, 10 (suppl H):38–42.
3. Brezis M, Rosen S, Epstein FH: Acute renal failure, in Brenner BM, Rector FC (eds): *The Kidney,* vol 1, ed 3. Philadelphia, WB Saunders Company, 1986, pp 735–799.
4. Wilkes BM, Mailloux L: Acute renal failure: Pathogenesis and prevention. *Am J Med* 1986; 80:1129–1136.
5. Epstein M: Calcium antagonists and the kidney. Future directions in the management of ARF. Presented at the Conference on Newer Aspects in the Treatment of Renal Failure, Geneva, 1989.
6. Whiteside-Yim C, Fitzgerald FT: Preserving renal function in surgical patients. *West J Med* 1987; 146:316–321.
7. Krian A: Incidence, prevention and treatment of acute renal failure following cardiopulmonary bypass. *Int Anesthesiol Clin* 1976; 14:87–101.
8. Abel RM, Buckley MJ, Austen WG, et al: Etiology, incidence, and prognosis of renal failure following cardiac operations. *J Thorac Cardiovasc Surg* 1976; 71:323–333.
9. Hilberman M, Meyers BD, Carrie BJ, et al: Acute renal failure following cardiac surgery. *J Thorac Cardiovasc Surg* 1979; 77:880–888.
10. Koning HM, Koning AJ, Defauw JJAM: Optimal perfusion during extra-corporeal circulation. *Scand J Thorac Cardiovasc Surg* 1987; 21:207–213.
11. German JC, Chalmers GS, Hirai J, et al: Comparison of nonpulsatile extracorporeal circulation on renal tissue perfusion. *Chest* 1972; 61:65–69.
12. Yeboah ED, Petrie A, Pead JL: Acute renal failure and open-heart surgery. *Br Med J [Clin Res]* 1972; 1:415–418.
13. Hilberman M, Derby GC, Spencer RJ, et al: Sequential pathophysiological changes characterizing the progression from renal dysfunction to acute renal failure following cardiac operation. *J Thorac Cardiovasc Surg* 1980; 79:838–844.
14. Koning HM, Leusink JA, Nas AA: Renal function following open-heart surgery: The influence of postoperative artificial ventilation. *Thorac Cardiovasc Surg* 1987; 36:1–5.
15. Kjellstrand CM, Berkseth RO, Klinkman H: Treatment of acute renal failure, in Schrier RW, Gottschalk CW (eds): *Diseases of the Kidney.* Boston, Little, Brown, & Company 1988, pp 1501–1540.
16. Zamora JL, Burdine JT, Karlberg H, et al: Cardiac surgery in patients with end-stage renal disease. *Ann Thorac Surg* 1986; 42:113–117.
17. Laws KH, Merrill WH, Hammon J, et al: Cardiac surgery in patients with chronic renal disease. *Ann Thorac Surg* 1986; 42:152–157.
18. Lange HW, Aeppli DM, Brown DC: Survival of patients with acute renal fail-

ure requiring dialysis after open heart surgery: Early prognostic indicators. *Am Heart J* 1987; 113:1138–1143.

19. Matsuda H, Hirose H, Nakano S, et al: Results of open heart surgery in patients with impaired renal function as creatinine clearance below 30 mL/min. *Thorac Cardiovasc Surg* 1986; 27:595–598.

20. Hackmann T, Gascoyne RD, Naiman SC, et al: A trial of desmopressin (1-desamino-8$_D$-arginine vasopressin) to reduce blood loss in uncomplicated cardiac surgery. *N Engl J Med* 1989; 321:1437–1443.

21. Salzman EW, Weinstein MJ, Weintraub RM, et al: Treatment with desmopressin acetate to reduce blood loss after cardiac surgery. *N Engl J Med* 1986; 314:1402–1406.

22. Burke JF Jr, Francos GC: Surgery in the patient with acute or chronic renal failure. *Med Clin North Am* 1987; 71:489–497.

23. Roth F, Wuthrich H: The clinical importance of hyperkalemia following luxamethonium administration. *Br J Anaesth* 1969; 41:311.

24. Jarrell BE, Burke JF: Surgery in the patient with chronic renal failure, in Grennfield LJ (ed): *Problems in General Surgery-The High Risk Patient.* Philadelphia, Lippincott Publishers, 1984, pp 421–431.

25. Rohrer CH, Winkler MH, Sharp DN: Concurrent dialysis during cardiopulmonary bypass. *J Extra-Corporeal Tech* 1984; 16:33–36.

26. Perico N, Benigni A, Zoja C, et al: Functional significance of exaggerated renal thromboxane A_2 synthesis induced by cyclosporine A. *J Am Physiol Soc* 1986; 251:F581–F587.

27. Moss NG, Rowell SL, Falk RJ: Intravenous cyclosporine activates afferent and efferent renal nerves and causes sodium retention in innervated kidneys in rats. *Proc Natl Acad Sci USA* 1985; 82:8222–8226.

28. Bantle JP, Nath KA, Sutherland DER, et al: Effect of cyclosporine on renin-angiotension system and potassium excretion in renal transplant recipients. *Arch Intern Med* 1985; 145:505–508.

29. June CH, Thompson CB, Kennedy MS, et al: Profound hypomagnesemia and renal magnesium wasting associated with use of cyclosporine with bone marrow transplantation. *Transplantation* 1985; 39:620–624.

30. Wideman CA: Pharmacokinetic monitoring of cyclosporine. *Transplant Proc* 1983; 15(suppl 1):3168–3175.

31. Burckart GJ, Canafax DM, Yee GC: Therapeutic monitoring. *Drug Intell Clin Pharm* 1986; 20:649–652.

Index

A

Acid-base management: during cardiopulmonary bypass, 29–30

Acyclovir: after pediatric heart transplantation, 164

Adenine
for myocardial protection, 98
nucleotide pool in myocardial ischemic injury, 78–79
nucleotide synthesis, de novo pathway of, 90
glutamate incorporated into, 93

Adenosine deaminase inhibitor: for myocardial protection, 100–101

Adenosine therapy: for myocardial protection, 97

Adenosine triphosphate
cerebral
changes in circulatory arrest and low-flow bypass, 36
changes during circulatory arrest interrupted by 30 minutes of full-flow reperfusion, 37
hypothermia effects on, 273
myocardial
contribution to ventricular dysfunction mediated by free radicals during reperfusion, 100–101
replenishment by metabolic intervention, 96–99
replenishment, role of mitochondria in, 99–100
synthesis, cessation of, 75
synthesis, de novo pathway, enhancement by 5-amino imidazole-4-carboxamide riboside, 91

Aerobic exercise: in atherosclerosis, 5

Albumin: in cardiopulmonary bypass, 14

Allopurinol
in cardiopulmonary bypass, 24
for myocardial protection, 101

Alpha-adrenergic blockers: in tetralogy of Fallot, 182–183

5-Amino imidazole-4-carboxamide riboside: enhancing de novo pathway synthesis of adenisone triphosphate, 91

Anastomotic stenosis: neoaortic, after arterial switch, 235–236

Anatomy: coronary artery, in tetralogy of Fallot, 181–182

Ancrod: in cardiopulmonary bypass, 15, 20

Anesthesia: and renal failure, 316

Aneurysm: intra-atrial septal, epicardial echocardiography of, 293

Angiocardiograms: in tetralogy of Fallot with pulmonary stenosis, 183, 184, 185

Angiography: retinal fluorescein, during cardiopulmonary bypass, 25–27

Angioplasty, percutaneous transluminal cardiopulmonary bypass support during, 39–41
after myocardial infarction, 60

Angiotensin
converting enzyme, effects of cardiopulmonary bypass on, 11
renin-angiotensin system and hypertension after cardiopulmonary bypass, 11

Anomaly: Taussig-Bing, arterial switch for, 226–229

Antibodies: anti-CD4, before pediatric heart transplantation, 173

Anti-CD4 antibodies: before pediatric heart transplantation, 173

Antioxidant therapy: in atherosclerosis, 6

Antiplatelet therapy: in atherosclerosis, 6

Aortic
coarctation after pediatric heart transplantation, 168
cross-clamp times, long, and warm blood cardioplegia, 149–150
sinuses, drawings showing convention for naming, 215
valve
echocardiography of, epicardial, 298–299
homograft disruption, epicardial echocardiography of, 306
leaflet avulsion, epicardial echocardiography of, 293
surgery, warm blood cardioplegia in, 147

Apolipoprotein B-containing lipoproteins: in atherosclerosis, 1

Aprotonin: in cardiopulmonary bypass, 14

Arrhythmias: postischemic ventricular, role of calcium in, 80–81

A Simple, Once-a-Year Dose!

Review the partial list of titles below. And then request your own FREE 30-day preview. When you purchase a Year Book, we'll also send you an automatic notice of future volumes about two months before they publish.

This system was designed for your convenience and to take up as little of your time as possible. If you do not want the Year Book, the advance notice makes it easy for you to let us know. And if you elect to receive the new Year Book, you need do nothing. We will send it on publication.

No worry. No wasted motion. And, of course, every Year Book is yours to examine FREE of charge for thirty days.

Year Book of **Anesthesia**® (22137)
Year Book of **Cardiology**® (22114)
Year Book of **Critical Care Medicine**® (22091)
Year Book of **Dermatology**® (22108)
Year Book of **Diagnostic Radiology**® (22132)
Year Book of **Digestive Diseases**® (22081)
Year Book of **Drug Therapy**® (22139)
Year Book of **Emergency Medicine**® (22085)
Year Book of **Endocrinology**® (22107)
Year Book of **Family Practice**® (20801)
Year Book of **Geriatrics and Gerontology** (22121)
Year Book of **Hand Surgery**® (22096)
Year Book of **Hematology**® (22604)
Year Book of **Health Care Management**® (21145)
Year Book of **Infectious Diseases**® (22606)
Year Book of **Infertility** (22093)
Year Book of **Medicine**® (22087)
Year Book of **Neonatal-Perinatal Medicine** (22117)
Year Book of **Neurology and Neurosurgery**® (22120)
Year Book of **Nuclear Medicine**® (22140)
Year Book of **Obstetrics and Gynecology**® (22118)
Year Book of **Occupational and Environmental Medicine** (22092)
Year Book of **Oncology** (22128)
Year Book of **Ophthalmology**® (22135)
Year Book of **Orthopedics**® (22116)
Year Book of **Otolaryngology – Head and Neck Surgery**® (22086)
Year Book of **Pathology and Clinical Pathology**® (22104)
Year Book of **Pediatrics**® (22088)
Year Book of **Plastic and Reconstructive Surgery**® (22112)
Year Book of **Psychiatry and Applied Mental Health**® (22110)
Year Book of **Pulmonary Disease**® (22109)
Year Book of **Sports Medicine**® (22115)
Year Book of **Surgery**® (22084)
Year Book of **Ultrasound** (21170)
Year Book of **Urology**® (22094)
Year Book of **Vascular Surgery**® (22105)

Mosby-Year Book, Inc. • 11830 Westline Industrial Drive • St. Louis, MO 63146